Fundamental
CARDIOVASCULAR
and PULMONARY
PHYSIOLOGY

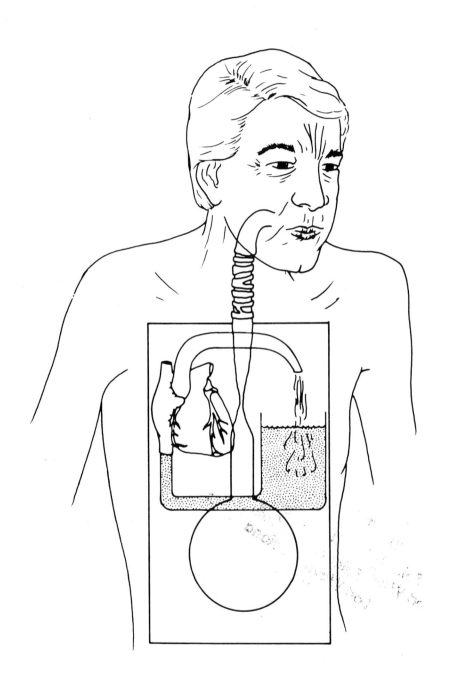

Fundamental
CARDIOVASCULAR
and PULMONARY
PHYSIOLOGY

JERRY FRANKLIN GREEN, Ph.D.

Professor
Department of Human Physiology
School of Medicine
University of California
Davis, California

Second Edition

LEA & FEBIGER

Philadelphia

1987

Lea & Febiger
600 Washington Square
Philadelphia, PA   19106-4198
U.S.A.
(215) 922-1330

Library of Congress Cataloging-in-Publication Data

Green, Jerry Franklin.
  Fundamental cardiovascular and pulmonary physiology.

  Bibliography: p.
  Includes index.
  1. Cardiovascular system. 2. Lungs.; I. Title.
[DNLM: 1. Cardiovascular System—physiology. 2. Lung—
physiology. WF 970 G796f]
QP102.G73   1987   612.1   86-21043
ISBN 0-8121-1068-4

1st Edition, 1982
2nd Edition, 1987

PRINTED IN THE UNITED STATES OF AMERICA

Print number: 5   4   3   2   1

To my mother,
HELEN RADESKY GREEN,
who inspired my academic interest.

PREFACE

The major objective of this book is to present a succinct summary of the basic concepts of the physiology of the circulatory and respiratory systems. A subsidiary objective is to point out parallel concepts as they recur in the discussion of both systems. This text is not meant to be the latest, up-to-date, critical review of each aspect in these fields, nor is it meant to be a clinical text. *Fundamental Cardiovascular and Pulmonary Physiology* was written primarily to introduce basic structure and function to the first-time reader and should prove useful to students of medicine, physiology, bioengineering, and the paramedical specialties such as nursing, anesthesia, respiratory therapy, and physical therapy.

In the interest of brevity, I have taken a moderately dogmatic approach and have avoided extensive documentation with research data. I have also attempted to avoid controversial areas and emphasize concepts that are widely accepted. Since this was a subjective judgement on my part, not all instructors will agree with my approach. I have referenced important historical articles where I felt such references were warranted and, for more advanced reading, have cited the latest pertinent chapters in the *Handbook of Physiology.* I have also reorganized relevant topics in a natural progression from structure to function and have introduced basic concepts in the chapter where they first apply.

Many colleagues have helped me prepare this text by providing their thoughts and careful criticisms. They include Drs. Barauch Bromberger-Barnea, Walter Ehrlich, Alan P. Jackman, Glen A. Lillington, Wayne Mitzner, Gibbe Parsons, Richard L. Riley, Theodore C. West, and Robert Wise. For their help I express my sincere thanks. I would also like to thank my numerous colleagues and students who encouraged me to undertake this second edition.

Davis, California   Jerry Franklin Green

CONTENTS

SECTION I—CARDIOVASCULAR PHYSIOLOGY

Chapter 1: The Heart and Circulation: A Brief Overview
Function of the heart and circulatory system   3
Basic anatomy of the heart   5
Properties of heart muscle   7
Basic anatomy of the circulatory system 10

Chapter 2: Electrophysiology of the Heart
Ionic basis of the cardiac action potential 17
Characterization of the action potential 19
Anatomy of the conductive system of the heart 25
Origin of the heartbeat 25
Velocity of conduction 28
Excitability of the heart 29
The electrocardiogram 32

Chapter 3: The Heart as a Pump
Cardiac muscle 39
Sliding filament model 40
Excitation-contraction coupling 43
Length-tension relationship 43
Determinants of cardiac performance 45
Pressure-volume curve of the heart 47
Ventricular function curve 48
Cardiac cycle 52
Heart sounds 56
Venous pulse 57
Normal pressure and flow as measured during the
   cardiac cycle 57

Chapter 4: Circulatory Mechanics
Volume-pressure relationships 59
Pressure-flow relationships 68
Conceptual model of circulatory system 75

Chapter 5: **Determinants and Distribution of Systemic Blood Flow**

Venous return 81

Cardiac output 85

Distribution of cardiac output 93

Chapter 6: **Determinants of Arterial Blood Pressure and Its Normal Value**

Arterial pressure-flow relationships 96

Concept of effective back pressure 98

Mean arterial blood pressure 100

Pulse pressure 101

Normal values of arterial blood pressure in the human 104

Chapter 7: **Control of the Cardiovascular System**

Determinants of vascular tone 105

Local control of vascular tone................... 108

Neurogenic control of vascular tone.............. 110

Control of cardiac function 115

Neural control of cardiovascular function 118

Chapter 8: **The Microcirculation**

Determinants of capillary pressure 128

Filtration-absorption 130

Chapter 9: **The Pulmonary Circulation**

Mechanical determinants of pulmonary blood flow   140

Neurogenic determinants of pulmonary blood flow   148

Local determinants of pulmonary blood flow....... 148

Chapter 10: **Other Regional Circulations**

Coronary circulation 150

Skeletal muscle circulation 153

Cerebral circulation 155

Splanchnic circulation.......................... 156

Cutaneous circulation.......................... 157

Chapter 11: **The Blood**

Composition 160

Normal values of blood volume in the human 164

Regulation of blood volume 164
Physical chemistry of blood 167

SECTION II—PULMONARY PHYSIOLOGY

Chapter 12: The Pulmonary System—A Brief Overview
Function....................................... 175
Basic anatomy 176
Lung volumes 181

Chapter 13: Pulmonary Mechanics
Volume-pressure relationships of the lung 183
Pressure-flow relationships of pulmonary airways .. 197
Work of breathing.............................. 205

Chapter 14: Pulmonary Gas Exchange
Gas exchange through the individual pulmonary
   capillary 206
Gas exchange through the lung as a whole 208
Quantifying the effects of the ventilation-perfusion
   relationship 210
The "effective" compartment 212
Calculating physiologic shunt 213
Determining ventilation-perfusion distributions 221

Chapter 15: Lung Water
Starling forces.................................. 225
Pulmonary edema 227

Chapter 16: Control of Respiration
Central control centers 229
Chemoreceptors................................. 231
Pulmonary receptors............................ 236
Effector organ.................................. 238

Appendix 1. Language.. 239

Appendix 2. Hemodynamics 240

Appendix 3. Ventilation-perfusion relationships 247

References   257

Index   263

CARDIOVASCULAR PHYSIOLOGY

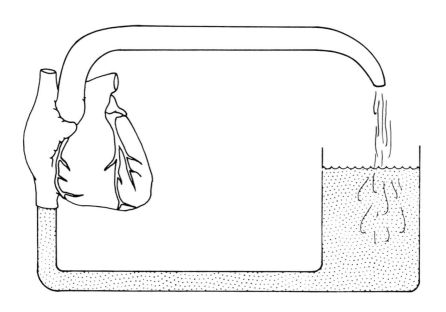

1

THE HEART AND CIRCULATION: A BRIEF OVERVIEW

FUNCTION OF THE HEART AND CIRCULATORY SYSTEM

Inspection, palpation, auscultation, and contemplation are the basic clinical tools of the cardiologist. The cardiologist must rely primarily on a sound knowledge of the physiology of the cardiovascular system and secondarily on experience and intuition. With this chapter we begin our discussion of the basic aspects of cardiovascular physiology.

Teleologically speaking, the function of the heart is to keep the body fluids in motion. Each of the 100 trillion cells in the body (give or take a few hundred million) is a living entity unto itself, capable of functioning and, in some cases, even regenerating, provided there is a relatively constant internal environment. The *homeostatic process*, termed *le milieu interieur* by Claude Bernard (1879), maintains this environment and depends on the transport of nutrients and waste products between the interstitial fluids of the body and the blood. The heart keeps the blood moving throughout the body and those specialized organs, such as the lungs, kidneys, and liver, allow for the adequate maintenance of nutrients and removal of waste products.

We like to think that the heart provides the pressure necessary for adequate tissue perfusion, but this is not strictly the case. The heart provides to the arterial system a given quantity of blood volume (the stroke volume). When this blood volume is forced on the arteries, which are highly elastic in composition and possess a low compliance (for definition see Chapter 4), a high pressure is produced by their elastic recoil. The high resistance to blood flow found in the "downstream" arteries prevents this elevated pressure from immediately dissipating. Thus, the pumping action of the heart *interacting* with the mechanical properties of the arterial system produces the pressure necessary to perfuse the tissues. Similarly, the pumping ability of the heart *interacting* with the mechanical properties of the veins provides the blood volume that the heart passes to the arteries.

This brief discussion of cardiac and circulatory *interdependence* is meant to emphasize an important point: the heart does not act alone in maintaining circulatory homeostasis. The heart is only one link (although an important and necessary link) in a circular chain of events that, by necessity, must interact to achieve the end result—the continued movement of body fluids.

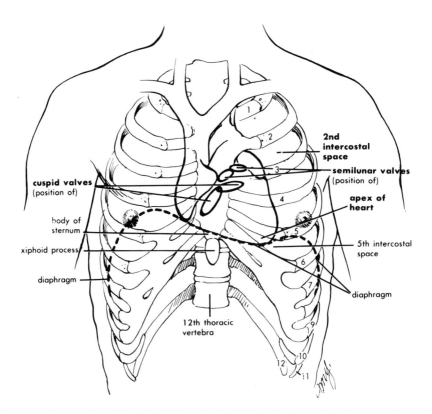

Fig. 1–1. Anterior view of the thorax showing the position of the heart in relationship to the ribs, sternum, and diaphragm, and the position of the heart valves. (From Crouch, J.E.: Functional Human Anatomy. 4th Ed., Philadelphia, Lea & Febiger, 1985.)

BASIC ANATOMY OF THE HEART

The human heart is a hollow, muscular organ about the size of the human fist. It lies obliquely in the *middle mediastinum* in the anterior inferior part of the thorax. The heart's position relative to the chest wall is shown diagrammatically in Figure 1–1. A venous angiocardiogram (Fig. 1–2a) and a sketch (Fig. 1–2b) identifying anatomic highlights are also presented. About two thirds of the heart lies to the left of the midsternal line. The apex of the heart is at the level of the fifth intercostal space, 7 to 9 cm to the left of the midsternal line.

The heart has four chambers. The two thin-walled *atria* are separated by the *interatrial septum,* and the two thick-walled ventricles are separated by the *interventricular septum* (Fig. 1–3). The boundaries of the cardiac chambers are indicated on the heart's surface by the *coronary sulcus,* which separates atria from ventricles, and by the *anterior* and *posterior longitudinal sulci,* which separate right and left ventricles. The vessels supplying the heart itself (*coronary arteries, sinus,* and *veins*) are located in these sulci.

The atria are the receiving chambers of the heart. The systemic veins empty into the *right atrium,* whereas the pulmonary veins empty into the *left atrium.* The ventricles are the pumping chambers of the heart. They receive blood from their respective atria and pump it into the pulmonary and systemic circulations. The right ventricle pumps into the *pulmonary artery* and the left ventricle into the *aorta.*

The atria and ventricles are joined by a fibrous *AV ring,* which is continuous on the right side with the *tricuspid valve* and on the left side with the *mitral valve.* These *atrioventricular valves* consist of three triangular flaps on the right side and two triangular flaps on the left side. *Chordae tendineae* are attached at the free edge of the valve cusps. These tendineae originate from *papillary muscles* arising from the inner surface of the ventricles. When the ventricles fill with blood and begin to contract, the valve cusps are forced closed by the increasing pressure. To prevent the valves from turning back into the atria and regurgitating blood, the chordae tendineae act like guy wires. When the atrial pressures exceed the pressure in the ventricles, the valves open, allowing blood to enter each ventricle.

The valves situated at the ventricular outflows are the *semilunar valves,* and each consists of three flaps. The *pulmonic valve* opens into the pulmonary artery, whereas the *aortic valve* opens into the aorta. These valves open during ventricular ejection and close when ventricular pressure falls below arterial pressure. The action of the cardiac valves during various stages of the cardiac cycle is illustrated in Figure 1–4.

The heart wall is mainly composed of cardiac muscle, which is thinnest in the atrial wall and thickest in the left ventricle. The *ventricular myocardium* (heart muscle) has a more complicated fiber arrangement than

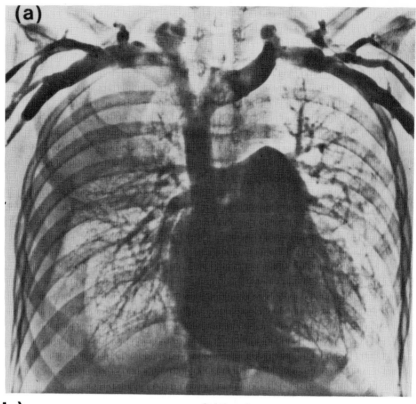

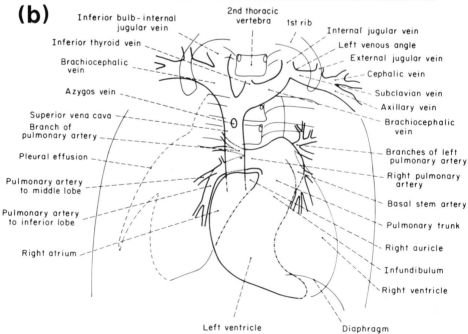

Inferior bulb - internal jugular vein	2nd thoracic vertebra 1st rib	Internal jugular vein
Inferior thyroid vein		Left venous angle
Brachiocephalic vein		External jugular vein
		Cephalic vein
Azygos vein		Subclavian vein
		Axillary vein
Superior vena cava		Brachiocephalic vein
Branch of pulmonary artery		
Pleural effusion		Branches of left pulmonary artery
		Right pulmonary artery
Pulmonary artery to middle lobe		Basal stem artery
Pulmonary artery to inferior lobe		Pulmonary trunk
		Right auricle
Right atrium		Infundibulum
		Right ventricle
	Left ventricle Diaphragm	

Fig. 1–2. Venous angiocardiogram. (From Wicke, L.: Atlas of Radiologic Anatomy. Baltimore, Urban & Schwarzenberg, 1979.)

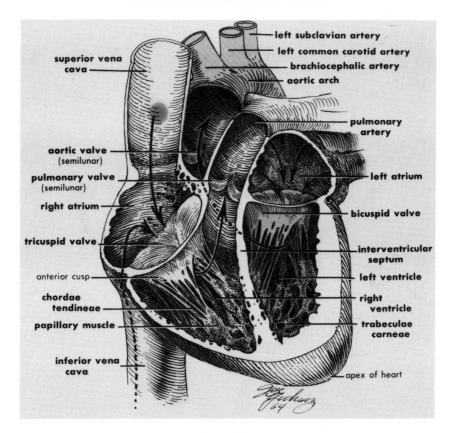

Fig. 1–3. Anterior view of the opened heart showing the cardiac chambers and valves. The arrows indicate the direction of flow through the heart. (From Crouch, J.E.: Functional Human Anatomy. 4th Ed., Philadelphia, Lea & Febiger, 1985.)

does the atrial myocardium. The muscle fibers are organized into spiral patterns and have both their origins and their insertions on the fibrous tissues at the bases of the ventricles. Therefore, their contraction results in a wringing-like action that does not completely empty the ventricles. After systole, a residual volume of blood remains. When the ventricles contract, their base is pulled downward as the heart rotates to the right so that the apex is pushed forward in the region of the fifth intercostal space. Changes in the dimensions of the heart during contraction can be seen in the x-ray films presented in Figure 1–5.

PROPERTIES OF HEART MUSCLE

The efficiency and ability of the heart to perform its task depend on sequential conduction of the cardiac impulse and the rapid sequential

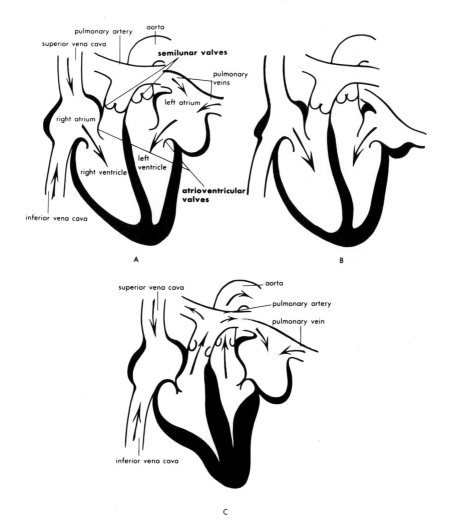

Fig. 1–4. Action of the cardiac valves during various stages of the cardiac cycle. *A:* Heart is relaxed; semilunar valves are closed; atrioventricular valves are open; atria and ventricles are filling with blood. *B:* Atria are contracted; ventricles are relaxed and filling; semilunar valves remain closed; atrioventricular valves are open. *C:* The atria are relaxed as the ventricles contract. The atrioventricular valves are closed; the semilunar valves are open; and blood is pumped into the pulmonary artery and the aorta. (From Crouch, J.E.: Functional Human Anatomy. 4th Ed., Philadelphia, Lea & Febiger, 1985.)

activation of the contractile apparatus. These actions are possible because all cardiac tissues exhibit four basic properties to varying degrees.

  1. *Excitability.* Like nervous tissues and other types of muscle fibers, all cardiac cells can respond to electrical, mechanical, or chemical stimuli or to changes in the electrical, mechanical, or chemical environments.

  2. *Inherent rhythmicity.* In contrast to skeletal muscle, cardiac muscle

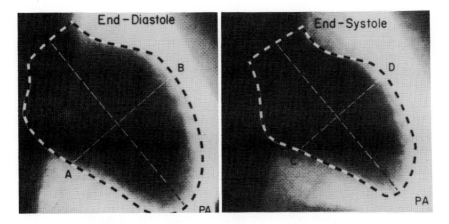

Fig. 1–5. Angiographic frames taken at end-diastole and end-systole. (From Grossman, W.: Cardiac Catheterization and Angiography. 3rd Ed. Philadelphia, Lea & Febiger, 1986.)

cells can originate an impulse that starts a chain reaction leading to a normal beat. This ability is especially developed in pacemaker or nodal tissue, such as the SA or AV nodes, but can occur in any cardiac tissue. The region of the heart with the fastest inherent rhythmicity initiates the heartbeat. Normally, inherent rhythmicity decreases from SA node downward to the ventricular myocardium, which has the lowest intrinsic (spontaneous) frequency.

3. *Conductivity.* All cardiac tissues can propagate impulses, although the rate of conduction varies with the type of tissue. Specialized conduction fibers, such as Purkinje's fibers, are the fastest-conducting tissues in the heart. Table 1–1 presents the rates of conduction occurring in the various types of cardiac tissues.

4. *Contractility.* All cardiac tissues possess the ability to contract in response to an impulse. Ventricular and atrial myocardial muscle cells are the major contracting tissues, but even the specialized cells, such as Purkinje's network and the nodal cells, are capable of contraction (see Table 1–1).

Table 1–1. Summary of Velocity of Conduction, Rhythmicity and Contractility of Various Cardiac Tissues

Tissue Type	Velocity (cm/sec)	Rhythmicity	Contractility	Cell Size (μ)
SA node	5	high	practically none	10–15
Atrium	80–100	little	maximal	10–20
AV node	5	high	very little	10–15
Bundle of His (Purkinje's fibers)	300–400	little	very little	50–70
Ventricles	30	little	maximal	15–25

BASIC ANATOMY OF THE CIRCULATORY SYSTEM

As previously mentioned, the basic function of the circulatory system is transport. The transport medium is, of course, the *blood,* which travels continuously in a closed circular system. A schematic illustration of the circulation is presented in Figure 1–6. The component parts of the circulation are the *heart;* the *arteries,* which conduct the blood away from the heart; and the *arterioles,* the small arteries that deliver the blood to the *capillaries* where exchange occurs. Downstream from the capillaries are the *venules,* which collect and store blood from the capillaries and

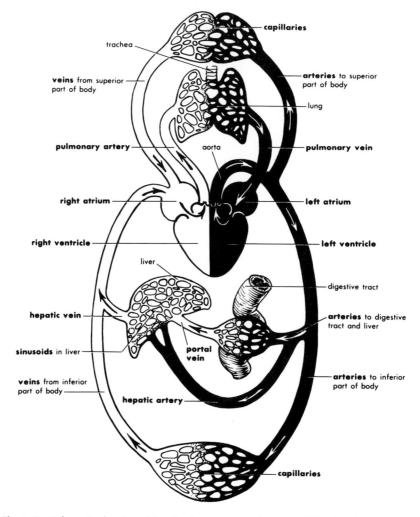

Fig. 1–6. Schematic drawing of the circulatory system. Oxygenated blood is shown in black and nonoxygenated blood in white. The arrows indicate the direction of flow. (From Crouch, J.E.: Functional Human Anatomy. 4th Ed., Philadelphia, Lea & Febiger, 1985.)

then deliver it to the large conducting *veins,* which carry it back to the heart.

Within the circulation are two major subdivisions, the *systemic circulation,* fed by the left ventricle, and the *pulmonary circulation,* fed by the right ventricle. The systemic circulation, sometimes called the *greater circulation,* supplies blood to most organs of the body, such as the brain, skeletal muscles, and gastrointestinal tract. The pulmonary circulation, called the *lesser circulation,* supplies blood to the lungs where oxygen is taken up and carbon dioxide is given off.

The walls of the arteries are composed of essentially three layers (Rhodin, 1980). The *tunica intima,* the innermost layer, is thin and has a surface of endothelial cells lying on a *basement membrane.* The *tunica media* is the thick middle layer that is composed mostly of smooth muscle and elastic connective tissue. The outer layer is the *tunica externa* (also called the *adventitia*) and contains mostly fibrous connective tissue. The three layers are usually separated by *internal* and *external elastic membranes.*

There are generally two types of arteries: *elastic* and *muscular.* There is no distinct separation between the two; rather, they grade into each other. The elastic arteries predominate near the heart. In these arteries, the tunica media possesses relatively more elastic than smooth muscle fibers. Distally, smooth muscle fibers tend to predominate in the tunica media. The most distal arteries, the arterioles, are highly muscular.

The capillaries are structurally the simplest and smallest of all the vessels. They vary in diameter from 6 to 10 μm. The capillary wall is simply one layer of endothelial cells lying on a delicate basal lamina rich in reticular fibers. The capillaries form a "vascular bed" arising from the arterioles and converging on the veins (Fig. 1–7). They penetrate nearly every tissue of the body. Within a capillary bed one can often distinguish between true capillaries and *thoroughfare channels.* The latter channels run directly between arteries and venules (see Fig. 1–7) and often have a few smooth muscle fibers. A ring of smooth muscle, the *precapillary sphincter,* is located at the beginning of most capillaries and helps to regulate capillary blood flow.

Three basic types of capillary walls have been distinguished (Fig. 1–8). In the *continuous capillaries,* the endothelial lining appears complete and, as seen from the lumen of the vessel, appears smooth and similar to the endothelium lining of the larger vessels. Functional studies, however, have demonstrated that these capillaries behave as porous membranes (Landis and Pappenheimer, 1963; Crone, et al., 1970). Recent ultrastructural studies have revealed the existence of intercellular pore-like channels in the continuous capillaries (Karnovsky, 1967). The *fenestrated capillaries* are found in such organs as the kidney and intestines, which are characterized by high levels of metabolism and active exchange of fluids. The endothelial cells of these capillaries show numerous intracellular

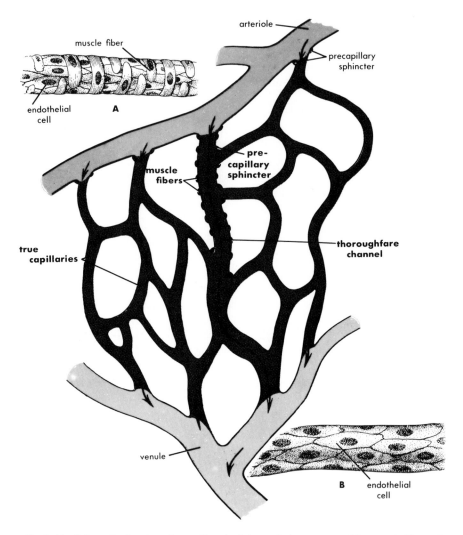

Fig. 1–7. Schematic drawing of a capillary bed. Insert A shows some of the muscle fibers of the proximal part of a thoroughfare channel. Insert B shows part of a true capillary. (From Crouch, J.E.: Functional Human Anatomy. 4th Ed., Philadelphia, Lea & Febiger, 1985.)

fenestrations, the functional dimensions of which are probably not much larger than those of the intercellular pores of continuous capillaries. Such organs as the liver and spleen possess capillaries known as *discontinuous* or intercellularly fenestrated. These capillaries possess an endothelial layer with obvious intercellular gaps. Scanning electron micrographs of the fenestrated and discontinuous types of capillaries are presented in Figure 1–9.

The venules closest to the capillaries are structurally similar to the

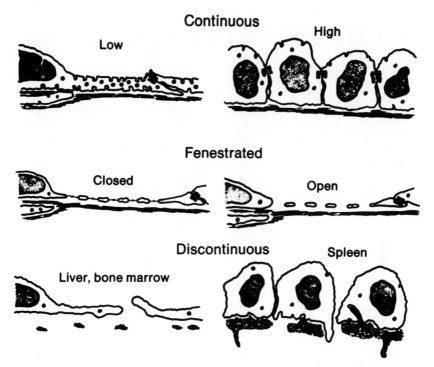

Fig. 1–8. Illustration of different types of capillaries. (From Majno, G.: Ultrastructure of the vascular membrane. Handbook of Physiology, Edited by F. Hamilton, Circulation, 3(2):2293, 1965.)

capillaries themselves, except their walls possess fibrous tissue outside the endothelial lining. The larger venules possess circularly arranged smooth muscle fibers. In larger veins, an outer tunica externa containing longitudinally arranged smooth muscle fibers can often be found. In general, the same layers as described for arteries can be found in large veins, but they are seldom as well defined. Veins, as a rule, have a greater diameter and thinner walls than do arteries.

Valves can be found in most large veins (exceptions are the venae cavae, portal system veins, and pulmonary veins). The valves are folds of tunica intima that allow the blood to flow to the heart but not backward (Fig. 1–10).

Closely associated with the circulatory system is the *lymphatic system*. Although this system is not anatomically a part of the circulation, its function is interconnected with that of the circulation. We must briefly consider its anatomy at this point. The lymphatic system is essentially a series of thin-walled vessels that provides an alternative route for the return of interstitial fluid to the vasculature. The lymphatic system begins as a network of *lymphatic capillaries*, which are simple endothelial

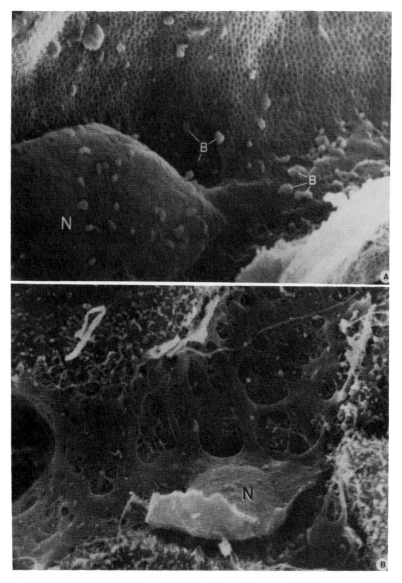

Fig. 1–9. *A:* Scanning electron micrograph of the endothelial surface of a finely fenestrated capillary such as is found in the kidney glomerulus. The pores are numerous and regularly arranged as in a sieve. They measure about 500 to 1000 Å in diameter. The nucleus (N) of this extremely thin cell bulges out into the lumen of the capillary. The cell surfaces are studded with small blebs (B) of unknown origin (×20,000; rat). *B:* Scanning electron micrograph of the inside of a liver sinusoid (discontinuous capillary). The endothelial cell is thickest in the region of the nucleus (N). From the nucleus, the cell extends out into thin margins that are fenestrated. The pores thus created are large, measuring as much as 2 μm in some instances. However, they vary greatly in size and shape (×11,000; rat). (From Motta, P., et al.: Microanatomy of Cell and Tissue Surfaces: An Atlas of Scanning Electron Microscopy. Philadelphia, Lea & Febiger, 1977.)

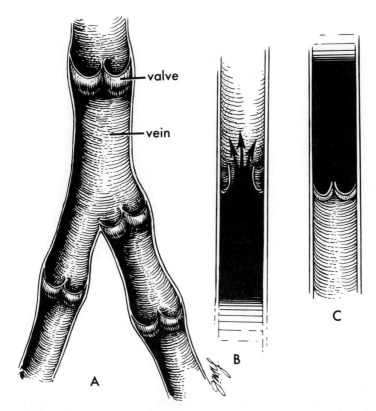

Fig. 1–10. Schematic drawing of venous valves. *A:* Veins opened to show structure and position of the valves. *B:* Valve opened as blood flows through. *C:* Valve closed as blood fills cusps and backflow of blood is prevented. (From Crouch, J.E.: Functional Human Anatomy. 4th Ed., Philadelphia, Lea & Febiger, 1985.)

vessels that begin "blindly." They collect the interstitial fluid directly from the interstitial spaces with relative ease (see Chap. 9). This collection can be accomplished because the endothelial cells of the lymphatic capillary are attached by thin anchoring filaments to the surrounding connective tissue. The junction of adjacent endothelial cells contains openings into the lymphatic capillary; the edge of one cell simply overlaps the edge of the other, thereby forming a small "valve" that opens into the capillary. Once interstitial fluid enters the lymphatic capillary (where it is called simply *lymph*), it cannot leave because any backflow closes the tiny inlet valves. The fluid then returns to the circulation by passing through a series of *lymph vessels* of increasing size, through *lymph nodes*, to the *right lymphatic duct* (also known as the *thoracic duct*). The thoracic duct empties its contents directly into the venous system at the point of junction of the left internal jugular and the left subclavian veins. The lymphatic vessels have many valves (similar to venous valves) and smooth muscle within their walls. When the lymph enters the lymphatic

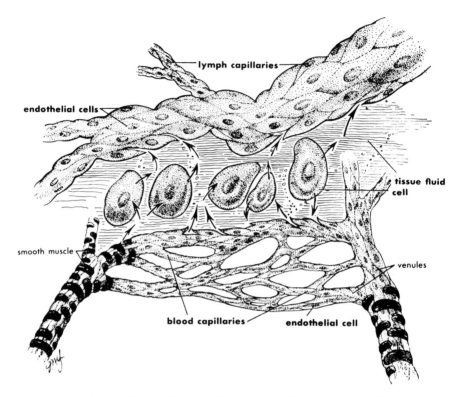

Fig. 1–11. Schematic drawing illustrating the movement of fluid from blood capillaries through the interstitial spaces into the lymphatic capillaries. (From Crouch, J.E.: Functional Human Anatomy. 4th Ed., Philadelphia, Lea & Febiger, 1985.)

system, it is propelled centrally by external compression on the lymph vessels by contracting muscles and arterial pulsation as well as by contraction of its own smooth muscle. Figure 1–11 illustrates the movement of fluid from blood capillaries, through the interstitial spaces, and into the lymphatic capillaries.

In addition to returning the interstitial fluid to the circulation, the lymphatic system is also the most important means of returning filtered protein from the interstitial spaces. The lymphatic system also filters the lymph at the lymph nodes, removing such foreign particles as bacteria and viruses. The thoracic duct also carries into the circulation substances absorbed from the gastrointestinal tract, mostly fats in the form of chylomicrons.

ELECTROPHYSIOLOGY OF THE HEART

IONIC BASIS OF THE CARDIAC ACTION POTENTIAL

Environment

The electrical activity of the heart is generated at the level of the individual cardiac muscle fiber. The electrical potential, which occurs within the cardiac fiber, and the changes in this potential result because of the ionic composition of the cell's environment and the semipermeable nature of the cell's membrane. The principal ions responsible for the electrical activity of the heart are sodium, potassium, calcium, chloride, and nondiffusible anions, which are found inside the cell and are mostly large proteins. Potassium and sodium are the most important diffusible ions. During resting conditions, the concentration of potassium ions inside the cell is around 130 mEq/L, whereas the extracellular potassium concentration is only around 5 mEq/L. A reverse concentration gradient exists for sodium ions (approximately 5 to 10 mEq/L inside the cell and approximately 130 mEq/L outside the cell).

Resting Potential

When a microelectrode is inserted into a resting cardiac muscle fiber and a reference electrode is placed in an electrolyte solution bathing the cell, a potential difference of between -70 to -90 mV (negative with respect to the outside of the fiber) is recorded in the muscle fiber. This *resting potential* depends primarily on the concentration differences of potassium and sodium ions across the cardiac muscle cell's membrane

and on the differential permeability of the cell membrane to these ions.*
A chemical force, based on the concentration gradient of each ion, results
in a net diffusion of that ion from a region of higher to lower concentration. To counter this chemical force, an electrostatic force develops.
If an equilibrium were established for any given ionic species, the chemical and the electrostatic forces would be equal and an *equilibrium potential*
for that ion would exist. The equilibrium potential for a given ion may
be defined as the membrane potential at which there is no *net* movement
of the ion across the cell membrane, i.e., the membrane potential that
just balances the ionic concentration difference across the membrane.
The equilibrium potential may be calculated, using the Nernst equation†
(Brown, 1974), as:

$$V_{ION} = -61.5 \log ([ION]_i([ION]_o). \qquad (2-1)$$

The brackets in this equation reflect the concentration of the ions, and
the subscripts, i and o, refer to inside and outside the cell, respectively.

The potassium equilibrium potential, V_K, is about -90 to -100 mV.
V_K is thus close to, but slightly more negative than, the resting potential
of the cell as actually measured with a microelectrode. This difference
represents a small potential of about 10 mV. It tends to drive potassium
out of the resting cell and is produced by a slow inward movement of
sodium.

The sodium equilibrium potential, V_{Na}, is about $+40$ to $+60$ mV. Both
chemical and electrical forces tend to pull sodium into the cardiac muscle
cell. However, because the permeability of the resting membrane to
sodium is small, the influx of sodium into the cell is also small. Nevertheless, this small influx of sodium moves the actual resting potential
away from the potassium equilibrium potential. Thus, the resting potential is less negative than the Nernst equation predicts.

One last point must be raised concerning the equilibrium potential.
A metabolic pump within the cell membrane actively transfers sodium
from the interior of the cell to the exterior while pumping potassium
into the cell. If this pump did not exist and if the exchange of sodium
for potassium were equal (actually, more sodium is pumped out than
potassium in), the steady inward diffusion of sodium would slowly
depolarize the cell, making the resting potential less negative.

The dependence of the resting membrane potential (Vm) on the intracellular and extracellular concentration differences of potassium and

---

*The permeability of a given ion may be defined as the net quantity of the ion that diffuses
across each unit area of membrane per unit concentration gradient and per unit membrane
thickness.

†The Nernst equation: $V_2 - V_1 = \dfrac{61.5 \text{ mv}}{z} \log (C_1/C_2)$, where C_1, V_1 and C_2, V_2 represent
the concentrations and potentials on both sides of the cell's membrane and z the net
number of charges on the solute particle.

sodium and on the respective membrane permeabilities (P_K and P_{Na}) to these ions is described by the *Goldman constant-field equation* as:

$$Vm = -61.5 \log \frac{[K^+]_I + (P_{Na}/P_K) [Na^+]_I}{[K^+]_O + (P_{Na}/P_K) [Na^+]_O}. \tag{2-2}$$

Because the relative permeability of sodium to potassium is small in the resting cardiac muscle cell ($P_{Na}/P_K = 0.01$), the value of Vm given by the Goldman equation approaches that of the potassium equilibrium potential as given by the Nernst equation for potassium.

In summary, the resting potential of the cardiac muscle cell depends primarily, but not entirely, on (1) the concentration difference of potassium ions across the muscle cell's membrane, (2) the selective permeability of the resting cell membrane predominantly to potassium ions, and (3) the diffusion of potassium ions down their concentration gradient from inside to outside the muscle fiber leaving the (negatively charged) anions inside the cell.

CHARACTERIZATION OF THE ACTION POTENTIAL

The onset of cardiac contraction is preceded by a change in the resting transmembrane electrical potential. This change is called a *depolarization.* The depolarization releases calcium ions into the myofibrils, thereby activating the contractile process (see Chap. 3). The relationship between depolarization and the onset of contraction is shown in Figure 2–1. Note

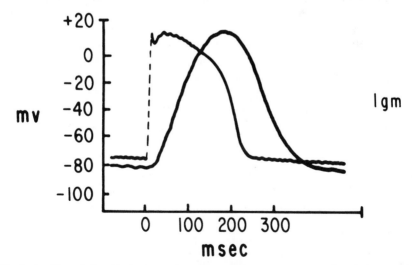

Fig. 2–1. The relationship between the transmembrane action potential and the onset of mechanical tension developed by a papillary muscle. The action potential is presented by the tracing with the rapid upstroke. Mechanical tension shows a uniform rise and fall. (Redrawn from Brooks, et al.: Excitability of the Heart. New York, Grune & Stratton, 1955. Reproduced by permission of the publisher.)

that rapid depolarization precedes tension development and return to the resting potential roughly coincides with peak tension development.

At the time of depolarization, the potential difference between the inside and outside of the cardiac cell falls to zero and actually reverses its sign for a brief period as the inside of the cell becomes positive relative to the outside. The depolarization of the cardiac cell represents a movement of the membrane potential away from the potassium equilibrium potential and toward the sodium equilibrium potential. Depolarization is caused by an increase in the conductance (permeability) of sodium.

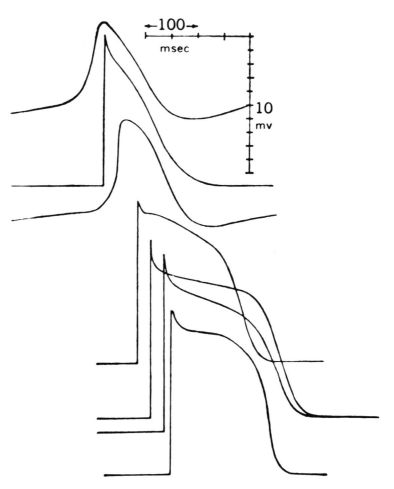

Fig. 2–2. Tracings of transmembrane action potentials recorded from the following sites (from top): sinoatrial node, atrium, atrioventricular node, bundle of His, Purkinje fiber in a false tendon, terminal Purkinje fiber, and ventricular muscle fiber. Note the sequence of activation at the various sites as well as the differences in the amplitude, configuration, and duration of the action potentials. (From Hoffman, B.F., and Cranefield, P.F.: Electrophysiology of the Heart. New York, McGraw-Hill Book Co., 1960.)

An increase in potassium conductance plays an important role in the return of the action potential toward its resting level in a process called *repolarization*. The time course of depolarization and repolarization varies from region to region within the heart, but essentially falls into two basic patterns (Fig. 2–2). The first pattern is referred to as the *pacemaker potential* because of the specific role played by this type of potential in generating the heartbeat. The pacemaker potential is found only in a few specific locations within the heart; most notably in the sinoatrial and atrioventricular nodes. The second pattern of electrical potential is that found in all other cardiac muscle fibers. This more widespread type is referred to as the *nonpacemaker potential*. Figure 2–3 schematically presents the two basic types of action potentials.

The nonpacemaker potential (upper tracing in Figure 2–3) is characterized by a rapid upstroke, designated phase 0. This upstroke is fol-

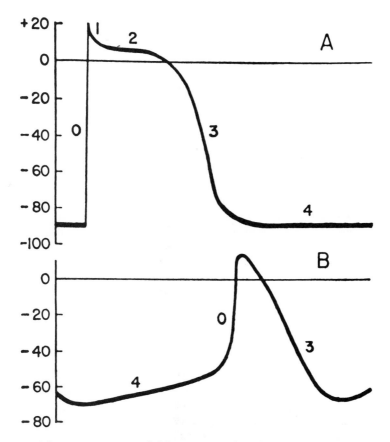

Fig. 2–3. Schematic tracing recorded from (A) ventricle and (B) sinoatrial node. See text for details. (From Hoffman and Cranefield: Electrophysiology of the Heart. New York, McGraw-Hill Book Co., 1963.)

lowed immediately by a brief period of partial repolarization termed phase 1. Phase 1 is, in turn, followed by a plateau (phase 2) that lasts from 0.1 to 0.2 seconds. The plateau phase is followed by a period when the potential becomes progressively more negative (phase 3) until, finally, the resting potential is again reached (phase 4).

The pacemaker potential (lower tracing in Figure 2–3) is characterized by a gradually depolarizing phase 4, a slower phase 0, an absent phase 1, and a phase 2 that is merged into phase 3. Thus, the plateau portion of this action potential is much reduced. Another important difference between the nonpacemaker and pacemaker action potentials is the magnitude of the resting potential. In the pacemaker cell, the resting potential is around -60 mV, about two thirds that of the nonpacemaker action potential. The lowest magnitude of the resting potential in the pacemaker cell is often called the *maximal diastolic potential* because, in this type of cell, the resting potential does not remain at rest very long.

Because the ionic basis for the two types of action potentials are somewhat different, we will discuss each separately.

Nonpacemaker Action Potential

Sodium and potassium are believed to diffuse through separate "pores" in the membrane called *sodium* and *potassium channels.* Furthermore, there are two types of sodium channels, the *fast* sodium channels and the *slow* sodium channels. The fast sodium channels are controlled by two types of "gates," the m gates and the h gates.* These gates are believed to be positive charges that are somehow fixed inside the channels, either at their openings or within the lipid matrix of the membrane adjacent to the channel. These charges create a positive electric field that blocks the channel from the movement of positive ions. When these positive charges ("gates") are pulled back from the channel, the channel's permeability to sodium increases. These electrical potentials are called *gating potentials.* Both the m and the h gates are controlled by the magnitude of the membrane potential. As the membrane potential becomes less negative (depolarizes), the m gates open and the h gates close. If the m gates opened at the same rate as the h gates closed, a distinction between these two gating potentials would not be necessary. However, such is obviously not the case. The m gate has a shorter time constant than does the h gate. Whereas the m gates open fully in less than 1 msec, the h gates require about 4 msec to close. Because the m gates open the fast channels to sodium diffusion, they are termed the *activation gates*, and because the h gates close the fast channel to sodium diffusion, they are termed the *inactivation gates.*

When a nonpacemaker type of cardiac muscle cell is at rest (resting

---

*The m and h designations were originally employed by Hodgkin and Huxley in their mathematical model of nerve conduction. J. Physiol., 117:500, 1952.

membrane potential about -90 mV), the m gates are closed and the h gates are open. Thus, even though both the electrostatic and the chemical forces tend to favor sodium diffusion into the cell, the permeability of the resting cell to sodium is low because of the obstructed channels (closed m gates). When the cell membrane is brought to a critical *threshold* level of about -60 to -70 mV, the m gates open, thereby activating the fast sodium channel (increasing the sodium permeability) and allowing sodium to diffuse into the cell. As sodium moves into the cell, the negative charges on the interior of the cell membrane are neutralized, and the transmembrane potential rapidly becomes less negative, i.e., depolarizes (phase 0 of the action potential). As soon as the membrane potential rises above -90 mV (becomes less negative), the h gates begin to close slowly, inactivating the fast sodium channels and decreasing sodium permeability. The h gates, however, do not close completely until sometime during phase 2.

At the end of phase 0, the cell is completely polarized with an inside voltage of about $+30$ mV. Although the concentration gradient for sodium still tends to force sodium into the cell, this diffusion is balanced (although not completely) by the positive electrostatic force now in the cell. This force tends to repel sodium from the cell.

During phase 1 and early phase 2 of the action potential, the closure of the h gates is completed, the sodium influx is tremendously reduced, and the membrane potential begins to fall. Merely closing the fast sodium channels would not in and of itself cause a change in the membrane potential unless the closure of these channels were accompanied by either an outward flux of some positive ion or an inward flux of some negative ion. The early repolarization that occurs during phase 1 of the fast type of action potential is believed to be caused by a transient influx of negatively charged chloride ions through some other type of channel and by an outflux of positively charged potassium ions.

During the plateau phase (phase 2) of the nonpacemaker action potential (when mechanical contraction begins, see Fig. 2–1), there is a slow inflow of both calcium and sodium ions through the *slow channels*. Although the activation and inactivation of these slow channels are not well understood, they are probably controlled by electrostatic gates opening and closing as the transmembrane potential reaches appropriate threshold voltages. The calcium that enters the myocardial cell during the plateau phase of the action potential is believed to be involved in the excitation-contraction coupling process by activating the contractile proteins that produce the contraction initiated by the action potential. As we shall see in the section on myocardial mechanics the contractile process can be enhanced by the administration of epinephrine. This enhancement may be caused by epinephrine's ability to increase the flow of calcium into the cardiac cell during the plateau phase of the action potential.

The exact mechanism responsible for the plateau phase of the action potential is not completely understood, but is related to changes in the permeability of the cell membrane to potassium. During the plateau phase of the action potential, the membrane potential is near zero. However, a concentration gradient for potassium remains, and tends to push potassium out of the cell. If this were allowed to occur, the efflux of potassium would make the inside of the cell more negative and repolarization would rapidly ensue. But, this does not occur; instead, the permeability of the cell membrane to potassium falls during phase 2. This reduction of potassium permeability has been termed *anomalous rectification* because we would expect a greater outflux of potassium that occurs as a result of the given chemical gradients. As a result of the reduced potassium permeability, there is only a small outward movement of potassium ions during phase 2. This outward movement almost balances the small inward movement of sodium and calcium ions, thereby tending to maintain the transmembrane potential near 0 mV.

During phase 3, the potassium permeability increases and the inward sodium and calcium ions traveling through the slow channels become inactivated. The net result is the final repolarization of the membrane and the return of the resting action potential.

Pacemaker Action Potential

The slower nature of this type of action potential is presumably related to its resting membrane potential and its effect on the fast sodium channels. Recall that the *h* gates begin to close at a transmembrane potential somewhat less than -90 mV. As the transmembrane potential approaches the level of approximately -55 mV, the *h* gates tend to close completely, inactivating the fast sodium channels. Thus, only the slow sodium channels are available for sodium diffusion at transmembrane potentials less negative than -55 mV. These slow channels appear activated (opened) when the transmembrane potential reaches around -40 mV, the same level as the pacemaker cell threshold. Thus, when the threshold potential is reached in the pacemaker cells, depolarization apparently proceeds (slowly) by diffusion of sodium primarily through the slow channels. This would explain the slower upstroke of phase 0 and the slower nature in general of the transmembrane potential of the pacemaker cell.

As far as the constantly decreasing potential in phase 4 is concerned, it is generally believed that a progressive reduction in the potassium permeability causes this phenomenon. As a consequence of the decreasing potassium permeability, the outward diffusion of potassium progressively decreases while sodium slowly but steadily leaks into the cells. These two ion fluxes, when taken collectively, slowly tend to make the inside of the cell less negative with respect to the outside, reducing the phase 4 potential.

ANATOMY OF THE CONDUCTIVE SYSTEM OF THE HEART

The normal adult heart contracts at a rhythmic rate of about 72 beats per minute. Under normal conditions, the heartbeat arises as a pacemaker potential in the specialized pacemaker region called the *sinoatrial (SA) node*, which lies in the sulcus terminalis on the posterior aspect of the heart where the superior vena cava joins the right atrium. This potential spreads from the sinoatrial node through the myocardium of the atrium like "fluid poured over a flat surface" (Lewis), causing the atrial muscle to contract. In the septal wall of the right atrium, near the orifice of the coronary sinus, another mass of nodal tissue, called the *atrioventricular (AV) node*, receives the traveling potential from the atrium and, after a slight pause, conducts it to the *atrioventricular bundle* (also called the *bundle of His*) with which the AV node is continuous. The atrioventricular bundle passes through the atrioventricular septum, the membranous interventricular septum, and finally divided into the *right and left branches*, which course down each side of the muscular interventricular septum. These branches pass under the endocardium of the right and left ventricles, respectively. Each branch divides into a number of branches (the *terminal conducting fibers* or *Purkinje's fibers*), which are continuous with the cardiac muscle fiber at their ends. Because the cardiac muscle is a functional syncytium (the intercalated discs provide low electrical resistance), the action potential spreads easily from the Purkinje's fibers to all ventricular muscle fibers. Here, the potential stimulates ventricular contraction to begin near the apex and to proceed to the base of the heart. The conducting system of the heart is schematically illustrated in Figure 2–4.

ORIGIN OF THE HEARTBEAT

Under normal conditions, the heartbeat arises in the sinoatrial (SA) node. The SA node contains two principal types of cells: (1) small, round cells that contain few organelles and myofibrils and are probably the pacemaker cells, and (2) thin, elongated cells, intermediate in appearance between the round and ordinary myocardial cells. These transitional cells probably begin the conduction process.

Although the heartbeat usually originates in the SA node, other *latent* pacemakers (called *ectopic foci*) elsewhere in the heart can assume pacemaker control under different conditions. Fibers located near the junction of the sinus node and atrial muscle are reserve pacemakers capable of driving the heart (at a lower frequency) in the event that the automaticity of the true sinoatrial pacemaker fibers are suppressed. In addition, fibers in the atrioventricular node and bundle of His can become active pacemakers when the activity of the pacemakers in the SA node is suppressed. In general, ectopic foci become pacemakers when (1) their

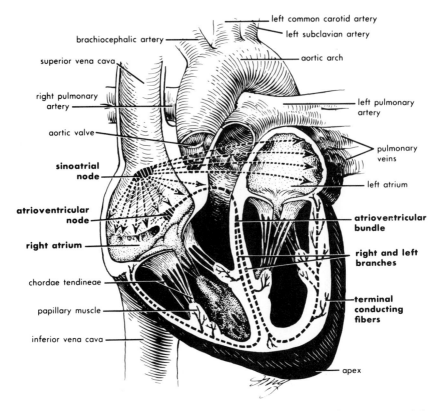

left common carotid artery

left subclavian artery

brachiocephalic artery

aortic arch

superior vena cava

right pulmonary
artery

left pulmonary
artery

aortic valve

pulmonary
veins

**sinoatrial
node**

left atrium

**atrioventricular
node**

**atrioventricular
bundle**

right atrium

**right and left
branches**

chordae tendineae

**terminal
conducting
fibers**

papillary muscle

inferior vena cava

apex

Fig. 2–4. Anterior view of the opened heart shows the intrinsic conducting system of the heart. Arrows indicate passage of impulses in the walls of the atria. (From Crouch, J.E.: Functional Human Anatomy. 4th Ed., Philadelphia, Lea & Febiger, 1985.)

own rhythmicity becomes enhanced; (2) the rhythmicity of the higher-order (SA or AV) pacemakers becomes depressed, in which case they drive the heart at a frequency lower than the normal sinus rhythm; or (3) all conduction pathways between the ectopic focus and higher order pacemakers become blocked.

A typical action potential as recorded from a pacemaker cell (SA node) is shown in the lower half of Figure 2–3. Note that the resting potential of the pacemaker cell is less than that of the potential as recorded from a ventricular myocardial cell (top half of Figure 2–3). Further comparisons reveal that phase 0 of the action potential has a much slower velocity, the plateau is absent, and repolarization (phase 3) is more gradual. However, the most important difference in the action potential of a pacemaker cell is phase 4. In the nonpacemaker cell, the transmembrane potential remains constant during this phase. However, in the pacemaker cell, there is a slow, steady depolarization called the *pacemaker potential*. Phase 4 depolarization proceeds at a steady rate until a threshold potential is reached. Afterward, an action potential is triggered.

Pacemaker cells can vary the frequency of discharge by any one of three mechanisms. First, the rate of depolarization during phase 4 can change (i.e., a change in the slope of the pacemaker potential). Second, the threshold potential can change. Third, the absolute value of the resting potential (lowest portion of the pacemaker potential) can change. Figure 2–5 illustrates how these mechanisms work. An increase in the rate of phase 4 depolarization (b to a in the top half of Fig. 2–5) causes an earlier threshold potential and a resultant increase in heart rate. A reduction in the threshold potential (from TP-2 to TP-1 in the lower half

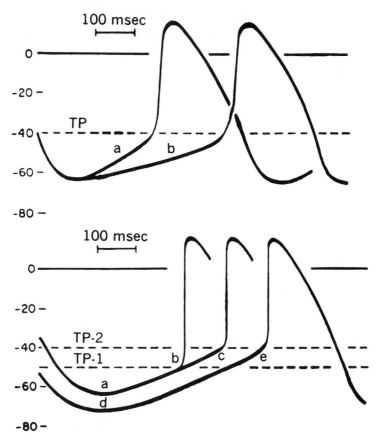

Fig. 2–5. Schematic drawing representing the important mechanisms responsible for changes in the frequency of discharge of a pacemaker fiber. The upper diagram illustrates the decrease in rate caused by a decrease in the slope of phase 4 from a to b and, thus, an increase in the time required for the transmembrane potential to reach the threshold potential (TP). The lower diagram illustrates the rate changes associated with a change in the level of the threshold potential from TP-1 to TP-2; also shown is a change in rate owing to an increase in resting potential. See text for further details. (From Hoffman, B.F., and Cranefield, P.F.: Electrophysiology of the Heart. New York, McGraw-Hill Book Co., 1960.)

of Fig. 2–5) accelerates the onset of phase 0 (from c to b) with a resultant increase in heart rate. Finally, a reduction in the magnitude of the resting potential (from d to a) accelerates the time to reach threshold TP-2 (from e to c) with a resultant increase in heart rate. Reversing the directional change of these three mechanisms decreases heart rate.

VELOCITY OF CONDUCTION

The speed by which the excitation wave of cardiac muscle travels through the heart is principally a function of the level of the resting membrane potential. There are at least two reasons why this is true. First, the resting potential determines the amplitude of the potential which, in turn, determines the rate of change of the potential (the slope of phase 0). The greater the rate of change of the potential, the shorter the time required to reach the threshold potential and the greater the conduction velocity. Second, the level of the resting potential determines the amount and kind of sodium channels that open when threshold is reached. It has been estimated that about one half of the fast sodium channels are inactivated (h gates closed) when the resting membrane potential is about -70 mV and that all fast channels are inactivated when the resting membrane potential is between -55 to -50 mV. Thus, the more negative the resting membrane potential, the greater the number of fast sodium channels available, the larger the magnitude of the sodium current, and the faster the upstroke of the action potential. It therefore stands to reason that, in regions of the heart where the resting membrane potential is more negative, such as in the ventricular my-ocardial cells and in the Purkinje's fibers, the velocity of conduction is relatively fast (1.0 to 4.0 m/sec). In the SA and AV nodes, where the resting membrane potential is low, the velocity of conduction is slower (around 0.02 to 0.1 m/sec). Thus, in general, the more negative the resting action potential, the greater the velocity of conduction.

The reason for these relationships lies in what is known as *local currents*. As a cell depolarizes, currents carried by the movement of cations in one direction and anions in the opposite direction flow from regions of higher to lower potentials. In the interior of the cell, anions flow in one direction and cations in the other, whereas, at the exterior of the cell, the opposite migration of ions occurs. The more negative the resting membrane potential, the greater the magnitude of these local currents. Because these local currents are the stimulus that shifts the membrane potential from its resting level to its threshold levels, they are the stimulus that depolarizes the adjacent resting portion of the cardiac fiber. Therefore, the greater the number of local stimuli (local currents), the more rapid the propagation of the wave of depolarization down the fiber.

EXCITABILITY OF THE HEART

As a wave of excitation passes over the heart, it produces a rhythmic synchronous contraction known as the *cardiac cycle*. The excitability of the heart varies with different time intervals within the cardiac cycle. Figure 2–6, taken from the classic work of Marey (1885), illustrates this time-honored principle of cardiac action. When a heart is contracting in normal sinus rhythm, the intervals (*diastole*) between ventricular contractions (*systole*) are evenly spaced. An electrical stimulus applied early in a systolic period does not elicit an extra contraction (record 2–3, Fig. 2–6). However, if the stimulus comes later in systole, an extra contraction, called an *extrasystole*, is evoked, but only after a considerable latency (crosshatched areas in records 4–6, Fig. 2–6). This latent period becomes shorter as the stimulus is applied farther into systole. If the stimulus comes during diastole, an extrasystole is evoked with little or no latency (record 8, Fig. 2–6). Finally, Figure 2–6 illustrates an abnormally long diastolic interval, known as a *compensatory pause*, which follows an extrasystole.

The information obtained from the early experiments of Marey and from the more recent studies clearly show that four states of excitability occur during the cardiac cycle. These states are represented schematically in Figure 2–7 and are (1) the effective refractory period, (2) the relative refractory period, (3) the period of supernormality, and (4) the period of normal excitability. The *effective (absolute) refractory* period is that period in the cardiac cycle during which no stimulus, however strong, can elicit a propagated action potential.* The *relative refractory period* is that period in the cardiac cycle during which a stimulus can elicit a propagated action potential; however, this stimulus must be greater than is normally needed to elicit a similar response in diastole. The *period of supernormality* follows the relative refractory period and is characterized by the fact that a propagated action potential can be elicited by a stimulus of less strength than is normally needed in diastole. Finally, the *period of normal excitability* extends from the end of the supernormal period throughout diastole.

The significance of these various refractory periods for cardiac muscle has already been inferred. Because the effective refractory period actually outlasts the peak of tension development (see Figs. 2–1 and 2–7), it is impossible to tetanize (a fusion of individual contraction into a prolonged sustained contraction) cardiac muscle. This property is important for cardiac muscle because a cardiac tetanization would be incompatible with life.

---

*What we now refer to as the effective refractory period was at one time called the absolute refractory period. However, recent evidence suggests there is no period in the cardiac cycle when a strong stimulus will not either initiate a local membrane response or in some way influence the repolarization process. Therefore, the term effective rather than absolute has been used to describe this particular part of the cardiac cycle.

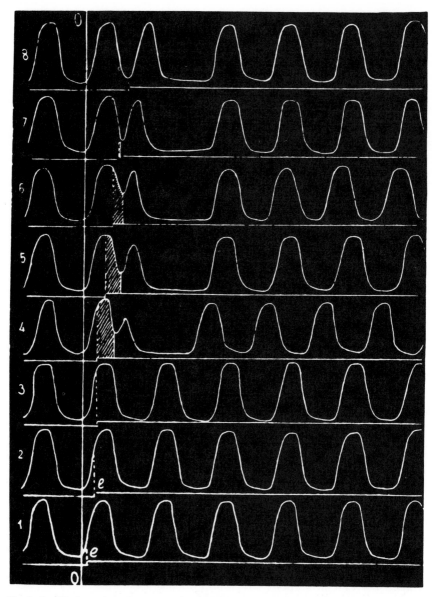

Fig. 2–6. Tracings of spontaneous and induced contractions of a frog's ventricle showing the refractory period, the latency of the evoked responses, and the compensatory pause. The lower line in each record shows the time of stimulation. An ineffective stimulus, e, indicates the effective refractory period. Line 0–0 shows the onset of spontaneous beats. The latency of the evoked responses during the relative refractory period is indicated by the crosshatched areas. (From Marey, E.J.: Excitations electriques du coeur physiologie experimentale. Travaux du Laboratoire de M. Marey. Paris, Masson and Cie, 2:63, 1876.)

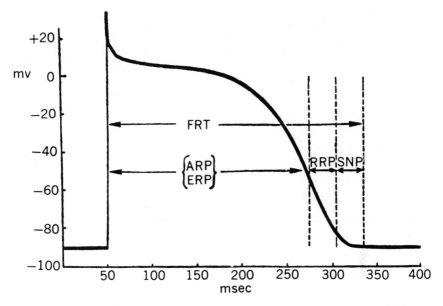

Fig. 2–7. Schematic drawing of the relationship between transmembrane potential from a single cardiac fiber and excitability of that fiber to stimulation. FRT = full recovery time; ARP/ERP = absolute refractory period/effective refractory period; RRP = relative refractory period; SNP = supernormal period. (From Hoffman, B.F., and Cranefield, P.F.: Electrophysiology of the Heart. New York, McGraw-Hill Book Co., 1960.)

The ionic basis for the effective refractory period is probably based on the fact that the fast sodium channels are completely closed (h gates closed) until repolarization of the membrane has proceeded to a level of approximately -55 mV. Thus, during this period, a stimulus, no matter how strong, cannot give rise to an action potential because there is little inward sodium diffusion. The mechanism responsible for the relative refractory period is also presumably related to the level of membrane potential during this period of the cardiac cycle. Recall that the local currents shift the membrane potential from its resting to threshold levels during a propagated response and that the more negative the resting membrane potential, the greater the magnitude of these local currents. Thus, early in the relative refractory period when the fast sodium channels are beginning to open, a greater amount of applied current is necessary to generate a propagated action potential. Also, the action potential itself is small and has a slow rising velocity characteristic of the low membrane potential from which it arises. Thus, the latency period between stimulus and contraction is longest when the stimulus comes early in the relative refractory period.

A Comment on Ionic Mechanisms

The descriptions given of the ionic mechanisms responsible for the cardiac membrane and action potentials currently seem the most reasonable. However, this area is being actively investigated and ideas are changing. As Brooks, et al. (1955), have pointed out, "Experimentation in this field has been cleverly conceived, skillfully executed and the results very adequately reported. Unquestionably the facts of observation can be accepted. Explanations and theories of function are quite another matter, and it is anticipated that they will be modified very frequently in the future." This statement is as true today as it was in 1955.

THE ELECTROCARDIOGRAM

The electrocardiogram has become one of the most important and widespread tools used in cardiology today. When used and interpreted properly by the well-trained professional, it becomes an especially useful diagnostic technique in identifying disturbances of cardiac rhythm and other specific cardiac abnormalities. Its development has been a direct outgrowth of our growing understanding of the electrophysiology of the heart.

Concept of the Dipole

As the wave of depolarization spreads over the heart, the excited (depolarized) portion of the myocardium becomes negative (at its surface) with respect to other (polarized) regions. Therefore, electrical currents flow from the resting portions (positive) through the surrounding conductive medium of the body and back to the excited (negative) regions of the myocardium. Because the entire body is a conductive medium (composed of electrolytes), the wave of cardiac excitation (negative potential preceded by a positive potential) can be viewed at any instant as an electrical *dipole* (something akin to a two terminal electrical generator). Figure 2–8 illustrates the type of electrical field generated by a dipole. An electrode placed on the skin can measure the change in potential produced by this advancing dipole. This measurement is the basis for the electrocardiogram. The potential difference measured by two electrodes placed within the electrical field produced by the dipole depends on (1) the voltage of the dipole generator, (2) the orientation of the electrodes with respect to a line parallel to the dipole, and (3) the distance of the electrodes from the dipole.

Standard Lead System

An electrocardiogram may be recorded by measuring the *potential difference* between any two points on the body. These two points, when

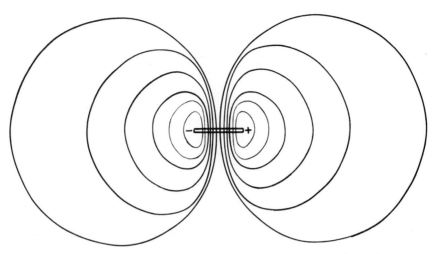

Fig. 2–8. Electrical field around a dipole. Circles represent isopotential lines. The greatest electrical differences exist along lines parallel to the dipole; the least on a line perpendicular to the dipole. (From Littmann, D.: Textbook of Electrocardiography. New York, Harper & Row Publishers, 1972.)

taken together, constitute an electrocardiographic *lead*. Three leads are commonly used today. The electrodes for these leads are placed on the right and left arms and usually on the left leg, although either leg is acceptable. Because arms and legs act as linear conductors to the torso, this lead system is equivalent to placing the electrode on the shoulders and on the abdominal region. By joining these points, an area resembling an equilateral triangle is covered. Lead I (right and left arm) represents the top of the triangle; lead II (right arm—left leg) represents the right side of the triangle (from the point of view of the patient); and lead III (left arm and leg) represents the left side of the triangle. This system is essentially the same as that introduced in 1913 by the Dutch physiologist Einthoven. The triangular arrangement of leads has since become known as *Einthoven's triangle*. The leads are bipolar, but are now simply referred to as the standard limb leads because of their extensive use. Figure 2–9 illustrates the standard lead configuration.

Electrocardiographic Deflections

The normal ECG tracing begins each cardiac cycle with a deflection called the *P wave*, which is produced by the depolarization of the atrial muscle (Fig. 2–10). The next major deflection is known as the *QRS*

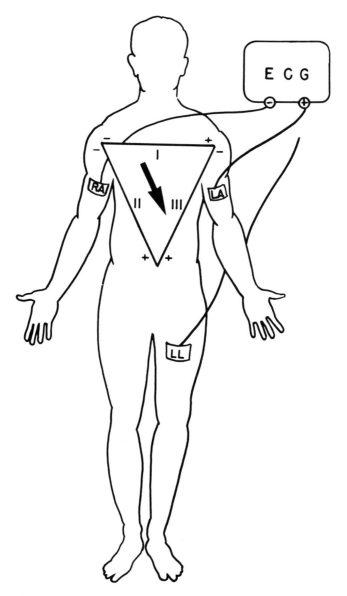

Fig. 2–9. The classic, standard bipolar leads. All switching is accomplished in the ECG machine. With lead I, illustrated, the left arm is connected to the positive terminal of the recorder and the right arm to the negative. The left leg, although joined to the instrument, makes no electrical contact and takes no part in the derivation of lead I. Lead II is obtained by removing the left arm from the circuit and connecting the left leg. In lead III, the left arm is rejoined in the position occupied by the right arm in the other two leads; the left leg remains in place. The arrow parallel to lead II demonstrates the electrical axis of the heart during a normal ventricular excitation. See text for further details. (Modified from Littmann, D.: Textbook of Electrocardiography. New York, Harper & Row Publishers, 1972.)

complex, which is produced by the depolarization of the ventricular muscle.*

Following the QRS complex is a wave of relatively large amplitude called the *T wave,* which represents ventricular repolarization. Occasionally, a *U wave* may follow the T wave in a normal ECG. The origin of this wave is unknown. Repolarization of the atria, which follows the P wave and continues into the QRS complex, produces a small electrocardiographic wave that can rarely be detected in the conventional leads.

During the interval between the P wave and QRS complex, excitation reaches the AV node and travels through the bundle of His and Purkinje's network. The *P-R interval* (or P-QRS interval) thus indicates the time between excitation of the atria and excitation of the ventricles, including conduction time, and ranges between 0.12 to 0.2 seconds in the normal adult. The duration of the QRS complex is approximately 0.08 seconds. The *Q-T interval,* which corresponds to the time required

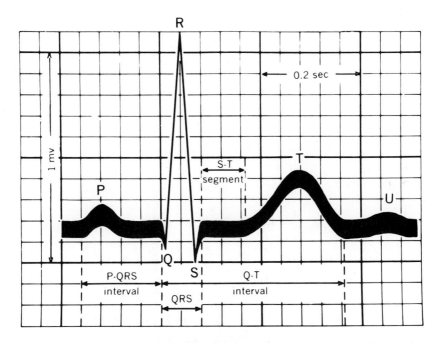

Fig. 2–10. Normal electrocardiographic deflections with conventional terms. (From Milnor, W.R.: The electrocardiogram. *In* Medical Physiology. Edition 14. Edited by V.B. Mountcastle. St. Louis, The C.V. Mosby Co., 1980.)

---

*The terminology here is purely arbitrary, but is fixed by convention. A positive deflection is termed an *R wave,* and any subsequent negative deflection is termed an *S wave.* If the ventricular complex begins with a negative deflection, it is termed a *Q wave.* The same cardiac event responsible for a Q wave in one lead may produce a simultaneous R wave in another.

for complete electrical excitation and recovery of the ventricles, averages about 0.35 seconds.

Electrical Axis of the Heart

During electrical activation of the heart, each individual fiber actually produces a dipole effect. Each dipole has its own direction and magnitude. When each of these individual dipoles are taken together, they produce what can be considered a single *equivalent dipole*. At any given instant, this equivalent dipole has its own orientation and direction. From the relative amplitudes and directions of the deflections in the individual standard ECG leads, it is possible to (1) determine the orientation vector representing the equivalent dipole of the heart and (2) establish the value of the equivalent dipole.

Under normal conditions, lead II gives the greatest deflection in the R wave during ventricular excitation (Fig. 2–11). Lead I is next, and lead III follows with the smallest deflection. Thus, under normal conditions, the electrical axis of the equivalent dipole during ventricular excitation is directed downward and toward the left. Because lead II almost parallels the axis, it should (and does) give the largest deflection (see Figs. 2–10 and 2–4). Such vectorial analysis can provide useful information to the physician on the anatomic orientation of the heart, the relative size of each ventricle, and electrical abnormalities.

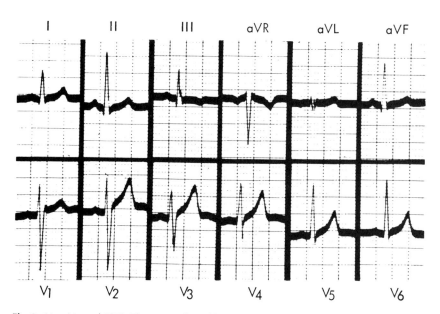

Fig. 2–11. Normal ECG. The numerals and letters above the tracing identify the lead. (From Littmann, D.: Textbook of Electrocardiography. New York, Harper & Row Publishers, 1972.)

Precordial Leads

The standard leads introduced by Einthoven give a kind of panoramic view of the myocardium. Standard practice today supplements the standard leads with so-called *precordial leads* (precordial means related to the anterior surface of the lower thorax). These leads give more direct information concerning the electrical activity of the heart. The precordial leads measure the potential difference between a reference electrode and an exploring electrode when placed at various positions on the chest (Table 2–1 and Fig. 2–12). This system consists of a central (reference) terminal connected through resistors that are parallel to the three points of Einthoven's triangle (both arms and one leg). The central terminal is supposed to be analogous to an electrode placed at a substantial distance from the heart because the potentials generated at the reference electrodes effectively cancel each other. Therefore, the voltage obtained by pairing the central and exploring electrode is dominated by the electrical changes at the exploring site. These electrodes are therefore called *unipolar*. Six unipolar electrodes are commonly used today and are designated with the letter V (for voltage). In addition, the central terminal electrodes are used to record unipolar extremity leads designated VR, VL, and VF (for voltage from right and left arms and foot, respectively). The information obtained from the precordial system of ECG leads is consistent with the conceptual representation of the heart as a dipolar generator. As such, the ECG leads supplement the standard leads of Einthoven by recording dorsoventral components of the three-dimensional electrical field of the heart. Although the theoretic basis for this system is debatable, its clinical value is unquestionable. An example of a normal ECG with both standard and precordial leads is presented in Figure 2–11.

Table 2–1. Position of the Unipolar Leads

Lead	Position
VR	Right arm
VL	Left arm
VF	Left leg
V_1	At level of fourth intercostal space on right side of sternum
V_2	At level of fourth intercostal space on left side of sternum
V_3	Midway between positions 2 and 4
V_4	In midclavicular line, fifth intercostal space
V_5	In left anterior axillary, fifth intercostal space
V_6	In left midaxillary, fifth intercostal space

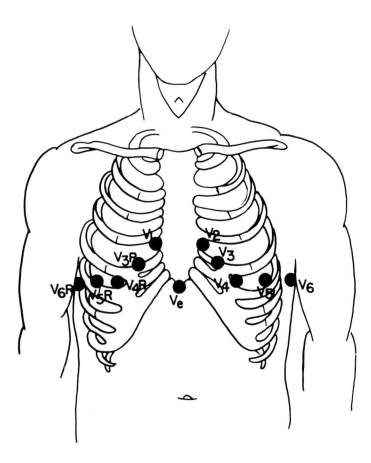

Fig. 2–12. Surface locations of the precordial leads. In this figure, several positions in addition to the standard leads are shown (V_3R, V_4R, V_e, etc.). Some laboratories routinely use these additional lead positions. They provide additional sampling from areas at varying distances from the source of electrical activity. (From Littmann, D.: Textbook of Electrocardiography. New York, Harper & Row Publishers, 1972.)

THE HEART AS A PUMP

CARDIAC MUSCLE

Before proceeding with our discussion of the heart as a pump, we need to emphasize that the heart is actually a muscle and that it derives its pumping ability from the contractile properties of the cardiac muscle. A brief description of the actual contractile unit is useful because our current understanding of the contractile process is based on the anatomy of the contractile unit itself, the *sarcomere*. Figure 3–1 presents a schematic drawing of cardiac muscle as seen under the light microscope. The myocardium, when viewed under the light microscope, consists of an arrangement of cylindrically shaped, striated muscle fibers ranging from 10 to 15 μ in diameter and 30 to 60 μ in length. The individual fibers are surrounded by a membrane called the *sarcolemma*. A rich supply of capillaries surrounds each fiber. The myocardial fibers branch and appear fused to other fibers by a thickening in the sarcolemma called the *intercalated disk*. Under the electron microscope, the intercalated disk appears to consist of two opposing membranes divided by a space. Although there is no actual connection between fibers, the intercalated disk is actually a low-resistance pathway for the easy transmission of electrical potentials from one fiber to another. Thus, from an electrophysiologic point of view, the myocardium functions as a genuine syncytium (this is not true from a strict anatomic point of view, however). Each muscle fiber consists of many longitudinal subunits, termed the *myofibrils,* that run the length of the fiber. A schematic illustration of a group of myofibrils is presented in Figure 3–2. The myofibril is composed of a serially repeated structure, the *sarcomere* (1.5 to 2.5 μ long), which contains the actual contractile proteins, the *myofilaments*. The sarcomeres of all the myofibrils are arranged adjacently so that the whole fiber has a striated appearance when viewed under a light microscope. The myofilaments are two specific types of proteins, actin and myosin. The chemical interaction of actin and myosin produces the force of contraction. The cell nucleus, many mitochondria, and the sarcoplasmic reticulum make up the remainder of the myocardial fiber.

SLIDING FILAMENT MODEL

The structure of the sarcomere has been analyzed in detail and forms the basis for the *sliding filament model of cardiac contraction* (Braunwald, et al., 1967). Although the actual ultrastructural interactions which occur in cardiac muscle are probably more complex than depicted here (Brady, 1979), the basic sliding filament model allows insight into mechanical properties of cardiac muscle. A single sarcomere is presented in Figure 3–1. The sarcomere is delimited by two adjacent dark lines, the Z *lines* (Figs. 3–2 and 3–3). The distance between Z lines varies with the state of muscle contraction, but is generally between 1.5 and 2.5 μ. When viewed under the electron microscope, the sarcomere contains alternating light and dark bands. In the center of the sarcomere is a dark

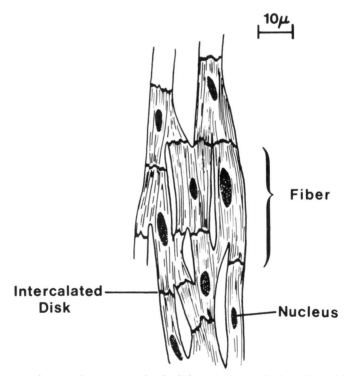

Fig. 3–1. Cardiac muscle as seen under the light microscope. The branching of fibers and the centrally located nucleus within each cell are evident. (Redrawn by permission from Braunwald, E., Ross, J., Jr., and Sonnenblick, E.H.: Mechanisms of contraction of the normal and failing heart. N. Engl. J. Med., 227(15):794, 1967.)

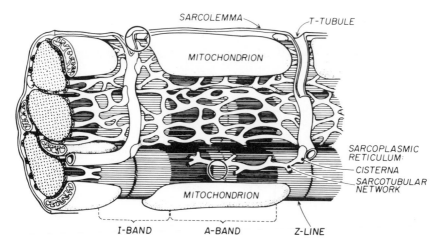

Fig. 3–2. Diagram of the ultrastructure of the working myocardial cell. Note the relationship of the intracellular membrane system to the sarcomere. (Reprinted by permission from Katz, A.M.: Congestive heart failure. N. Engl. J. Med., *293*:1184, 1975.)

band of constant width (1.5 μ) called the *A band*, which consists of filaments (10 mμ in diameter) of the protein, myosin. On both sides of the A band are the light-colored *I bands* made of actin protein (5 mμ in diameter). Because the actin filaments usually overlap the myosin filaments, the I bands can vary in length, depending on the degree of overlap. In the center of the A band is the *H band*, which comprises a thickening of the myosin filament known as the *M line*. Each thick myosin filament in the A band is surrounded by six thin actin filaments. The myosin has two important biochemical properties. First, it can split ATP into ADP and inorganic phosphate. Second, it combines reversibly with actin to form actomyosin. The actual contractile process occurs (in the presence of calcium ions) when actin and myosin combine to form actomyosin. The interaction of actin and myosin produces cross-bridges at specific sites between the filaments. The cross-bridges draw the actin and myosin filaments past each other in a longitudinal fashion. Remember that both the thick myosin filament and the thin actin filament remain constant in length during the actual contractile process; thus, as the cross-bridges are made, the Z lines come together, thereby shortening the sarcomere (see Fig. 3–3).

Because the force for shortening occurs when cross-bridges are formed between the actin and myosin, the greatest force logically occurs when the number of cross-bridges is greatest. This occurs in the myocardium when the sarcomere length is 2.2 μ, the length at which the actin and myosin myofilaments provide the greatest number of force-generating sites. When the sarcomere is stretched beyond 2.2 μ, the force decreases as the myofilaments disengage and fewer sites become active. At a length

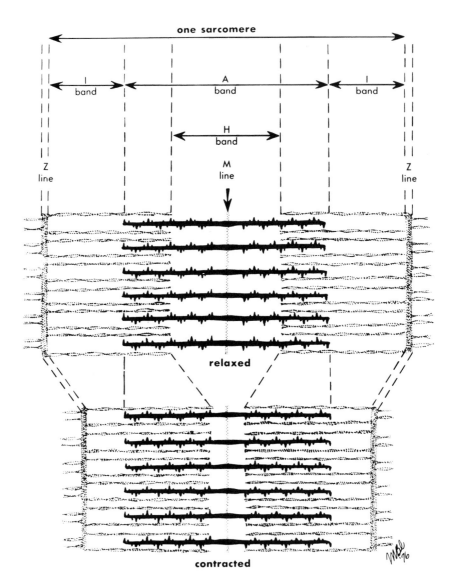

Fig. 3–3. Schematic drawing of a single sarcomere shows the changing relationships of the I, A, and H bands as contraction takes place. Note that the thin actin filaments slide between the dark myosin filaments and the I and H bands partially disappear. The A band remains constant in length. (From Crouch, J.E.: Functional Human Anatomy. 4th Ed. Philadelphia, Lea & Febiger, 1985.)

of 3.65 μ, the two types of myofilaments are completely disengaged, and the tension falls to zero. The developed tension is also less than maximum when the sarcomere length is less than 2.2 μ. At this length, the actin myofilaments pass over each other and break the cross-bridges.

EXCITATION-CONTRACTION COUPLING

The contractile process depends on a complicated *excitation-contraction coupling mechanism* which, in turn, depends on the anatomy of the sarcolemma and the fiber's intracellular membrane systems. The first system is a channel-like invagination of the sarcolemma that extends into the myocardial fiber and is filled with interstitial fluid. These *transverse tubules* are called the *t-tubules* (see Fig. 3–2). In contrast to the t-tubules of skeletal muscle, those in the myocardium run longitudinally as well as transversely. The t-tubules open freely to the extracellular space. The second type of structure is the *sarcoplasmic reticulum,* which consists of a series of interconnecting longitudinal membrane tubules located near the surface of the individual sarcomeres. These tubules surround the bundles of contractile proteins, but are not directly connected to the outside of the cell. As the longitudinal components spread along the surface of the individual sarcomere toward the Z line, they form what is generally referred to as the *subsarcolemmal cisternae,* which abut directly against but have no contact with the T system (see Fig. 3–2). The area consisting of the subsarcolemmal cisternae and the adjacent region of either the sarcolemma or t-tubule is called the *dyad.*

These membrane systems function in the excitation-contraction coupling as follows. Depolarization of the sarcolemma produces an electrical potential that travels along the t-tubule to the interior of the cell where it depolarizes cisternal membranes of the sarcoplasmic reticulum. These membranes communicate closely with the t-tubules. Once depolarized, the cisternae release calcium ions into the myofibrils. The calcium activates the myosin which, in turn, splits the ATP. The hydrolysis of ATP by myosin provides the energy to form the cross-bridges between actin and myosin and, thus, produces the contraction of the muscle. The sarcoplasmic reticulum then takes up the calcium that was previously released, returning the sarcomere to a relaxed state.

LENGTH-TENSION RELATIONSHIP

One of the most important conclusions of the sliding filament model of cardiac contraction is that the developed or active tension of the cardiac muscle is proportional to the number of cross-bridges between the actin and myosin myofilaments. The number of cross-bridges, in turn, is proportional to the length of the sarcomere. This apparent property of cardiac muscle forms the basis of the *length-tension relationship,* which

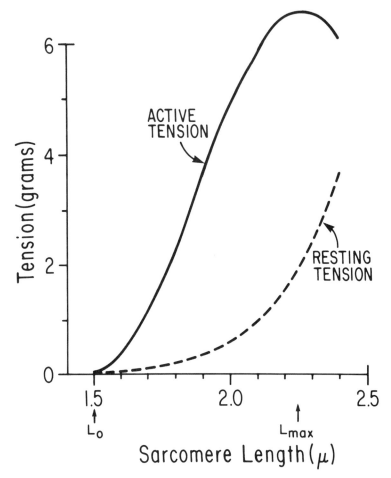

Fig. 3–4. The relationship between papillary muscle sarcomere length, resting tension, and the developed (active) tension. The active tension increases up to a sarcomere length of 2.2 μ and then decreases while the resting tension increases markedly above a sarcomere length of 2.2 μ. This sarcomere length generally corresponds to an end-diastolic pressure of about 10 mm Hg. (Redrawn by permission of The American Heart Association from Sonnenblick, E.H., Spotnitz, H.M., and Spiro, D.: Role of the sarcomere in ventricular function and the mechanism of heart failure. Circ. Res., *15*(Suppl. 11):70, 1964.)

has been carefully studied in isolated strips of papillary muscle. Figure 3–4 shows the results of one such study. One end of the papillary muscle was fixed to a firm support; the other end was fixed to a force transducer that measured the developed tension. The apparatus was constructed so that the length of the muscle could be adjusted; however, once the length was set, it was held constant so that the muscle contraction was isometric.* As the muscle was stretched (when not contracting), a resting tension developed (dashed line, see Fig. 3–4) suggesting that the behavior of a resting muscle is similar to that of a nonlinear spring. When the muscle was electrically stimulated, an active isometric tension developed as a function of the muscle length. The active tension of this muscle (see Fig. 3–4) increased to a maximum sarcomere length of 2.2 μ (known as L_{max}) and then decreased. Recall that 2.2 μ is the length of a myocardial sarcomere at which the actin and myosin myofilaments produce the greatest number of force-generating sites. Stretching the muscle beyond a sarcomere length of 2.2 μ decreased the developed force because the myofilaments become partially disengaged and fewer cross-bridges were formed. At sarcomere lengths of less than 2.2 μ, the actin myofilaments passed each other and, again, fewer cross-bridges were developed. It is interesting to note that a sarcomere length of 2.2 μ in the intact heart occurs with a ventricular pressure of about 10 to 12 mm Hg. This range is usually the upper limit of ventricular filling pressure.

DETERMINANTS OF CARDIAC PERFORMANCE

From the length-tension relationship of cardiac muscle (Fig. 3–4), one can easily see that the initial length of the cardiac muscle fiber immediately preceding contraction determines its isometric tension and therefore should influence its performance. This initial stretch of cardiac muscle is called the *preload*. Another important determinant of cardiac performance is the force which the heart must pump against, called the *afterload*. *Heart rate* is another obviously important determinant of cardiac performance primarily because the greater the frequency of contraction the greater the blood flow.† Finally, the force which the heart muscle itself contracts, called the *contractility*, is a major determinant of cardiac performance.

The concept of myocardial contractility is easy to understand but extremely difficult to adequately define. In the intact heart, a change in contractility can be easily recognized as an increase or decrease in the work performed per beat at constant end-diastolic volume. But, what has changed and how can it be best measured? All definitions of contractility fall short of their goal at this point because contractility is really the net effect of all mechanisms that influence the contracting proteins. In the absence of an adequate definition of myocardial contractility, we can at least begin to appreciate the concept by recognizing that a change in contractility appears to be related to a *qualitative* change in the force generated at the cross-bridge sites; whereas, a change in fiber length

---

*Isometric: isos = same; metron = measure.
†An increase in heart rate has also been shown to increase contractility.

(the preload) appears to influence *quantitatively* the number of active force generating sites. The contractility of the myocardium can be increased with certain drugs, such as digitalis and epinephrine. The increase in contractility produced by these drugs is generally referred to as an *inotropic** effect and is manifest as an increase in the end-systolic pressure-volume curve (see below). The increase in heart rate which can occur with certain drugs such as epinephrine is referred to as a *chronotropic†* effect.

To summarize, the four major determinants of cardiac performance are:

1. preload
2. afterload
3. contractility
4. heart rate

The effects these determinants have on cardiac performance can best be studied in the intact beating heart by evaluation with the ventricular *pressure-volume curve* and the *ventricular function curve.*

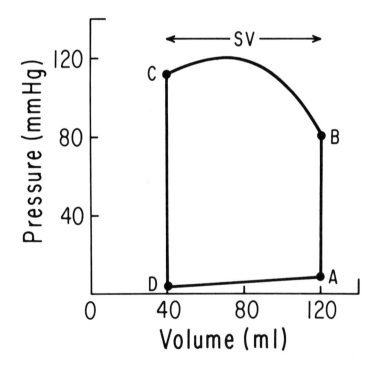

Fig. 3–5. Ventricular pressure-volume diagram. See text for details. SV = stroke volume.

---

*Inotropic: ino = fiber; tropos = influencing
†Chronotropic: chrono = time; tropos = influencing

PRESSURE-VOLUME CURVE OF THE HEART

The work of the heart (e.g., the left ventricle) can be defined as the product of ventricular pressure and ventricular volume, or the area of the pressure-volume curve. Figure 3–5 presents a pressure-volume curve of a left ventricle during a single cardiac cycle (see below). Line segment D-A represents diastolic filling of the ventricle. The reciprocal of this line is equal to the diastolic compliance of the left ventricle. On the pressure axis, $\dfrac{D + A}{2}$ represents the mean left atrial or left ventricular diastolic pressure. The ventricle begins to contract (point A) at a measurable end-diastolic pressure that represents the initial load of the ventricle or *preload*. As the ventricular myocardium develops tension, ventricular pressure rises, thereby closing the mitral valve (point A). Until the aortic valve opens (point B), the contraction is isovolumic. Ejection begins at point B, and the ventricular pressure at this point (equal to aortic pressure) represents ventricular *afterload*. Ejection continues until point C, where the ventricular pressure falls below aortic pressure. The volume ejected during this period is the stroke volume (SV). The initial phase of ventricular relaxation (line segment C-D) is isovolumic. As pressure in the left ventricle falls below that in the left atrium (point D), blood begins to flow into the ventricle during the period of diastolic filling (line segment D-A). This inflow of blood stretches the ventricular wall and produces the preload for the next contraction.

The effect that successive changes in preload have on the pressure-volume curve of the left ventricle and, therefore, on left ventricular work is illustrated in Figure 3–6. As the mean left atrial pressure increases, diastolic filling increases, thereby increasing preload (point a′). If afterload does not change, ejection begins at the same ventricular pressure (point b′). The initial phase of ventricular relaxation now begins at point c′. An increase in preload increases the area of the pressure-volume curve (increases left ventricular work). Notice that successive increases in preload cause the initial point of relaxation (point c′) to fall on a linear line. Because this straight line does not change, except by interventions that produce changes in contractility, its slope can be used as a measure of contractility (see the following). For want of a better name, we can call this line the *end-systolic pressure-volume curve*.

The effect on the ventricular pressure-volume curve of changes in afterload is presented in Figure 3–7. Two examples are illustrated. A change in afterload per se (curve 1) increases the ventricular pressure where ejection begins. If contractility does not change, the initial phase of relaxation moves up the end-systolic pressure-volume curve. As a result, stroke volume decreases and the work of the heart usually increases. Example 2 illustrates the result of the heart's attempt to compensate for an increase in afterload to maintain a constant stroke volume.

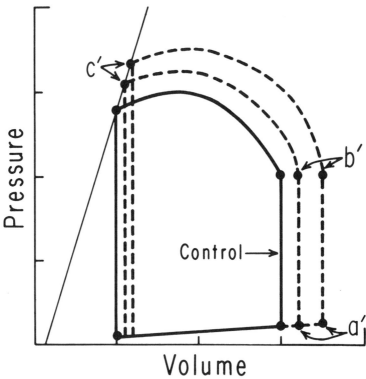

Fig. 3–6. Ventricular pressure-volume diagrams illustrating the effects of changes in *preload* on ventricular work. See text for details.

The heart compensates for an increase in afterload by allowing an increase in preload. The end result is a larger pressure-volume curve and an increase in ventricular work.

Changes in contractility are illustrated in Figure 3–8. An increase in contractility can be represented by an increase in the slope of the end systolic pressure-volume curve (curve 1). A decrease in contractility can be represented by a decrease in the slope of this curve (curve 2). Because contractility changes so profoundly affect the slope of the end systolic pressure-volume curve, this relationship is often measured as an index of the contractile state of the myocardium.

VENTRICULAR FUNCTION CURVE

The effects of preload, afterload, contractility, and heart rate on pumping ability of the heart can also be evaluated with the aid of the *ventricular function curve*. The physiologic basis of this relationship is *Starling's law of the heart*. Briefly, Starling's law states that an increase in the stretch of the ventricles immediately before contraction (end-diastole) results in an increase in stroke volume. In terms of the length-tension relationship,

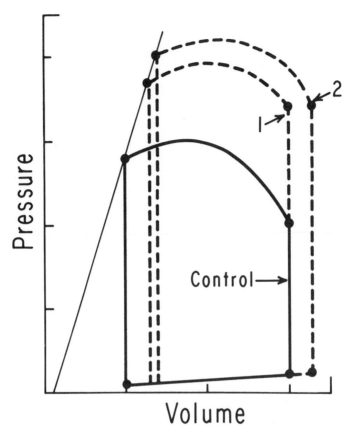

Fig. 3–7.   Ventricular pressure-volume diagrams illustrating the effects of changes in *afterload* on ventricular work. See text for details.

increasing the initial muscle length (the preload) results in a more force-ful contraction and leads to an increase in stroke volume. Because di-rectly quantitating the amount of ventricular stretch (preload) is difficult, indirect measurements of preload are made. These measurements in-clude ventricular end-diastolic volume, ventricular end-diastolic trans-mural pressure, or transmural atrial pressure. Figure 3–9 shows the type of relationship obtained when stroke volume is plotted against an index of ventricular stretch. Such a relationship is generally referred to as a *ventricular* or *cardiac function curve* and represents the length-tension re-lationship applied to the whole heart.

Although a stroke volume function curve may adequately describe the heart's ability to pump a certain amount of blood per beat, its use-fulness is limited. Other indexes of ventricular performance, such as stroke work, minute work, or cardiac output, are often more informative, especially if we wish to assess the pumping ability of the heart over a

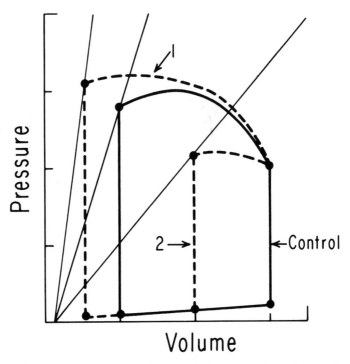

Fig. 3–8. Ventricular pressure-volume diagrams illustrating the effects of changes in *contractility* of ventricular work. See text for details.

period of time. If we wanted to study the heart's ability to pump the venous return we would select cardiac output as the index of ventricular performance. On the other hand, if we were interested in the amount of work the heart can do we would use stroke work or minute work as an index of ventricular performance. A commonly used *cardiac output function curve* is shown in Figure 3–10. Right atrial transmural pressure is used as the index of ventricular stretch. The reasoning is as follows: the greater the right atrial transmural pressure, the greater the ventricular filling, and the greater the end-diastolic volume, the greater the ventricular stretch. If the heart rate remains constant, the increased cardiac output results solely from the increased ventricular stretch.

Patterns of Ventricular Performance

An infinite number of cardiac function curves is possible. At any given degree of stretch, a normal heart should be able to pump more blood and do more work than a *hypoeffective* heart (i.e., diseased heart). Similarly, a *hypereffective* heart should give a better performance than a normal heart. Figure 3–11 demonstrates the basic patterns of the cardiac function curves. At constant heart rate and afterload, the slope of the cardiac function curve is a function of the contractile state of the myo-

The Heart as a Pump

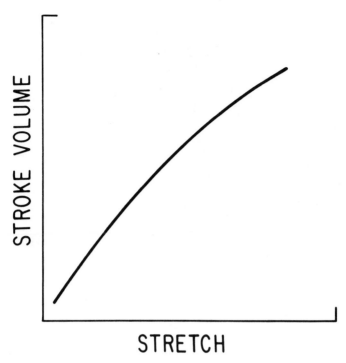

Fig. 3–9. The Frank-Starling relationship—stroke volume as a function of ventricular end-diastolic stretch. An increase in the stretch of the ventricles immediately before contraction (end-diastole) results in an increase in stroke volume. Note that ventricular end-diastolic stretch is synonymous with the concept of preload. (From Green, J.F.: Mechanical Concepts in Cardiovascular and Pulmonary Physiology. Philadelphia, Lea & Febiger, 1977.)

cardium, i.e., the *contractility*. An increased contractility produces a hypereffective heart and increases the slope of the cardiac function curve. A decrease in contractility produces a hypoeffective heart and decreases the slope of the curve. At any given state of contractility, a change in preload (heart rate and afterload remaining constant) simply causes the heart to "move" up or down its existing function curve, i.e., the slope does not change. An increase in afterload (at constant contractility and heart rate) depresses the curve, leading to a hypoeffective heart. A decrease in afterload pushes the cardiac function curve in the opposite direction. When cardiac output is used as the index of pumping ability (as in Fig. 3–11), an increase in heart rate increases the slope of the curve, whereas a decrease in heart rate does the opposite. To summarize, changes in afterload, contractility, and heart rate change the slope of the cardiac output function curve; changes in preload cause the heart to "move" up or down its existing curve. These changes are illustrated in Figure 3–12.

Common factors that can lead to a hypereffective heart are (1) an increase in the sympathetic nerve activity to the heart, (2) an increase

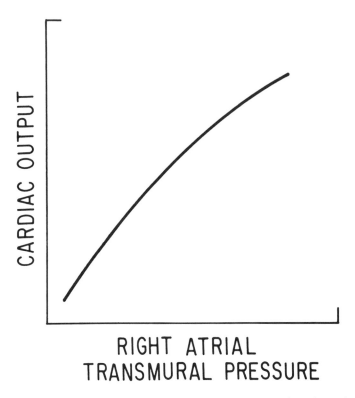

Fig. 3–10. A right ventricular cardiac function curve. An increase in the right atrial pressure results in an increase in right ventricular stretch and then in ventricular (cardiac) output. This relationship assumes heart rate is constant. (From Green, J.F.: Mechanical Concepts in Cardiovascular and Pulmonary Physiology. Philadelphia, Lea & Febiger, 1977.)

in the level of circulating catecholamines, or (3) the administration of an exogenous positive inotropic agent, e.g., one that strengthens muscular action, such as the cardiac glycosides and isoproterenol. Other factors that can lead to a hypoeffective heart are decreased sympathetic nerve activity to the heart, physiologic depressants (such as myocardial hypoxia, hypercapnia, and acidosis), pharmacologic depressants (such as barbiturates), and loss of myocardium, as occurs following an infarction.

CARDIAC CYCLE

In the preceding sections of this chapter we discussed the heart's ability to pump blood. We will now turn our attention to the inevitable result of that ability, i.e. the hemodynamic events which occur during the cardiac cycle. Figure 3–13 is a schematic representation of the hemodynamic events that occur during the cardiac cycle. The values presented are expected in a normal adult human with a heart rate of 75 beats per minute. The period of ventricular relaxation is called *diastole*, and the

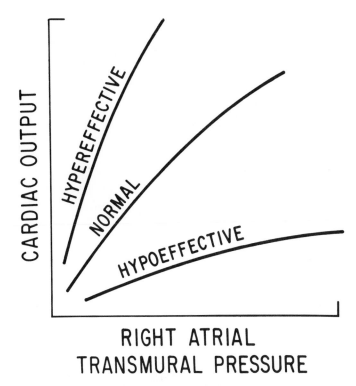

Fig. 3–11. Basic patterns of ventricular function curves. For a hypereffective heart, a given increase in right atrial pressure results in a greater than normal increase in cardiac output. For a hypoeffective heart, the same increase in right atrial pressure results in a less-than-normal increase in cardaic output. (From Green, J.F.: Mechanical Concepts in Cardiovascular and Pulmonary Physiology. Philadelphia, Lea & Febiger, 1977.)

period of ventricular contraction is called *systole*. This discussion of the cardiac cycle will begin during late diastole at the start of the P wave of the electrocardiogram. During diastole, the ventricles are filling with blood. The P wave signals the electrical excitation of the atria. In approximately 0.1 seconds, as the excitation spreads over most of the atrial muscle, atrial contraction commences, causing a slight rise in both atrial and ventricular pressures. This rise in pressure occurs in both cardiac chambers because the atrioventricular (mitral and tricuspid) valves are open. Because most of the ventricular filling occurs early in diastole, relatively little increase in ventricular volume (20 percent or less) occurs as a result of atrial contraction. The rise in ventricular pressure with atrial contraction cannot always be demonstrated. It is most pronounced during periods of prolonged diastole (with slow heart rates). During episodes of elevated heart rates, when the diastolic period is reduced, there does not appear to be enough time to allow the atrial contraction to be manifest as a rise in ventricular pressure. Sometimes, the AV valves

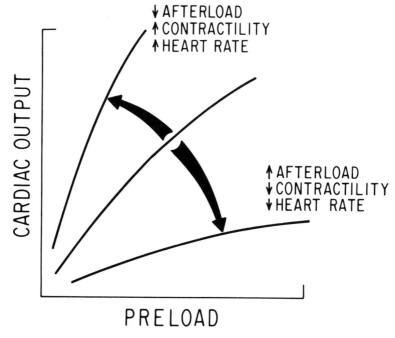

Fig. 3–12. Illustration of how preload, afterload, contractility, and heart rate affect the cardiac output function curve.

(mitral and tricuspid) close during diastole as a result of blood attempting to flow backward into the atria from the ventricles. More often, however, these valves close with the onset of ventricular contraction.

Late in diastole, the ventricles are invaded by the electrical excitation process as it spreads over the atrial muscle from the SA node and then via the bundle of His and the Purkinje network. Ventricular depolarization during this period is marked by the beginning of the QRS complex. Ventricular contraction begins shortly after the onset of the QRS complex. As the ventricles begin to contract, the intraventricular pressures begin to rise, thereby closing the AV valves, if they are not already closed (causing the first heart sound). During this early period of ventricular contraction (immediately following AV valve closure), the ventricles become an isolated chamber because the pulmonic and aortic valves are also closed. Because blood is incompressible, this period of ventricular contraction (lasting about 0.05 seconds) is termed the *isovolumic phase of contraction.* As the isovolumic contraction phase continues, the intraventricular pressure rises rapidly until the intraventricular pressures exceed the pressure in the pulmonary artery and aorta. Once this occurs, the semilunar valves (pulmonic and aortic) open, systole begins, and blood is ejected from the ventricles. Ejection is rapid at first and declines during the later stage of systole. During ejection, the arterial

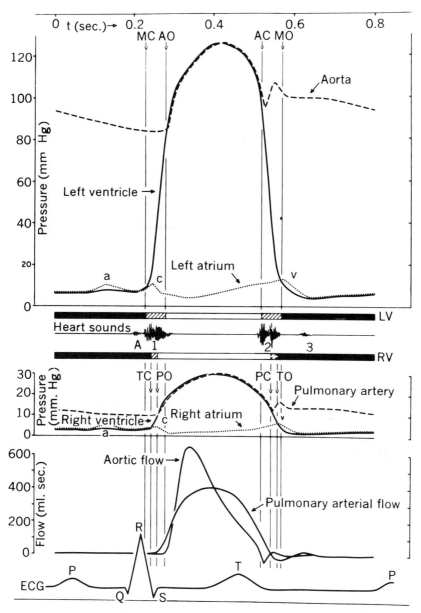

Fig. 3–13. Schematic representation of the hemodynamic events that occur during the cardiac cycle. From the top downward: pressure in the aorta, left ventricle, and left atrium; duration of left ventricular diastole (heavy shading), isovolumic periods (diagonal lines), and systole; pressure in the pulmonary artery, right ventricle, and right atrium; blood flow in the aorta and pulmonary artery; and electrocardiogram. Aortic valve opening and closure are indicated by AO and AC, respectively; MO and MC for the mitral valve; PO and PC for the pulmonic valve; and TO and TC for the tricuspid valve. (From Milnor, W.R.: The heart as a pump. *In* Medical Physiology. Edition 14. Edited by V.B. Mountcastle. St. Louis, The C.V. Mosby Co., 1980.)

and ventricular pressures are essentially equal because of the low resistance offered by the semilunar valves. Ventricular systole lasts approximately 0.3 seconds. At the end of this period, the ventricles begin
to relax and their pressures drop rapidly, closing the aortic and pulmonic
valves (causing the second heart sound). A tracing of changes in aortic
pressure shows a sharp notch where the aortic valve closes, known as
the *dicrotic notch*. This notch is followed by a slow decline of pressure
back to the diastolic level. The dicrotic notch is caused by a temporary
backflow of blood from the aorta into the left ventricle following the
initial period of ventricular relaxation. When the aortic valve closes, this
backflow suddenly stops. The end of backflow causes a sharp recoil of
the walls of the aorta, which produces a brief rise in aortic pressure.
The zenith of the aortic pressure occurs when aortic inflow equals the
peripheral runoff. When aortic inflow stops with the closure of the aortic
valve, peripheral flow continues as a result of the elastic recoil of arterial
walls. The recoil maintains a pressure gradient. The end of the period
of maximal ejection is marked by the beginning of ventricular repolarization and is signaled by the T wave of the electrocardiogram.

After the semilunar valves close, the *isovolumic relaxation phase* continues for approximately 0.08 seconds (isovolumic because the ventricles
are again isolated and the volume remains constant). The isovolumic
relaxation phase ends with the opening of the AV valves, which occurs
when ventricular pressures fall below atrial pressures.

A *phase of rapid filling* begins when the AV valves open. During systole,
blood accumulates in the atria and elevates their pressures. When ventricular pressure falls below atrial pressures, blood rushes down the
pressure gradient between atrium and ventricle. The ventricles fill even
though the pressure in both chambers continues to fall because of the
continuing relaxation of the ventricles. The rapid filling phase lasts
slightly more than 0.1 seconds.

The final part of the cardiac cycle is known as the *phase of slow filling*
or *diastasis*. This phase lasts about 0.2 seconds and is caused by continued
venous return. The period of diastasis is terminated by atrial systole.

HEART SOUNDS

Four heart sounds can be heard at the surface of the chest with the
aid of a stethoscope. Although four heart sounds can be heard, the first
two are the most audible and make up the classic "lubb-dub" sequence.
The first heart sound ("lubb") is composed of irregular vibrations of
frequency between 30 to 45 cps and lasts about 0.05 seconds. These
sounds are believed to have three origins: (1) vibrations of the AV valves
during and after closure, (2) vibrations set up by the blood ejecting
through the aortic orifice, and (3) vibrations in the cardiac muscle itself.
The component of the first heart sound that is caused by closure of the

tricuspid valve is best heard at the right sternal border in the fourth intercostal space; the mitral component is best heard at the apex of the heart.

The second heart sound ("dub") develops as a result of closure of the aortic and pulmonic valves. The vibrations of the second sound are usually higher than those of the first (approximately 50 to 70 cps) and are of shorter duration (about 0.025 seconds). Because the two valves rarely close at exactly the same time, the second sound may be split. The second sound usually occurs at the end of the T wave, although this relationship varies considerably. The part of the second sound associated with pulmonic valve closure is best heard in the parasternal line in the second left intercostal space. The component of the second sound associated with aortic valve closure is best heard in the second intercostal space near the right side of the sternum.

A third heart sound is usually audible in young adults, but is rarely heard in older people except in pathologic conditions. This sound develops about 0.2 seconds after the second sound and is believed to be caused by vibrations of the cardiac walls produced by rapid filling of the ventricles. The third heart sound is particularly well marked when blood flow is rapid, such as during exercise.

A fourth heart sound of low frequency and low amplitude occurs during atrial systole. It is the least important sound and is generally inaudible.

VENOUS PULSE

Pressure fluctuations similar to those occurring in the right atrium may be recorded in the jugular vein. There are three positive waves, conventionally labeled a, c, and v. The *a wave* of the venous pressure pulse is produced by the contraction of the right atrium. The *c wave* is produced at the start of ventricular systole when the tricuspid valve closes and bulges back into the atrium. The *v wave* is produced by the pressure built up within the right atrium as a direct result of continued venous return.

NORMAL PRESSURE AND FLOW AS MEASURED DURING THE CARDIAC CYCLE

Even though the amount of blood flow is essentially the same, the pressure measured in the systemic arteries is about five or six times greater than that in the pulmonary arteries. The reason for this increase is the difference in segmental resistances and compliances of these two segments of the cardiovascular system (see Chap. 4). The left ventricular output may be slightly greater than the right ventricular output because of a small amount of bronchial flow. There are tremendous variations

Table 3–1. Hemodynamic Variable Recorded During the Cardiac Cycle in a Normal Adult Human at Rest*

Variable	Mean	Range
Cardiac output (L/min)	5.0	4.0–6.4
Cardiac index (L/min·m²)	2.9	2.3–3.7
Brachial artery pressure (mm Hg)		
systolic	130	90–140
diastole	70	60–90
mean	85	70–105
Left ventricular pressure (mm Hg)		
systolic	130	90–140
end-diastolic	7	4–12
Mean left atrial pressure (mm Hg)	7	4–12
Pulmonary artery pressure (mm Hg)		
systolic	24	15–28
diastolic	10	5–16
mean	16	10–22
Right ventricular pressure (mm Hg)		
systolic	24	15–28
end-diastolic	4	0–8
Mean right atrial pressure (mm Hg)	4	−2–+8

*weight = 70 kg; surface area = 1.7 m²

in "normal" values between "normal" individuals. These variations must be expected and the limits of "normal" recognized. For this reason, Table 3–1 presents the normally expected values (means and ranges) of various hemodynamic variables that can be measured during the cardiac cycle. Measurements (especially cardiac output) are often expressed in terms of square meters of body surface area so that comparisons can be made between individuals of different sizes. The cardiac output is expressed in this way as the *cardiac index* (L per min per sq m of body surface area).

4

CIRCULATORY MECHANICS

VOLUME-PRESSURE RELATIONSHIPS

The Basics

The systemic and pulmonary blood vessels, like numerous other structures throughout the body (e.g., the chest wall, the abdominal wall, the lungs, the urinary bladder), are elastic structures. The fundamental property of an elastic structure is its inherent ability to offer resistance to a stretching force and to return to its resting or unstressed length or volume after the stretching force has been removed. Elastic elements, elastin and collagen within the walls of elastic structures are responsible for the recoil phenomenon of most organs. Hooke's law (Burton, 1954) is the basic principle defining elastic behavior; it states that, when an elastic substance is stretched, a tension develops that is proportional to the degree of deformation produced. Hooke's law, in its most usual form, is applied to longitudinal elements (e.g., a wire or a rubber band) and is expressed by the equation:

$$\frac{F}{A} = Y \left[\frac{L - L_0}{L_0} \right]. \tag{4-1}$$

The tension developed by stretching is defined as a force per cross-sectional area of the element stretched, F/A (dynes/cm^2); L is the stretched length (cm); and L_0 is the resting or "unstressed" length (cm). The quantity, Y, is the constant of proportionality, termed Young's modulus, and is a quantitative measure of an element's elasticity.

The term *elasticity* has been interpreted in different ways. However, the proper physical definition of elasticity is "the property of materials which enables them to resist deformation by the development of a resisting force or tension" (Burton, 1954). The popular usage of the term connotes the opposite meaning. If a material is easily stretched (e.g., has a low Young's modulus), it is popularly said to be highly elastic, whereas a material that resists stretch (e.g., has a high Young's modulus) is similarly regarded as less elastic. As will be shown, the popular concept actually refers to the compliance of an elastic object (i.e., its ability to be stretched) rather than to its elasticity in the true sense (i.e., its ability to resist stretch by developing a resistive tension or force).

The confusion between the proper and popular understanding of the term "elasticity" is so widespread that an author's meaning must be carefully considered. In this volume, the physical definition of elasticity is used. Thus, if Y is high, relative to some normal value, the element resists stretch and is considered to be elastic (or, in the popular sense, less elastic). A steel wire has a high Young's modulus, whereas a rubber band has a low Young's modulus. Figure 4–1 illustrates the relationship defined by Hooke's law.

Because Hooke's law must be applied to longitudinal elements, it is difficult to use this relationship to define elastic behavior of anatomic structures. Most such structures are not longitudinal elements, but are more akin to sacs (i.e., the lung) or cylinders (i.e., the blood vessels). Some physiologists investigating elastic behavior of certain selected blood vessels have tried to circumvent this problem by cutting helical strips of vessel and measuring the length-tension relationship of these strips. However, this approach has limited applicability. For example,

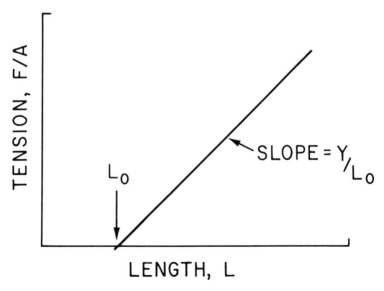

Fig. 4–1. Length-tension relationship of an elastic element as defined by Hooke's law. (From Green, J.F.: Mechanical Concepts in Cardiovascular and Pulmonary Physiology. Philadelphia, Lea & Febiger, 1977.)

it is misleading to cut a lung into strips to investigate its elastic behavior because such behavior results, in part, from its sac-like structure.

Concept of Compliance

Because obtaining strips of elastic structures is not always practical, physiologists have quantitated the degree of elasticity of an anatomic structure by measuring volume changes resulting from a given distending pressure. To understand this principle, let us consider the case of the three elastic balloons pictured in Figure 4–2. The coiled lines around the balloons represent the elastic elements within the walls. The arrows represent the degree of recoil produced by the elastic elements, i.e., the force with which the balloons collapse when the distending pressure is withdrawn. The pressure distending each balloon is the difference between the pressure within the balloon and the pressure outside the balloon and is called the *transmural pressure,* symbolized by P_{TM}. Thus,

$$P_{TM} = \text{transmural pressure} = P_{inside} - P_{outside}.$$

This basic relationship will be discussed in more detail later in the text.

Even though the volume of each balloon in Figure 4–2 is the same, the transmural pressure in each is markedly different. Thus, the transmural pressure in balloon A is greater than that in balloon B, and the transmural pressure in balloon C is less than that in balloon B. This is true because there is a greater amount of elastic substance within the wall of balloon A, causing a greater inward-acting recoil force and, therefore, requiring a greater internal pressure to maintain the same degree

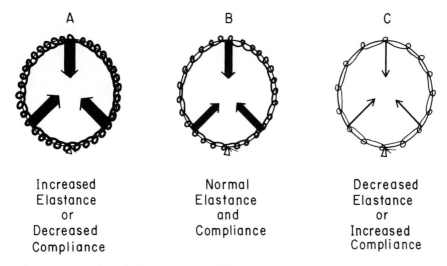

A	B	C
Increased	Normal	Decreased
Elastance	Elastance	Elastance
or	and	or
Decreased	Compliance	Increased
Compliance		Compliance

Fig. 4–2. Hypothetic balloons possessing different elastic content. (From Green, J.F.: Mechanical Concepts in Cardiovascular and Pulmonary Physiology. Philadelphia, Lea & Febiger, 1977.)

of distension. In contrast, the lesser amount of elastic substance in balloon C results in a lesser recoil force. This example suggests that, to quantitate the elasticity of an elastic structure, we must know the distending pressure and the absolute volume of the structure; to compare the elasticities of different structures, we need only adjust the volume of each structure to obtain some given volume (the same for all structures) and note the different distending pressure. This procedure would be difficult to carry out for most physiologic systems. The desired information, however, could be obtained by simply changing the volume and observing the changes in pressure. The ratio of the change in pressure to the change in volume, i.e., the slope of the volume-pressure curve, is called the *elastance* and serves as a quantitative measure of the elasticity of the structure in question. We do not need to know the absolute values; only the relative changes of these parameters are necessary.

Although the term elastance is extremely descriptive, i.e., an increased elastance means greater elasticity, most physiologists prefer to define elastic behavior in terms of *compliance*. Compliance is nothing more than the reciprocal of elastance and can thus be defined as:

$$C = \frac{\Delta V}{\Delta P},\qquad(4\text{--}2)$$

where C is compliance, ΔV is change in volume, and ΔP is change in transmural pressure. Compliance, therefore, expresses the change in volume resulting from a change in the distending pressure. It is inversely proportional to the elastance, which is the change in pressure resulting from a change in volume.

To summarize, we may state that elastance is an index of the ability of a structure to resist deformation by stress, whereas compliance describes the ability of a structure to give way (undergo deformation) to a stress. An easily inflatable balloon has high compliance and low elastance, whereas a stiff balloon that strongly resists inflation has low compliance and high elastance.

Figure 4–3 illustrates the volume-pressure relationships we would obtain from the balloons pictured in Figure 4–2. Notice that the slope of the volume-pressure curve for balloon A is much steeper than that for the other balloons, indicating that for a given change in volume a greater pressure results. This relationship is exactly what would be expected considering the greater elasticity in balloon A. Balloon A is thus "stiff" relative to normal (balloon B) and has decreased compliance, whereas balloon C is "flabby" relative to normal and has increased compliance.*

---

*Note that the concept of compliance avoids much of the confusion produced by the terms elasticity and elastance. Consequently, it is preferred.

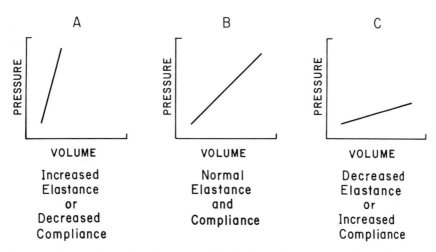

Fig. 4–3. Volume-pressure relationships of the balloons illustrated in Figure 4–2. (From Green, J.F.: Mechanical Concepts in Cardiovascular and Pulmonary Physiology. Philadelphia, Lea & Febiger, 1977.)

Although compliance is usually defined as the ratio of the change in volume to the change in pressure, a more specific definition is often needed (Green, 1979). Thus,

$$C = \frac{V - V_o}{P - O},\qquad(4\text{–}3)$$

where V_o is the resting or *unstressed volume* (i.e., the volume contained within the compliant structure when the pressure, P, within the compliant structure is zero, 0), and V is the volume above the unstressed volume. This relationship is demonstrated in Figure 4–4. Notice the similarity between this figure and Figure 4–1, which illustrates the relationship defined by Hooke's law. The unstressed volume (V_o) is analogous to the unstressed length (L_o), the reciprocal of the compliance coefficient ($1/C$) is analogous to Y/L_o, and pressure is analogous to tension. Thus, even though it may be difficult or even impossible to quantitate the elastic properties of an anatomic structure by measuring the length-tension relationships, the same kind of information can be obtained by measuring the volume-pressure relationships and by using the compliance as an index of elasticity.

The units of pressure used by most physiologists are cm H_2O or mm Hg; therefore, compliance is most often expressed as ml/cm H_2O or ml/mm Hg. Because 1 cm H_2O equals 0.738 mm Hg, the preceding units can be interconverted by multiplying ml/cm H_2O by 1/0.738 or ml/mm Hg by 1/1.355. Volume is frequently normalized on the basis of body weight; thus, compliance can be expressed as ml $\cdot$ kg $\cdot^{-1} \cdot$ mm Hg^{-1}.

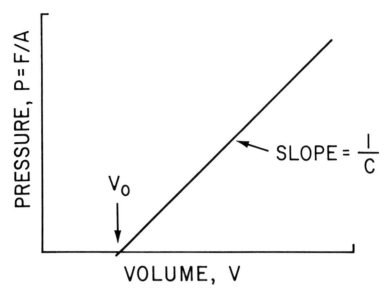

Fig. 4–4.   Graphic solution of Equation 4–3 illustrating how the volume-pressure relationship of an elastic structure is analogous to the length-tension relationship defined by Hooke's law (Eq. 4–1) and illustrated in Figure 4–1. (From Green, J.F.: Mechanical Concepts in Cardiovascular and Pulmonary Physiology. Philadelphia, Lea & Febiger, 1977.)

Vascular Compliance

Since systemic and pulmonary blood vessels are elastic structures, they demonstrate an inherent ability to recoil after a deforming stress is removed (Gow, 1980; Rothe, 1983). The deforming stress is an increase in the intravascular fluid volume. Such increases in the vascular volume stretch the walls of the vessels, and the recoil of the elastic vessel walls increases the intravascular pressure. The relationship of vascular volume to vascular transmural pressure is called *vascular compliance,* which measures the inherent elasticity of the vascular system in much the same way as alveolar compliance measures lung elasticity (see Chap. 14). When a vascular segment has a large compliance (relative to some other segment), it has less recoil ability and consequently has the capacity to hold large amounts of blood (relative to other segments) with little change in pressure.

Systemic Vascular Compliance

The total lumped compliance of the systemic circulation (the compliances of the arteries, capillaries, and veins) can be measured in experimental animals by momentarily stopping the circulation (usually by electrically fibrillating the ventricles) and rapidly equalizing the arterial and venous pressures by pumping blood from arteries to veins (Guyton, 1973; Green, 1979). The intravascular pressure that is measured when arterial and venous pressures are equal is the static transmural pressure of the system at that blood volume and is called the *mean systemic pressure* (P_{MS}). The circulation is reestablished by an electrical shock to the heart, and the total blood volume is increased by a known amount. The mean systemic pressure is again measured by the stop-flow procedure. The ratio of the change in volume to change in mean systemic pressure is the lumped compliance of the systemic circulation, C_s. Values of C_s in the dog have ranged from 1.4 to 4.2 ml $\cdot$ kg^{-1} $\cdot$ mm Hg^{-1} (Table 4–1).

Independent measurements of arterial compliance, C_a, of the dog have been measured as 0.067 ml $\cdot$ kg^{-1} $\cdot$ mm Hg^{-1} by rapidly removing a known quantity of blood from the arterial system at constant cardiac output and recording the fall in arterial pressure (Shoukas and Sagawa, 1973). C_a is 30 to 60 times less than C_s. Because the compliance of the arterial system is so small, compared with the compliance of the total systemic circulation, the venous compliance, C_v, is considered, as a first approximation, to be equal to C_s.

The relative differences between systemic, arterial, and venous compliances are graphically illustrated by their respective volume-pressure curves. These curves are illustrated in Figure 4–5 and were drawn from reported values for both arterial and venous compliances as presented in Table 4–1. None of these values, obviously, is entirely correct; the range can probably by accounted for by experimental error and the slight difference in measurement techniques. The values presented in Table 4–1 demonstrate relative differences between venous and arterial compliances in the systemic circulation. Consider the following example: If 100 ml of blood were rapidly injected into the arterial system of a 70-kg man (assuming compliance values presented in Table 4–1), the arterial pressure would rise approximately 21 mm Hg; however, if that same

Table 4–1.   Reported Values for Systemic Arterial, Lumped Systemic, and Lumped Pulmonary Compliance

Compliance Value (ml·kg^{-1}·mm Hg^{-1})	Reference	
Systemic arterial		
0.067	Shoukas and Sagawa,	1973
Lumped systemic (systemic venous)		
1.4	Guyton, et al.,	1973
1.8	Caldini, et al.,	1974
2.3	Richardson, et al.,	1961
2.4	Shoukas and Sagawa,	1971
3.3	Green and Attix,	1974
4.2	Drees and Rothe,	1974
2.57 (average)		
Lumped pulmonary		
0.217	Guyton, et al.,	1973
0.213	Engelberg and Du Bois,	1959
0.366–0.627	Maseri, et al.,	1972

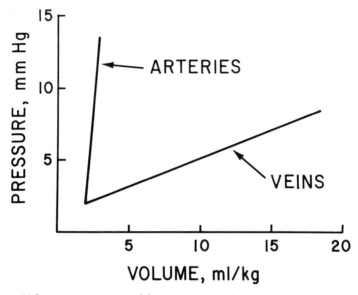

Fig. 4–5. Volume-pressure curves of the systemic arterial and venous systems. These curves were drawn from the average data presented in Table 4–1. A given change in volume results in a much smaller change in venous pressure than in arterial pressure because of a greater venous compliance. (From Green, J.F.: Mechanical Concepts in Cardiovascular and Pulmonary Physiology. Philadelphia, Lea & Febiger, 1977.)

volume were rapidly injected into the venous system, the venous pressure would rise less than 1 mm Hg. This example simply illustrates that the veins, because of their large compliance (relative to the arteries), have a greater capacity to hold blood volume than do the arteries. This basic difference in the volume-pressure relationship of the arterial and venous systems, which is related to anatomic differences in these two basic types of vessels, has a profound influence on overall circulatory mechanics.

Pulmonary Vascular Compliance

Pulmonary vessels, like those in the systemic circulation, are elastic; however, their compliance is quantitatively different. Historically, the pulmonary circulation has been considered a highly distensible system. When the basis for this conclusion is analyzed, most authors believe that the pulmonary arterial system (usually the pulmonary artery) is more compliant than the systemic arterial system (usually the aorta). Yet, when the lumped compliance of the pulmonary system (arteries, capillaries, and veins) is compared with the lumped compliance of the systemic system, the pulmonary system is significantly less compliant than the systemic bed. The lumped compliance of the pulmonary vascular bed has been measured in the dog as $0.217 \text{ ml} \cdot \text{kg}^{-1} \cdot \text{mm Hg}^{-1}$ (Guyton, 1973). Thus, for an average 12-kg dog under static conditions (i.e., when the circulation has been stopped and pressures throughout the pulmonary vascular bed have been equalized), an increase in volume of 2.6 ml causes the pressure to rise 1 mm Hg. This value for the compliance of the whole pulmonary vascular bed is substantially lower than the compliance values reported for the entire systemic vascular bed (Table 4–1). Other studies of pulmonary vascular compliance have yielded similar values.

The relative differences in the compliance of the systemic and pulmonary vascular beds are most dramatically illustrated by comparing the volume-pressure curves in Figure 4–6. The systemic curve was drawn from the average compliance calculated from the data presented in Table 4–1.

The compliance of the serial sections of the pulmonary vascular bed is distributed differently from that of the systemic circulation. The compliance values of large pulmonary arteries and veins are about equal, each accounting for about 15 percent of the total pulmonary vascular compliance. The small pulmonary vessels, small veins, venules, and capillaries account for the rest of the pulmonary vascular compliance (Engelberg and Du Bois, 1959).

Thus, we see that the blood vessels of both the systemic and pulmonary circulations are elastic structures and, as such, recoil inwardly when a volume stress is applied. The total compliance of the systemic circulation is greater than that of the pulmonary circulation, and the venous systems of both circulations possess the greatest compliance.

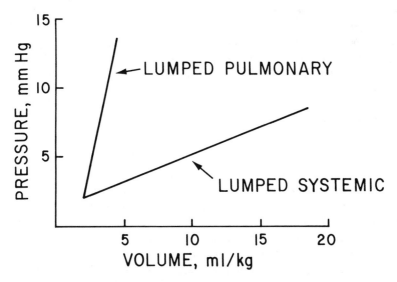

Fig. 4–6. Volume-pressure curves of the systemic and pulmonary vascular beds. These curves were drawn from the data presented in Table 4–1. (From Green, J.F.: Mechanical Concepts in Cardiovascular and Pulmonary Physiology. Philadelphia, Lea & Febiger, 1977.)

The functional significance of these volume-pressure relationships is discussed below.

PRESSURE-FLOW RELATIONSHIPS

The Basics

The physical principles that govern the flow of blood through the circulatory system, as well as the passage of air into and out of the lungs, are derived from the general laws of hydrodynamics (Whitaker, 1968). Before we discuss the basic principles that describe the flow of blood through vessels, we will discuss the flow of fluids, in general, through rigid and collapsible tubes. In this discussion, the fluid will be considered a liquid (like blood), but the same principles apply to air flow (as occurs in the lungs).

The basic expression for the flow of fluid through *rigid tubes* is Poiseuille's law, which states that the volume of fluid flowing past a point in the tube per unit time ($\dot{Q}$) is proportional to the difference in pressure between the inflow and outflow end of the tube ($P_I - P_O$) and the fourth power of the radius (r) of the tube, and is inversely proportional to the length of the tube (L) and viscosity of the fluid (η). (A derivation of Poiseuille's law, with certain other basic laws of hydrodynamics, can be found in Appendix 2.)

In mathematical terms, Poiseuille's law may be expressed for conditions of horizontal flow as follows:

$$\frac{P_I - P_O}{\dot{Q}} = \frac{8\eta L}{\pi r^4} = R. \qquad (4\text{-}4)$$

The quantity $8\eta L/\pi r^4$ represents factors that tend to retard flow and is referred to as the *resistance* to flow, R. The ratio of the difference in driving pressure to flow is used as an empiric way of defining the resistance to flow. Because L and η remain constant in most physiologic systems, a change in R is interpreted as a change in the radius of the tube (i.e., blood vessel or airway). The unit for resistance in the centimeter-gram-second (cgs) system is dynes $\cdot$ sec/cm^5; pressure is expressed as dynes/cm^2 and flow as cm^3/sec. Because in practice pressure is measured as mm Hg and flow as liters/minute (L/min), resistance is usualy expressed as mm Hg per L/min (mm Hg $\cdot$ L^{-1} $\cdot$ min).

The most commonly used form of the Poiseuille equation is obtained by rearranging Equation 4-4 as follows:

$$\dot{Q} = \frac{1}{R} (P_I - P_O). \qquad (4\text{-}5)$$

Two possible ways of graphically displaying Equation 4-5 are presented in Figure 4-7. Horizontal flow is assumed. The slope of the pressure-

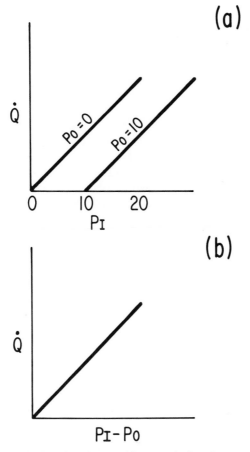

Fig. 4–7. Pressure-flow relationships for a rigid horizontal tube. The zero reference point for pressure is taken at the level of the tube. (*a*): Pressure-flow relationships obtained with two different outflow pressures (P_O) when flow ($\dot{Q}$) is plotted as a function of inflow pressure (P_I). (*b*): Pressure-flow relationship obtained for all outflow pressures when flow is plotted as a function of the driving pressure ($P_I - P_O$). This figure assumes that resistance is independent of pressures. Note the invariance of the slope (characteristic of the tube and viscosity of fluid) and the fact that the pressure surrounding the tube is irrelevant (compare with Fig. 4–4). (From Green, J.F.: Mechanical Concepts in Cardiovascular and Pulmonary Physiology. Philadelphia, Lea & Febiger, 1977.)

flow curve is equal to the reciprocal of the resistance (1/R); the steeper the slope, the less the resistance. The linearity of the pressure-flow relationship derived from Poiseuille's law implies constant radius, length, viscosity, and laminar flow (see Appendix 2). The pressure surrounding a rigid tube has no effect on the pressure-flow relationship; however, this is not the case with a collapsible tube.

An ideal *collapsible tube* is any tube made of material with characteristics such that any finite positive transmural pressure causes it to open fully and any finite negative transmural pressure at the outflow end causes it to collapse (at the outflow end). The pressure-flow relationships of such a tube are governed primarily by Poiseuille's law under conditions where the tube has a positive transmural pressure throughout, i.e., flow is proportional to the difference between the inflow and outflow pressure, and the pressure surrounding the tube has no effect on flow. When a finite negative transmural pressure develops at the outflow end, the tube becomes partially constricted (collapsed) at the outflow end, and the pressure surrounding the tube becomes most significant because it now replaces the outflow pressure as the back pressure to perfusion. A schematic drawing of an ideal collapsible tube (Starling resistor) is presented in Figure 4–8.* In this illustration, the pressure at the outflow end of the tube (P_O) is equal to atmospheric pressure. Because the pressure surrounding the tube (P_S) is greater than P_O, flow is proportional to the difference between the inflow pressure (P_I) and P_S, i.e., $\dot{Q} \, \alpha P_I - P_S$. The resistance to flow, at constant viscosity, is a function of the length and diameter of the tube up to, but not including, the area of collapse.

The pressure-flow relationships through an ideal Starling resistor may be succinctly summarized by the following three statements: (1) When the surrounding pressure is greater than the inflow pressure, no flow occurs through the tube. (2) When inflow pressure is greater than surrounding pressure and surrounding pressure is greater than outflow pressure, flow is proportional to the difference between inflow pressure and surrounding pressure, and changes in outflow pressure have no influence on flow. (3) When inflow pressure is greater than outflow pressure and outflow pressure is greater than surrounding pressure,

---

*Knowlton and Starling (1912) first used such a device in their heart-lung preparation as a means of controlling "peripheral resistance." They employed a thin-walled collapsible tube to traverse a chamber. The pressure in the chamber surrounding the tube could be set at any desired level. Since the time of Starling, a collapsible tube used in this manner has been known as a Starling resistor. Although the Starling resistor has been widely used in physiologic laboratories since the time of Starling, quantitative studies of the pressure-flow relationships through such tubes were not undertaken until 1941, when the physiologic significance of these relationships was recognized. Holt (1941), studying flow through collapsible tubes, found that lowering the outflow pressure did not significantly change flow when the outflow pressure was less than the pressure surrounding the collapsible segment of the tube. Reasoning from this model, he concluded that the collapse of systemic veins as they entered the chest accounted for the fact that atrial pressure may change independently of a change in peripheral venous pressure. In a theoretic discussion of energy and hydraulic gradients along systemic veins, based on a model of flow through collapsible tubes, Duomarco and Rimini (1954) pointed out an unusual independence of flow and pressure; this independence explains why negative intrathoracic pressure does not directly alter venous return. Rodbard (1955) compared the pressure-flow relationships of a rigid tube with a collapsible Penrose drain of the same dimensions. He demonstrated that the flow was markedly influenced by the pressure surrounding the collapsible drain and that the addition of an outflow resistance when the drain was collapsed had no influence on flow. He suggested that the special dynamics of collapsible drains or tubes could account for certain paradoxic findings in blood flow through partially stenosed vessels.

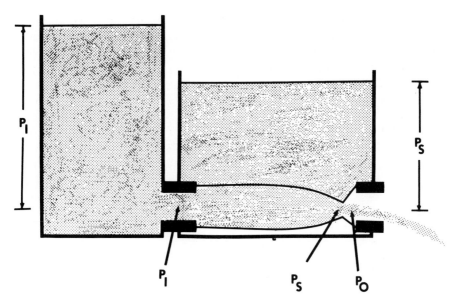

Fig. 4–8. Schematic drawing of an ideal Starling resistor. P_I = inflow pressure, P_S = surrounding pressure, and P_O = outflow pressure = atmospheric pressure. Flow is proportional to the difference between the inflow pressure and the surrounding pressure. (From Green, J.F.: Mechanical Concepts in Cardiovascular and Pulmonary Physiology. Philadelphia, Lea & Febiger, 1977.)

flow is proportional to the difference between inflow pressure and outflow pressure, and changes in surrounding pressure have no influence on flow. The three possible conditions of a Starling resistor are depicted as hydraulic models in Figure 4–9.

An intuitive understanding as to why P_S functions as a back pressure to perfusion when P_S is greater than P_O may be obtained by considering what happens at the downstream end of a Starling resistor (the area of collapse). The pressure at the downstream end can never deviate significantly above or below P_S. If the pressure rose above P_S, the tube would be wide open, and the pressure would then be dissipated into the lower pressure system at the outflow end of the tube, P_O. (The outflow pressure is the pressure distal to the area of collapse.) If the pressure at the downstream end of the tube were less than P_S, the tube would shut completely and flow would cease. Thus, pressure at the downstream end of an ideal Starling resistor becomes equal to P_S and independent of flow and, as such, functions as a *pressure load* and not as a resistance (resistance is related at constant viscosity, according to Poiseuille's law, to the length and diameter of the tube upstream from the point where P_S acts). For this reason P_S becomes the back pressure

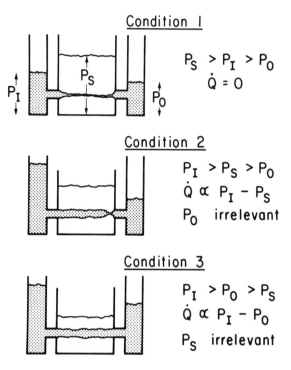

Fig. 4–9. Hydraulic models depicting the three conditions of a Starling resistor. (From Green, J.F.: The pulmonary circulation. *In* The Peripheral Circulation. Edited by R. Zelis. New York, Grune & Stratton, 1975. Reproduced here with permission of the publishers.)

to perfusion whenever P_I is greater than P_S and P_S is greater than P_O; hence:

$$\dot{Q} = \frac{1}{R} (P_I - P_S). \tag{4–6}$$

A change in P_O has no influence on $\dot{Q}$ unless P_O is greater than or equal to P_S. If this situation occurred, the transmural pressure at the distal end of the tube would become positive, the tube would open, and P_O would replace P_S in Equation 4–6 (P_O would then be the back pressure). Similarly, a change in flow would not influence P_O when P_S is greater than or equal to P_O. These unique relationships, where a change in flow has no influence on the pressure drop across the outflow constriction ($P_S - P_O$) and a change in this pressure drop has no influence on flow, are accomplished by the automatic control of the cross-sectional area of the outflow constriction, as described by Permutt and Riley (1963). Note that P_S acts as a pressure load and not as a resistance. Thus, the term "Starling resistor" is actually a misnomer. Misinterpretation of this critical point can lead to much confusion. The pressure-flow relationships of Starling resistors are plotted in various ways in Figure 4–10. The three examples presented were chosen because they are identical to the pressure-flow relationships obtained in different physiologic systems: the pulmonary airway, the pulmonary circulation, the systemic arteries, and the systemic veins. Careful study and thought about this figure will assure the reader of a complete understanding of the hydrodynamics of collapsible tubes.

Measure of Resistance

In most physiologic systems, an increase in the resistance to flow, calculated as the ratio of the driving pressure to flow, is generally interpreted as a decrease in the radius of the conduit(s) through which the flow occurs because the length and viscosity tend to remain constant. Although this interpretation is accurate under most conditions, there are situations in which an increase in the resistance ratio is best interpreted as simply an indication of an increased dissipation of potential energy somewhere throughout the flow circuit. A classic example of such a situation can be found in the pulmonary vascular bed. As we shall discuss in a later chapter, the pulmonary capillaries are believed to function as Starling resistors. That is, whenever the alveolar pressure (the pressure surrounding the pulmonary capillaries) is greater than the pulmonary venous pressure (outflow pressure), the pressure at the outflow end of the pulmonary capillaries becomes equal to alveolar pressure and alveolar pressure functions as the back pressure. Whenever alveolar pressure rises, as with positive pressure ventilation, pulmonary vascular resistance, calculated as the difference between pulmonary arterial and left atrial pressure divided by cardiac output, also rises. Because the increase in alveolar pressure functions as an increased pressure load and not as an increased resistance, the increase in the calculated pulmonary vascular resistance results from an increased dissipation of energy across the downstream end of the pulmonary capillaries and does not reflect changes in the upstream dimensions of the vessel or in the viscosity of the blood. Therefore, before an adequate interpretation of resistance measurements ($\Delta P/\Delta \dot{Q}$) can be made, the investigator must be keenly aware of the type of system that is measured (rigid versus collapsible) and of the effective back pressure used in the resistance equation.

Vascular Resistance

The blood pressure that develops in the arterial vessels of the systemic and pulmonary circulations is dissipated in large part by the time the blood arrives in the atria. This fact suggests that the blood vessels have a resistive function in addition to their capacitive function. The magnitude of their resistance is, however, different at different levels of the circulation. The ratio of driving pressure (e.g., arterial minus atrial pressure) to flow (e.g., cardiac output) is called *vascular resistance* and is a

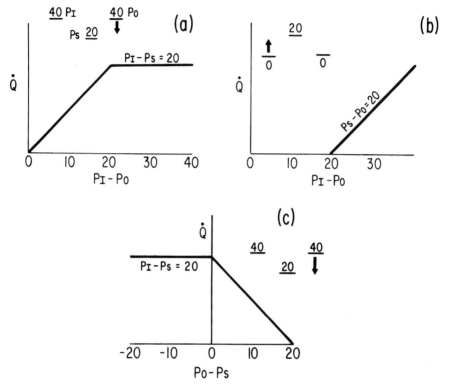

Fig. 4–10.   Pressure-flow relationships for a thin-walled horizontal collapsible tube. The zero reference point for pressures is taken at the level of the tube. Note the invariance of the slope (characteristic of the tube and viscosity of the fluid) and the fact that the surrounding pressure (P_S) is not irrelevant. The inserts represent the relative levels of P_I, P_S, and P_O. (a): The pressure-flow relationship obtained when flow ($\dot{Q}$) is plotted as a function of the difference between inflow (P_I) and outflow (P_O) pressures. The example is given for $P_I = P_O = 40$ and $P_S = 20$. As P_O is lowered at constant P_I and P_S, $\dot{Q}$ increases until P_O becomes equal to P_S ($P_I - P_O = P_O - P_S$). As P_O is lowered below P_S, P_S becomes the effective back pressure and flow remains constant. Once $P_O \leq P_S$, $\dot{Q}$ is unaffected by P_O. (b): The pressure-flow relationship obtained when $\dot{Q}$, as in (a), is plotted as a function of $P_I - P_O$; however, in this example $P_I = P_O = 0$, $P_S = 20$, and the pressure-flow relationship is obtained by raising P_I at constant P_S and P_O. As P_I is raised, no flow occurs until P_I exceeds P_S ($P_I - P_O = P_S - P_O$); thereafter $\dot{Q}$ increases as P_I exceeds P_S. Again, changes in P_O have no effect on $\dot{Q}$ as long as $P_O \leq P_S$. Note that with the Starling resistor different types of pressure-flow relationships can be obtained by either lowering P_O at constant P_I and P_S or by raising P_I at constant P_O and P_S. This is to be contrasted with the rigid system where the same relationship (Fig. 4–1) is obtained by either raising P_I or lowering P_O at constant (and irrelevant) P_S. (c): The pressure-flow relationship obtained when $\dot{Q}$ is plotted as a function of $P_O - P_S$. In this example, as in example (a), $P_I = P_O = 40$ and $P_S = 20$. As P_O is lowered (decreasing $P_O - P_S$), $\dot{Q}$ increases until $P_O \leq P_S$ ($P_I - P_O = P_I - P_S$); thereafter $\dot{Q}$ remains constant because the driving pressure $P_I - P_S$ is constant. Again, changes in P_O, when $P_O \leq P_S$, have no effect on $\dot{Q}$. (From Green, J.F.: Mechanical Concepts in Cardiovascular and Pulmonary Physiology. Philadelphia, Lea & Febiger, 1977.)

measure of the amount of pressure energy that is dissipated by the blood vessels under dynamic flowing conditions.

Systemic Vascular Resistance. At a normal cardiac output of 5.0 L/min for an adult human, the mean systemic arterial pressure* is approximately 100 mm Hg, the pressure in the small veins and venules (capacitance vessels) is about 10 mm Hg, and the right atrial pressure is approximately 0 mm Hg. Thus, in the systemic circulation, the major pressure drops and, therefore, the largest amount of resistance occurs upstream of the veins (i.e., in the arteries) and only a small amount (one tenth of the total) occurs in the veins. This information is presented graphically in Figure 4–11. The solid line marked "aortic-right atrial pressure" represents the pressure drop occurring across the entire systemic circulation, whereas the solid line marked "small vein-right atrial pressure" represents the pressure drop occurring across the venous system only. Because the slope of such a *pressure-flow curve* is equal to the reciprocal of the resistance, a comparison of these slopes immediately provides a graphic evaluation of the difference in magnitude of arterial versus venous resistance. Remember that the slope of the "aortic-right atrial pressure" curve (1/TPR) is influenced by the resistance of the total system: arteries, capillaries and veins. The slope of the curve marked "small vein-right atrial pressure" is influenced only by the venous resistance (R_v). Note that, by tradition, the resistance across the entire systemic circulation is termed the *total peripheral resistance (TPR)*.

Pulmonary Vascular Resistance. At the normal cardiac output of 5 L/min, the mean pulmonary artery pressure is usually around 15 mm Hg, whereas the left atrial pressure is about 4 mm Hg. The pressure in the pulmonary capillaries (at the midpoint of the pulmonary vascular bed) is nearly midway between the pulmonary artery and the left atrial pressures at a value of 6 mm Hg. Thus, unlike the situation in the systemic circulation, the distribution of vascular resistance in the pulmonary system is divided about equally between artery and veins. Also, unlike the systemic circulation, the total pulmonary vascular resistance is considerably less than the total resistance across the systemic bed. This conclusion is illustrated by the dashed line in Figure 4–11, which is much closer to the pressure-flow curve of the systemic venous system than to the entire systemic circulation.

CONCEPTUAL MODEL OF CIRCULATORY SYSTEM

We will now develop a conceptual scheme of the circulatory system to use as a framework on which to hang much of the minutia (gee-whiz

---

*Do not confuse the "mean (systemic) arterial pressure" with the "mean systemic pressure." The former is the mean pressure in systemic arteries whereas the latter is the pressure observed throughout the systemic circulation when cardiac output is zero. The mean systemic pressure is very close to the pressure within the small veins and venules under *dynamic* conditions (normal cardiac output) (see Chapter 6).

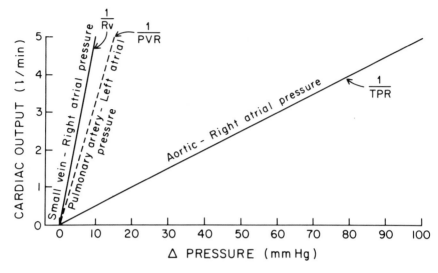

Fig. 4–11. Pressure-flow curves of the systemic and pulmonary vascular beds. See text for details.

numbers) presented elsewhere in this textbook. For the purpose of simplicity, the coronary and bronchial circulations are not considered.

The cardiovascular system can be conceptually divided into two major subdivisions: (1) the central circulation (the heart and the pulmonary circulation) and (2) the systemic circulation (loosely defined as all vascular beds fed from the aorta). This breakdown is to the reader's advantage because it is helpful to study the two major subdivisions of the system separately and then to put this knowledge together for a complete picture of the cardiovascular system. The heart, of course, functions as the body's vascular pump, transferring blood from the low-pressure systemic veins to the high-pressure systemic arteries. In this process, the heart pumps the blood through the pulmonary circulation where gas exchange occurs.

Although the heart is usually described in singular terms, there are actually two separate hearts, the left and the right. However, they are in intimate proximity to each other, sharing a common wall (see Chap. 1). The right heart, interposed between the systemic veins and the pulmonary artery, pumps blood from the systemic circulation into the pulmonary circulation. Except for minor beat-to-beat variations, the blood pumped by each heart per minute must be equal, as can be expected from a closed-circuit system. Indeed, at any given time, the flow at each and every point in the circulation must be equal. This is an inevitable consequence of a closed system.* Because the left and right hearts pump the same quantity of blood under steady-state conditions, we can conceptually lump the two hearts and the pulmonary circulation together into a single unit usually referred to as the central circulation.

The two principal mechanical properties of the circulatory system that must be considered in any conceptual schema are compliance and resistance, i.e., the volume-pressure and pressure-flow relationships. All vessels have both compliance and resistance. However, each function is not equally important at each serial segment of the circulation because of anatomic differences from aorta to vena cava (or from pulmonary artery to pulmonary vein). These anatomic differences have profound functional significance.

Table 4–2 summarizes the basic properties of the various serial sections of the systemic circulation (Burton, 1954). The aorta and large distributing arteries possess a great deal of elastic tissue. Therefore, their elastance is high and their compliance is low (*see above*). The function of the aorta is principally conductance; the function of the distributing arteries is resistance. The arterioles also possess elastic tissue, although less than that possessed by the aorta and distributing arteries. What the arterioles may lack in elastic tissue they more than make up with a thick coat of vascular smooth muscle. When contracted, this smooth muscle produces what is generally referred to as vascular or arteriolar tone. The arterioles have low compliance and their function is principally resistance. However, many physiologists have suggested that the arterioles also produce the effective back pressure for the arterial system (see Chap. 7). The

Table 4–2. Summary of the Basic Properties of the Various Serial Sections of the Systemic Circulation

Vessel	Mean Pressure (mm Hg)	Amount of Elastic Tissue	Primary Function
Aorta	90–110	+ + + +	Conductive
Distributing arteries	80–90	+ + + +	Resistive
Arterioles	40–60	+ + (mostly smooth muscle)	Resistive (effective back pressure)
Capillary	15–25	0	Exchange
Small veins and venules	5–10	0–+ (reappears in large venules)	Capacitive
Large veins and vena cava	0–2	+ + +	Resistive

*Although the flow at each point in the circulation at any given point in time must remain constant, the velocity (v) must vary at each point in the system depending upon the cross-sectional area (A), i.e., $v = \dot{Q}/A$.

smallest venules do not possess elastic tissue. However, small amounts of elastic tissue begin to reappear in the larger venules and small veins. As a group, the small veins and venules have little elastance and a large compliance. Toward the downstream end of the systemic circulation, in the large veins and vena cava, elastic tissue is found in large amounts. The compliance of this segment of the venous system is less than that of the small veins and venules, and its function is resistance. Thus, only one serial section of the systemic circulation (the small veins and venules) has significant compliance. Because the veins (principally the small veins and venules) can hold large volumes of blood, they are called the capacitance vessels. The arterial vessels on the other hand are called conductance (e.g., the aorta) or resistance (e.g., small arteries and arterioles) vessels, depending on their size.

Although the primary function of the venous system is capacitive, the resistance to flow within the large veins is nevertheless most significant. The function of the venous resistance is entirely different from that of the arterial resistance. Whereas the arteriolar tone maintains an elevated arterial blood pressure and distributes flow between parallel channels, the venous resistance is a major determinant of the amount of blood returning to the heart. This venous function is important and will be discussed in greater detail in the next chapter.

The reasons for conceptually placing the venous resistance downstream from the major systemic capacitance area are based not only on the relatively low compliance of this venous segment (large veins and vena cava), but also on functional evidence (Bartlestone, 1960; Caldini et al., 1974). If the arterial flow into the systemic circulation were suddenly stopped (e.g., by clamping the aorta), blood entering the right atrium would not stop instantly. It would continue to flow for several minutes, but the rate would decrease in an exponential manner. This behavior can be accounted for only by a significant resistance to flow between the capacitance area (*the vascular reservoir*) and the right atrium.

Although the resistance and compliance values of the pulmonary circulation are quantitatively different from those of the systemic circulation,* evidence suggests that the same basic conceptual schema can be applied. Thus, the pulmonary arteries and large pulmonary veins are considered primarily resistance vessels, whereas the small pulmonary veins and venules are considered the capacitance vessels.

In developing this conceptual schema of the circulation, the capillary segment of the systemic circulation was ignored because its primary

---

*Representative values of the pulmonary and systemic resistance and compliances determined in the dog are as follows. Systemic arterial resistance = 58.1 mm Hg $\cdot$ L^{-1} $\cdot$ min; pulmonary arterial resistance = 9.4 mm Hg $\cdot$ L^{-1} $\cdot$ min; lumped systemic compliance = 2.6 ml $\cdot$ kg^{-1} $\cdot$ mm Hg^{-1}; lumped pulmonary compliance = 0.1 ml $\cdot$ kg^{-1} $\cdot$ mm Hg; systemic venous resistance = 4.4 mm Hg $\cdot$ L^{-1} $\cdot$ min; and pulmonary venous resistance = 0.6 mm Hg $\cdot$ L^{-1} $\cdot$ min.

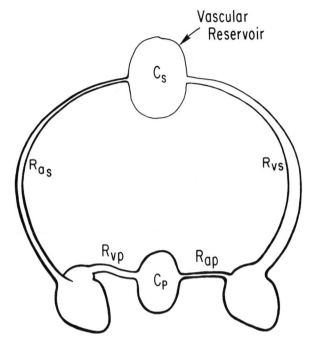

Fig. 4–12. Lumped parameter model of the circulatory system. R_{as} = systemic arterial resistance, R_{ap} = pulmonary arterial resistance, R_{vs} = systemic venous resistance, R_{vp} = pulmonary venous resistance, C_s = systemic vascular compliance, and C_p = pulmonary vascular compliance. (From Green, J.F.: Mechanical Concepts in Cardiovascular and Pulmonary Physiology. Philadelphia, Lea & Febiger, 1977.)

function is exchange. The capillaries have little effect on the overall hemodynamics of the circulation except that volume can leave or enter the circulation through the capillaries.

A schematic drawing of the circulatory system, known as a lumped parameter model, is presented in Figure 4–12. It is based on the mechanical properties of the circulatory system previously discussed. The term, *lumped parameter*, indicates that the many parallel vascular beds have been conceptually lumped together into a single equivalent channel. This circulatory system has been further lumped together into its two major subdivisions: the systemic circulation and the central circulation (composed of the two hearts and the pulmonary circulation). Each serial segment is considered to have only its primary hemodynamic function. Thus, the arterial system and large veins and vena cava are depicted as tubes, whereas the small veins and venules are depicted as a compliant sac. The corresponding segments of the pulmonary system are depicted similarly. Because this conceptual model is designed to illustrate the important nontransport characteristics of the circulatory system, the capillary beds have been excluded. A comparable hydraulic model of the circulatory system is presented in Figure 4–13.

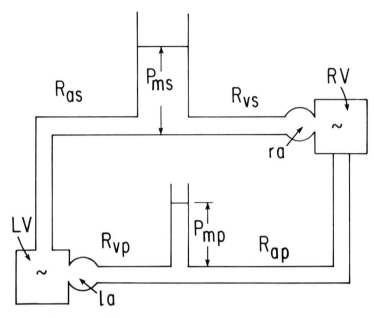

Fig. 4–13. Hydraulic model of the circulatory system. R_{as} = systemic arterial resistance, R_{ap} = pulmonary arterial resistance, R_{vs} = systemic venous resistance, R_{vp} = pulmonary venous resistance, P_{ms} = mean systemic pressure, P_{mp} = mean pulmonary pressure, ra = right atrium, RV = right ventricle, la = left atrium, and LV = left ventricle. (From Green, J.F.: Mechanical Concepts in Cardiovascular and Pulmonary Physiology. Philadelphia, Lea & Febiger, 1977.)

Although these models may seem unrealistic, that is, they lump all the many parallel channels together and exclude the capillaries, they nevertheless possess many of the significant characteristics of the cardiovascular system, as shown in the next chapter. Thus, they provide a useful conceptual framework on which to hang modifying bits and pieces of information.

To summarize, both systemic arteries and veins have resistive and capacitive functions; the relative magnitudes of these functions depend principally on structural differences. The function of resistance may be found within the arterial system and at the outflow of the venous system. The function of capacitance is dominant at the level of the small veins and venules.

The next chapter will begin to deal with the hemodynamic consequences arising from the structure of the systemic circulation.

5

DETERMINANTS AND DISTRIBUTION OF SYSTEMIC BLOOD FLOW

VENOUS RETURN

Vascular Reservoir

A description of the determinants of venous return should begin with the importance of the reservoir function of the veins. In order for any pump to operate, there must be some fluid to pump! This relationship is fundamentally significant. Consider the example illustrated in Figure 5–1. If the inflow and outflow ends of a simple hand pump, such as a sailboat bilge pump which operates on the stroke-volume principle,* were attached to the same single rigid tube (Fig. 5–1), fluid could not be pumped because there would be no fluid for the pump to take up; the system would be rigid. If, however, the rigid tube were cut in half and a reservoir interposed between the cut ends from which the pump could obtain fluid, not only would the pump be operable, but the amount of fluid that could be pumped would be limited only by the number of strokes per minute. The heart is not really any different from the bilge pump. It needs a reservoir of blood from which it can draw the blood to be pumped. Fortunately, the highly compliant veins (the small veins and venules) provide this necessary *vascular reservoir.*

---

*Fluid is taken up into the pumping chamber during a period of relaxation, then ejected during a period of activation.

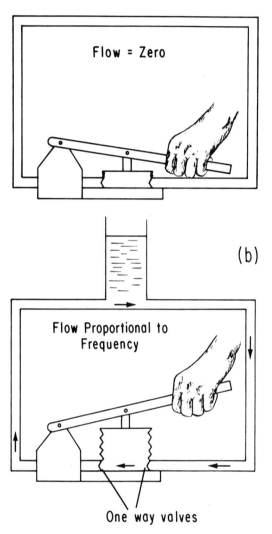

(a)

Flow = Zero

(b)

Flow Proportional to
Frequency

One way valves

Fig. 5–1. Schematic drawing illustrating the operating mechanism of a stroke-volume pump. (a): When the pump is connected in series with a rigid system, fluid is not available to prime the pump; therefore, flow is zero. (b) When the pump is connected in series with a reservoir, fluid may be taken into the pumping chamber from the reservoir during the relaxation phase of the pumping cycle and ejected into the reservoir during the active phase of the cycle. In general, the greater the frequency of the pumping cycle, the greater the flow, until the frequency becomes high enough to limit the period of inflow to such an extent that the chamber is not filled completely during the relaxation phase. (From Green, J.F.: Mechanical Concepts in Cardiovascular and Pulmonary Physiology. Philadelphia, Lea & Febiger, 1977.)

Pressure Gradient For Venous Return

As was discussed in Chapter 4, a pressure gradient, i.e., an upstream pressure minus a downstream pressure, is necessary for flow. The upstream driving pressure for venous return is the pressure at the inflow to the venous system, or the pressure within the small veins and venules, which is equal to the static mean systemic pressure, P_{MS}. That is, under static conditions (when venous return equals zero), the downstream (right atrial) pressure rises to equal the upstream driving pressure (the mean systemic pressure, i.e., the pressure within the small veins and venules) for venous return. The mean systemic pressure is determined by the blood volume and the elastic properties of the systemic circulation (see Chap. 4) and is defined as follows:

$$P_{MS} = \frac{V - V_o}{C_S}, \tag{5-1}$$

where C_S is systemic vascular compliance, mostly that of the small veins and venules (ml/mm Hg); V_o is unstressed vascular volume (ml), which is the volume contained in the vascular reservoir when the mean systemic pressure is atmospheric; and V is the total vascular volume (ml) (compare with Eq. 4–3, Chap. 4). $V - V_o$ is thus the stressed volume of the circulatory system (volume above V_o).

The downstream pressure for venous return is the pressure at the outflow to the venous system. When right atrial pressure, P_{RA}, is greater than atmospheric pressure. P_{ATM}, right atrial pressure is the effective downstream pressure. (For convenience, the atmospheric pressure is always considered to be zero.) When right atrial pressure falls to a subatmospheric value, the great veins entering the chest collapse at their point of entry, isolating the right atrium from the rest of the splanchnic circulation. Under these conditions, the great veins, at their point of entry into the chest, function as Starling resistors, i.e., their internal pressure becomes fixed at the effective surrounding pressure, which is atmospheric pressure. Atmospheric pressure, therefore, becomes the effective downstream pressure whenever the right atrial pressure falls to subatmospheric values.

Knowing the driving pressures, we can write an expression describing the pressure-flow relationship of the venous system as follows:
Whenever

$$P_{RA} > P_{ATM},$$

$$\tag{5-2}$$

$$\dot{Q} = \frac{P_{MS} - P_{RA}}{R_{VS}},$$

and whenever

$$P_{RA} \leq P_{ATM},$$

(5–3)

$$\dot{Q} = \frac{P_{MS} - P_{ATM}}{R_{VS}}.$$

In these equations, $\dot{Q}$ is venous return (L/min); R_{VS} is systemic venous resistance, i.e., the resistance to flow of the large veins and vena cava (mm Hg · L^{-1} · min); P_{MS}, P_{RA}, and P_{ATM} (mm Hg) are defined as previously described. Graphic solutions to Equations 5–2 and 5–3 are presented in Figure 5–2 for both positive (Eq. 5–2) and negative (Eq. 5–3) values of right atrial pressure. The resulting curve, known as the *venous return curve*, represents all possible combinations of venous return and right atrial pressure. If one understands the shape and position of the venous return curve, one understands the determinants of venous return.

Because volume and the elastic characteristics of the systemic circulation are the determinants of the mean systemic pressure, any consideration of the determinants of venous return must also entail the consideration of the volume-pressure relationship of the systemic circulation. Thus, an increase in V increases P_{MS} and, therefore, venous return. A decrease in V_O and C_S also increases P_{MS} and venous return. An increase in V can be accomplished simply by a transfusion. A decrease in V_O or C_S requires a contraction of the vascular smooth muscle located within the walls of the small veins and venules. This contraction can be accomplished either by vasoconstrictor agents circulating in the blood or by direct action of the sympathetic nerves. The effects that changes in the mean systemic pressure have on the venous return curve are illustrated in Figure 5–3.

The systemic venous resistance (R_{VS}) also has a profound effect on venous return. An increase in this resistance decreases venous return, whereas a decrease in resistance increases venous return. An increase in the systemic venous resistance can be achieved either by a contraction of the smooth muscles within the walls of the large veins or by external compression, such as may occur with an abdominal tumor or a pregnancy. The effects that changes in the systemic venous resistance have on the venous return curve are illustrated in Figure 5–4.

Thus, contraction of the systemic veins can have opposite effects on venous return, depending on whether the small veins and venules or the large veins contracted. A contraction of the small veins and venules decreases V_O and C_S, increasing $\dot{Q}$. A contraction of the large veins increases R_{VS} and decreases $\dot{Q}$.

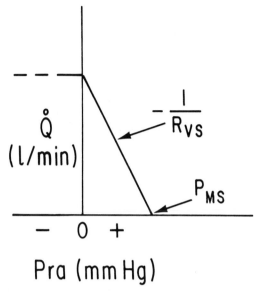

Fig. 5–2. Graphic solutions to Equation 5–2 (solid line) and Equation 5–3 (dashed line). Right atrial pressure (P_{ra}) is plotted on the abscissa and venous return ($\dot{Q}$) on the ordinate. The resulting curve, known as the venous return curve, describes the pressure-flow relationships of the venous system. The slope of the venous return curve equals minus the reciprocal of the systemic venous resistance (R_{vs}). When $\dot{Q}$ equals zero, P_{ra} (the downstream pressure) rises to equal P_{MS} (the upstream driving pressure for venous return). As P_{ra} is lowered, the pressure gradient for venous return ($P_{MS} - P_{ra}$) increases as does venous return. When P_{ra} falls below zero (the dashed line), the great veins entering the chest collapse at their point of entry into the chest. At this point, the pressure within the veins becomes fixed at atmospheric pressure (O), and the pressure gradient for venous return becomes fixed at its maximal value. Venous return, therefore, does not increase, even when P_{ra} is lowered to a negative (subatmospheric) value. For venous return to increase further when $P_{ra} \leq O$, either P_{MS} must increase (Fig. 5–3) or R_v must decrease (Fig. 5–4). (From Green, J.F.: Mechanical Concepts in Cardiovascular and Pulmonary Physiology. Philadelphia, Lea & Febiger, 1977.)

CARDIAC OUTPUT

Duality of Cardiac Output Control

In many respects, the terms *cardiac output* and *venous return* are unfortunate semantic choices because they suggest entirely different flows. But, as we have seen, because of the closed and circular nature of the cardiovascular system, they must remain equal except for minor transient periods.* Therefore, both the circuit and the heart should obviously play important roles in determining the total systemic flow. Because there is a natural inclination to associate cardiac output control with the heart, most physiologists are unaware of the contribution made by the systemic blood vessels, despite the accomplishment of much important

---

*Perhaps a better choice of terms would be total systemic flow.

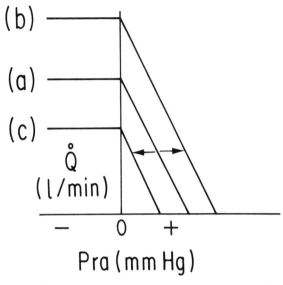

Fig. 5–3. This figure illustrates the effects that changes in mean systemic pressure, P_{MS} (P_{ra} at zero $\mathring{Q}$), can have on the venous return curve. Increasing P_{MS} (curve b) shifts the venous return curve to the right, thereby increasing venous return (Q) at any level of P_{ra}. Decreasing P_{MS} (curve c) shifts the venous return curve to the left, thereby decreasing $\mathring{Q}$ at any level of P_{ra}. An increase in P_{MS} can be brought about by an increase in the stressed vascular volume, a decrease in the unstressed vascular volume, or a decrease in systemic compliance (Eq. 5–1). Similarly, opposite changes in these parameters decrease P_{MS} and, therefore, $\mathring{Q}$. (From Green, J.F.: Mechanical Concepts in Cardiovascular and Pulmonary Physiology. Philadelphia, Lea & Febiger, 1977.)

and significant work (Caldini, et al., 1974; Guyton, 1973; Starling, 1897; Krogh, 1912). Nevertheless, cardiac output control rests as much with systemic factors as with cardiac factors because as Grodins (1967) succinctly states, ". . . mechanical coupling between heart and circuit dictates that cardiac output is a function of both heart and circuit parameters." A full appreciation of this statement is indispensable in understanding the operation of the cardiovascular system.

Right Atrial Pressure as a Coupler

The right atrial pressure is a unique pressure in the cardiovascular system. It is not only the back pressure to the systemic circulation, but is also the simultaneous inflow pressure for the heart. The right atrial pressure is, thus, a function of the amount of blood returned to the heart and the pumping ability of the heart. If the heart were a perfect pump, the right atrial pressure would always be maintained at an atmospheric or slightly subatmospheric value. This would establish a maximum gradient for venous return. If the heart were anything less than a perfect pump, the right atrial pressure would rise to a positive value, thereby reducing the pressure gradient for venous return. In essence,

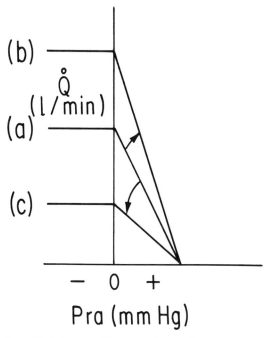

Fig. 5–4. This figure illustrates the effects that changes in systemic venous resistance (R_{vs}) have on the venous return curve. Increasing R_{vs} (curve c) decreases the slope of the venous return curve, thereby decreasing venous return ($\dot{Q}$) at any level of right atrial pressure (P_{ra}). Decreasing R_{vs} (curve b) increases the slope of the venous return curve, thereby increasing $\dot{Q}$ at any level of P_{ra}. An increase in R_{vs} can be achieved by a contraction of vascular smooth muscles within the walls of the large veins or by external compression. A decrease in R_{vs} occurs with an elevated blood volume, which increases transmural pressure of the veins, thus increasing their radius. (From Green, J.F.: Mechanical Concepts in Cardiovascular and Pulmonary Physiology. Philadelphia, Lea & Febiger, 1977.)

the right atrial pressure couples the pumping ability of the heart to the systemic circulation by directly affecting the pressure gradient for venous return. Such mechanical coupling between heart and circuit is absolutely essential if cardiac output is to remain equal to venous return.

The coupling nature of the right atrial pressure is best seen with the aid of the cardiac function and venous return curves. Figure 5–5a presents a cardiac function curve with right atrial pressure measured relative to atmospheric pressure as the independent variable. (This figure and all subsequent figures were originally obtained from animal experiments [Guyton, et al., 1973] and extrapolated to the human.) The magnitude of the right atrial pressure at zero cardiac output is equal to the pleural pressure because the transmural pressure is zero at this point. A venous return curve, identical to those discussed earlier (see above), is presented in Figure 5–5b. The cardiac function curve represents all possible combinations of cardiac output and right atrial pressure. The venous return curve represents all possible combinations of venous return and right

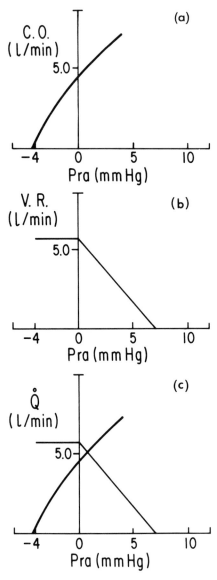

Fig. 5–5. (a): Cardiac function curve—output as a function of right atrial pressure, measured relative to atmospheric pressure. (b): Venous return curve—venous return as a function of right atrial pressure, measured relative to atmospheric pressure. The cardiac function curve represents all possible combinations of cardiac output and right atrial pressure. The venous return curve represents all possible combinations of venous return and right atrial pressure. Because cardiac output and venous return must be equal, there can only be one possible combination of total systemic flow ($\dot{Q}$) and right atrial pressure. This combination can be determined by the intersection of the cardiac function and venous return curves when plotted on the same coordinates (c). (From Green, J.F.: Mechanical Concepts in Cardiovascular and Pulmonary Physiology. Lea & Febiger, 1977.)

atrial pressure. At any one moment under steady-state conditions, one and only one cardiac output must be equal to venous return and to one and only one right atrial pressure. The exact combination of flow and right atrial pressure can be obtained by combining the cardiac function curve and venous return curve on the same axis. Figure 5–5c represents a graphic analysis of the determinants of cardiac output. Given any constant blood volume, systemic compliance, venous resistance, cardiac contractility, heart rate, afterload, and pleural pressure, the resulting cardiac output, venous return, and right atrial pressure may be determined by the intersection of the cardiac function and venous return curves.

Cardiac Factors Influencing Venous Return

Figure 5–6 presents a graphic analysis with three function curves corresponding to the normal, hypoeffective, and hypereffective heart and further illustrates the coupling nature of the right atrial pressure. Point A represents a normal cardiac output of 5 L/min and a right atrial pressure of about 1 mm Hg. Blood is returned to the heart with a pressure gradient ($P_{MS} - P_{RA}$) of 6 mm Hg. If the heart suddenly became hypoeffective without any significant changes in the systemic blood vessels, it would be unable to pump 5 L/min. Venous inflow to the heart would exceed the heart's ability to remove blood from the veins for a brief period. Right atrial pressure would rise until the pressure gradient for venous return (3 mm Hg) reduced venous return to match cardiac

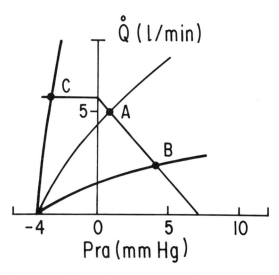

Fig. 5–6. Graphic analysis of the cardiovascular system illustrating the effect of a normal (A), hypoeffective (B), and hypereffective (C) heart. (From Green, J.F.: Mechanical Concepts in Cardiovascular and Pulmonary Physiology. Philadelphia, Lea & Febiger, 1977.)

output. The circulation would once again be balanced, and the steady-state cardiac function curve would move from point A to point B along the venous return curve (see Fig. 5–6). The rise in right atrial pressure couples the venous return to cardiac output. If the heart's pumping ability suddenly increased, it could not actually pump more blood unless the venous return increased. The increased pumping action of the heart lowers right atrial pressure, which increases the pressure gradient (P_{MS} − P_{RA}) and increases venous return. Further decreases in P_{RA} continue to increase venous return until P_{RA} falls below atmospheric pressure. At such a point, the great veins collapse, and venous return becomes fixed at its maximum pressure gradient (7 mm Hg). At point C, the heart potentially could pump more blood. This is a perfect example of the truism, "The heart cannot pump more blood than it receives." To increase cardiac output under these conditions (curve C), the systemic factors influencing venous return must actively change.

Systemic Factors Influencing Cardiac Output

Until now, we have considered only how cardiac output could be varied by changing cardiac factors (inotropic and chronotropic properties of the heart) while maintaining constant circuit parameters (volume, compliance, etc.). However, cardiac output also can be varied by altering circuit parameters while keeping cardiac factors constant. Figure 5–7 presents a graphic analysis of the circulatory system with three different

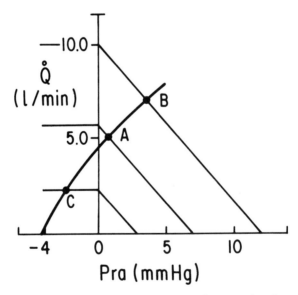

Fig. 5–7. Graphic analysis of the cardiovascular system illustrating the effect of a normal (A), increased (B), and decreased (C) mean systemic pressure. (From Green, J.F.: Mechanical Concepts in Cardiovascular and Pulmonary Physiology. Philadelphia, Lea & Febiger, 1977.)

venous return curves representing a normal (A), increased (B), and decreased (C) mean systemic pressure. When the mean systemic pressure is suddenly increased from its normal value of 7.0 mm Hg to 12.0 mm Hg, venous return increases, raising right atrial pressure. The rise in right atrial pressure increases the filling of the heart, thereby stretching the ventricles, and increases cardiac output through the Starling mechanism to match the venous return. The venous return curve shifts to the right, changing the intersection with the ventricular function curve from point A to point B. A reduction in mean systemic pressure shifts the venous return curve to the left, intersecting the cardiac function curve at point C. In these examples, right atrial pressure also serves as the coupling mechanism between venous return and cardiac output.

The preceding illustration shows that the control of cardiac output does not rest exclusively with heart factors, but also with systemic factors. Consider the important example of exercise. Exercise increases the cardiac output from the normal resting value of 5 L/min to well over 25 L/min. If the inotropic and chronotropic properties of the heart were the only factors to change during exercise, cardiac output would not significantly increase. The normal right atrial pressure is only about 1 mm Hg. Increasing the pumping ability of the heart lowers right atrial pressure, but, as soon as the right atrial pressure is reduced to atmospheric pressure, the veins entering the chest collapse, limiting the venous return (Fig. 5–8). If only cardiac factors were operative in exercise, the equilibrium point would move only from A on the normal curve to B, increasing cardiac output by only a few hundred cubic centimeters per minute. A significant increase in cardiac output relies on active changes on the part of the systemic blood vessels, i.e., a decrease in systemic compliance or venous resistance. In other words, to obtain a fivefold increase in cardiac output, it is not enough to augment the slope of the cardiac function curve. The venous return curve must also shift to the right and increase its slope, thereby shifting the equilibrium point from A to C (see Fig. 5–8).

Controlling Mechanisms of Cardiac Output

The mechanisms responsible for changes in mean systemic pressure, the resistance to venous return, and the contractile properties of the heart are also responsible for the shape and position of the venous return and cardiac function curves. The parameters that affect the mean systemic pressure essentially determine the static volume-pressure relationship of the systemic circulation (see Chap. 4), the stressed volume (V), the unstressed volume (V_o), and the compliance (C). The most immediate way to increase or to decrease V is by transfusion or hemorrhage. C and V_o can be indirectly changed through reflex adjustment of vascular smooth muscle tone or can be directly altered by direct stimulation of the vascular smooth muscle by such agents as epinephrine or

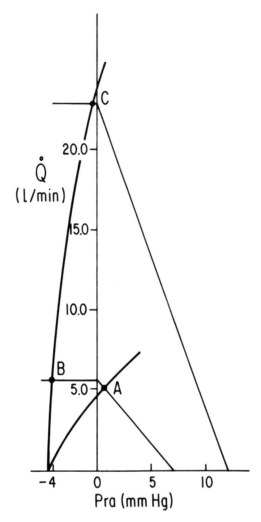

Fig. 5–8.   Graphic analysis of the cardiovascular system illustrating response to exercise. See text for details. (From Green, J.F.: Mechanical Concepts in Cardiovascular and Pulmonary Physiology. Philadelphia, Lea & Febiger, 1977.)

exogenous drugs. R_v can similarly be changed by indirect reflex adjustment and direct chemical stimulation. In addition, R_v can be altered by changes in the transmural pressure of the venous resistance vessels, which usually occur because of volume shifts into and out of these vessels. Changes in cardiac parameters sufficient to alter the slope of the cardiac function curve usually alter the inotropic and chronotropic properties of the myocardium (see Chap. 3). The cardiac function curve is shifted along the pressure axes by changes in pleural pressure.

   In summary, cardiac output is controlled not only by how well the heart can pump blood but also by the ability of the systemic blood vessels to return blood to the heart. A significant increase in cardiac output, as that which occurs during exercise, requires active alterations in both heart and circuit parameters.

DISTRIBUTION OF CARDIAC OUTPUT

Throughout the systemic circulation are numerous parallel vascular beds, e.g., splanchnic, renal, cerebral, coronary, skeletal muscle, skin, and others. The distribution of cardiac output to any given channel is determined by a direct application of Poiseuille's law (Eq. 4–4) to the individual channel. If either the pressure drop or the resistance of the individual channel changes, the flow through the channel also changes.* If, for example, the pressure drop and the arterial resistances remained constant in each channel, except the skeletal muscle where the arterial resistance fell, the flow in all channels would remain constant while skeletal muscle blood flow would increase. Such a scenario necessitates an increase in cardiac output, not only because total flow increases (the result of the increase in skeletal muscle flow), but also because an increase in cardiac output is necessary to hold arterial pressure constant in the face of a falling resistance in one of the parallel channels. If cardiac output remained constant as skeletal muscle arterial resistance fell (all other resistances remaining constant), arterial pressure would fall, reducing flow in all other channels. The end result would be a rise in skeletal muscle blood flow accompanied by a fall in blood flow in all other channels; however, total circuit flow (cardiac output) would remain unchanged. In other words, the flow in any one channel is linked to the flow in any other channel because (1) the sum of all parallel flows must equal the cardiac output and (2) the arterial driving pressure for all channels is the same.

Distribution of Cardiac Output According to Metabolic Requirements

The actual flow that any channel has at any time is determined by its specific metabolic requirements. This relationship is best illustrated by considering cardiac output and its distribution at rest and during maximum exercise. Figure 5–9 shows the relationship between cardiac output, oxygen consumption, and work during exercise. Cardiac output

---

*Note that the total "lumped" arterial resistance for the entire systemic circulation (R_a) is determined by summing the individual arterial resistances of all the parallel channels as *reciprocals*. Thus,

$$\frac{1}{R_a} = \frac{1}{R_{a_1}} + \frac{1}{R_{a_2}} + \frac{1}{R_{a_3}} + - - - - - \frac{1}{R_{a_n}},$$

where $R_{a_1} \ldots \ldots R_{a_n}$ represent the arterial resistances of individual channels.

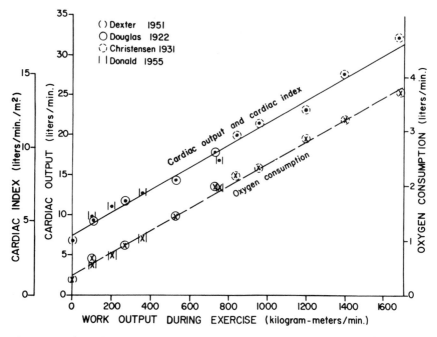

Fig. 5–9. Relationship between cardiac output and work output (solid curve) and between oxygen consumption and work output (dashed curve) during exercise. The data were derived from studies by Douglas and Haldane (1922), Christensen and Mitteilung (1931), Dexter, et al. (1951), and Donald, et al. (1955). (From Guyton, A.C., Jones, C.E., and Coleman, T.G.: Circulatory Physiology I: Cardiac Output and its Regulation. Philadelphia, W.B. Saunders, 1973.)

and oxygen consumption increase linearly as exercise increases. Because both oxygen consumption and cardiac output increase during exercise, the increase in cardiac output can be related to an increase in metabolism. Table 5–1 presents the distribution of cardiac output in a normal human subject at rest and during exercise.* Note that, at rest, blood flow is distributed equally between the splanchnic bed, the kidneys, and the skeletal muscles. At rest, the brain has a blood flow of 750 ml/min or about 13 percent of the cardiac output. During maximal exercise, cardiac output increases fivefold. The skeletal muscles are obviously the most active metabolically because their flow increases from slightly more than 1 L/min to 22 L/min, or an increase from 21 to 88 percent of the cardiac

---

*As with arterial blood pressure, one would expect that cardiac output and its distribution would vary widely within any given homogeneous group of individuals and that the best way to determine normal values is statistically. Unfortunately, the procedures that are available today to measure cardiac output and its distribution are so complicated and often dangerous (requiring invasive interventions, such as cardiac catheterization) that the large number of measurements necessary to establish normal values statistically are not available. The figures presented in Table 5–1 are, however, believed to be reasonable approximations of "normal."

Table 5–1.   Estimated Distribution of Cardiac Output in a Normal Human Subject* at Rest and During Maximal Exercise†

Region	Rest Blood Flow		Maximal Exercise Blood Flow	
	ml/min	% total	ml/min	% total
Splanchnic	1,400	24.1	300	1.2
Renal	1,100	19.0	250	1.0
Cerebral	750	12.9	750	3.0
Coronary	250	4.3	1,000	4.0
Skeletal muscle	1,200	20.7	22,000	88.0
Skin	500	8.6	600	2.4
Other organs	600	10.3	100	0.4
	5,800		25,000	

*Weight = 70 kg; body surface area = 1.7 sq m
†From: Wade and Bishop (1962).

output. The heart muscle also works actively, and its flow increases fourfold. On the other hand, the blood flow to the brain remains constant at 750 ml/min; the flow to all other regions falls. This fall in blood flow to the nonexercising regions is a compensatory mechanism that shifts the blood to the regions that are metabolically more active. As we will see in the next chapter, this redistribution of cardiac output is partially caused by a reflex increase in the arterial resistance of the nonexercising regions and by the massive decrease in arterial resistance of the skeletal muscle. The brain, however, cannot afford to have its blood flow compromised, even for a short time; therefore, an elaborate local mechanism (called autoregulation) prevents a decrease in its flow. Thus, both local and reflex mechanisms determine the flow to an individual region in relation to its metabolic needs. In addition, these same mechanisms augment venous return and interact with the intrinsic and extrinsic mechanisms governing cardiac performance to augment the flow through the heart.

6

DETERMINANTS OF ARTERIAL BLOOD PRESSURE AND ITS NORMAL VALUE

The systemic circulation primarily provides nutrients to and removes waste products from the various organs and tissues of the periphery. (Consequently, the systemic circulation is often called the peripheral circulation.) Because this is accomplished by the perfusion with arterial blood of the systemic vascular beds down a pressure gradient (see Chap. 4), one should understand how this pressure gradient is established. In the preceding chapter, we discussed the determinants of cardiac output. In this chapter we will discuss how the cardiac output interacts with the mechanical properties of the systemic circulation to produce the systemic arterial pressure, which becomes the upstream perfusion pressure for the systemic circulation.

ARTERIAL PRESSURE-FLOW RELATIONSHIPS

The pressure-flow relationships of the arterial system can be described by an application of the Poiseuille equation (Eq. 4–5),

$$\dot{Q} = \frac{1}{R} (P_I - P_O). \tag{4–5}$$

The inflow pressure (P_I) is the arterial pressure (P_a). The outflow pressure (P_O), however, depends on the exact pressure gradient one wishes to measure. If we define the inflow pressure of the venous system (mean systemic pressure) as the outflow pressure of the arterial system, we may use the following equation to describe arterial pressure-flow relationships:

$$\dot{Q} = \frac{1}{R_a} (P_a - P_{MS}), \tag{6-1}$$

where $\dot{Q}$ is cardiac output, P_a is arterial (aortic) pressure, P_{MS} is mean systemic pressure (the pressure in the vascular reservoir), and R_a is the arterial resistance (the resistance to blood flow between the aorta and the small veins and venules).

From a strict anatomic point of view, the arterial system ends at the beginning of the capillaries. R_a, as defined by Equation 6–1, includes the resistance of the capillaries and the resistance of the arteries. However, on a practical basis, this need not concern us because the resistance of the short capillary segment is so small, relative to the arterial resistance, that R_a can be considered equal to the arterial resistance.

Frequently, one finds a pressure-flow equation written to define the pressure-flow relationship for the entire systemic circulation. In this expression, the arterial pressure is the inflow pressure whereas the right atrial pressure is taken as the back pressure,

$$\dot{Q} = \frac{1}{TPR} (P_a - P_{RA}). \tag{6-2}$$

The resistance, TPR (total peripheral resistance), represents the resistance to blood flow across the entire systemic circulation from aorta to right atrium. Because the largest pressure drop across the systemic circulation occurs within the arteries, the total peripheral resistance term (TPR) of Equation 6–2 largely reflects this pressure drop; however, unlike the arterial resistance term (R_a) of Equation 6–1, TPR also reflects changes in venous resistance. For this reason, many physiologists in recent years have preferred to use Equation 6–1 to describe arterial pressure-flow relationships.

Rearranging Equation 6–1 yields

$$P_a = \dot{Q} R_a + P_{MS}. \tag{6-3}$$

This relationship defines the determinants of arterial pressure. At a normal cardiac output of 5 L/min, R_a equals 18.6 mm Hg $\cdot$ L^{-1} $\cdot$ min^{-1} whereas P_{MS} equals 7 mm Hg. This yields a *mean* arterial pressure (P_a) of 100 mm Hg. Because the pressure in the small veins and venules (the mean systemic pressure) amounts to only about 7 percent of the arterial pressure, the principal determinants of arterial pressure are therefore the cardiac output ($\dot{Q}$) and arterial resistance (R_a). It is important at this point not to confuse the mean systemic pressure, which is the pressure in the small veins and venules, with the mean systemic *arterial* pressure, which is the mean pressure in the arteries, usually measured in the aorta or its major branches. The factors that change cardiac output (e.g., a change in venous return or a change in the ionotropic properties of the heart) also change arterial pressure at constant arterial resistance. Similarly, the factors that change arterial resistance at constant cardiac output also change arterial pressure.

CONCEPTS OF EFFECTIVE BACK PRESSURE

In Equation 6–1, the mean systemic pressure was defined as the back pressure for arterial perfusion. The use of this particular back pressure implies that the arterial system functions as a rigid tube. In recent years, several studies have suggested that *small* arterial vessels probably function more as collapsible tubes (Permutt and Riley, 1963; Ehrlich, et al., 1975; Jackman and Green, 1977). Permutt and Riley (1963) first extended the principles of the Starling resistor (see Chap. 4) to arterioles by suggesting that active tension in the smooth muscles in the walls of arterioles functioned as an inward-acting pressure, analogous to the pressure surrounding a collapsible tube. In their model, under conditions where $\dot{Q}$ equals 0, this inward-acting pressure manifests itself as a critical closing pressure,[*] as suggested by Burton (1951), much as P_I equals P_S in the Starling resistor when $\dot{Q}$ equals zero (see Eq. 4–6). Under conditions of flow, when the capillary pressure (P_O) is less than the critical closing pressure, this inward-acting pressure manifests itself as the "effective" back pressure to perfusion, P_c', much as the surrounding pressure does in a Starling resistor when the outflow pressure is less than the surrounding pressure. The pressure-flow relationships through the arterial system, therefore, can be described by Equation 6–1 by allowing P_c' to replace P_{MS} as the back-pressure. Thus:

$$\dot{Q} = \frac{P_a - P_c'}{R_a}. \tag{6–4}$$

The resistance to flow in this case depends on the dimensions of the vessel up to, but not including, the area of critical closure.

Because various resistances have been used to describe arterial pressure-flow relationships, confusion may result. Remember that a resistance is defined by a pressure drop divided by a flow. Establish which pressure drop is used, and the resistance will be defined.

---

[*]Because the critical closing pressure of a vascular bed is defined as the arterial pressure when $\dot{Q}$ equals zero, critical closing pressure can be measured in isolated vascular beds by occluding arterial inflow and measuring arterial pressure distal to the occlusion. After flow is occluded, arterial pressure rapidly falls to a plateau value greater than venous pressure. Critical closing pressures as high as 30 to 40 mm Hg are not unusual.

Burton (1951) defined the critical closing pressure (P_c') by an application of Laplace's law, as follows:

$$P_c' = \frac{T_A}{r_0},$$ (6–5)

where T_A is active tension (vascular smooth muscle tone) and r_0 is unstretched radius. (Units of T_A/r_0 are dynes/cm^2, which is a pressure.) Substituting Equation 6–5 into Equation 6–4 yields:

$$\dot{Q} = \frac{1}{R_a}\left(P_a - \frac{T_A}{r_0}\right).$$ (6–6)

This equation allows one to predict the pressure-flow relationships that a vascular bed with tone would have if it behaved in a manner analogous to a Starling resistor with the active tone of small arterial vessels acting as an equivalent surrounding pressure, i.e., the effective back pressure. To illustrate this, Equation 6–6 is solved graphically in Figure 6–1A for the relationship between P_a and $\dot{Q}$ at constant T_A and r_0. R_a and R_0 were held constant at 1, while T_A was assigned the values of 10, 20, and 30. P_O was assumed to remain at atmospheric pressure. When $\dot{Q}$ equals 0, P_a equals P_c'. Note that no flow occurs until P_a is greater than P_c'; thereafter, flow increases linearly with P_a. An increase in the active tone of small arterial vessels (T_A) shifts the pressure-flow curve to the right without affecting the slope, which is the reciprocal of the large arterial vessel resistance. Figure 6–1B, replotted from Nichol et al., (1951), serves as an example of the pressure-flow relationships of a typical vascular bed under conditions of increasing vascular tone. These data were obtained from a rabbit's hind limb when the venous pressure was zero. Curves 1 to 4 represent increasing vasomotor tone produced by electrical stimulation of sympathetic nerves at increasing frequencies. Notice that an increase in the vasomotor tone of the small arterial vessels leads to a shift of the pressure-flow curves to the right. The slopes change only slightly until high degrees of tone are produced. That is, increasing the vasomotor tone leads to an increase in the effective back pressure.

With the introduction of the concept of the effective back pressure and the resultant arterial pressure-flow relationship (Eq. 6–4), the reader may wonder which conceptual approach to the arterial system should be used (e.g., Eq. 6–1 or 6–4). The answer to so many questions in physiology and medicine today also applies to this situation: use the approach that you find most useful. The concept of the effective arterial back pressure allows one to distinguish between what is happening in the larger arterial vessels from what is happening in the small arterioles solely on the basis of the arterial pressure-flow relationship. On the other hand, the more traditional approach (Eq. 6–1) is easier to com-

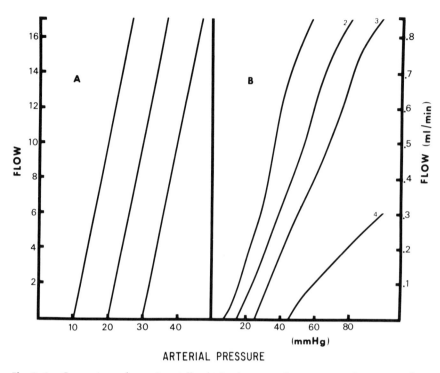

Fig. 6–1. Comparison of experimentally obtained pressure-flow curves to the pressure-flow relationships theoretically expected if a vascular bed behaved analogously to a Starling resistor with the active tone acting as an equivalent surrounding pressure. In (A), theoretically derived curves are drawn and, in (B), actual data curves obtained from the rabbit's hind limb by Nichol et al. (1951) are replotted. The abscissa is the arterial pressure. (From Green, J.F.: Mechanical Concepts in Cardiovascular and Pulmonary Physiology. Philadelphia, Lea & Febiger, 1977.)

municate and, as a first approximation, is quite adequate (e.g., a change in tone of either the large or the small arterial vessels is reflected as a change in the parameter, R_a; that is, a change in the amount of potential energy dissipated by the arterial system).

MEAN ARTERIAL BLOOD PRESSURE

In the preceding discussion we pointed out that the arterial blood pressure is a function of cardiac output, arterial resistance, and effective arterial back pressure, be it P_{MS} or P_c'. Because cardiac output is blood volume per unit time, we were implicitly referring to a time-averaged pressure; i.e., the *mean arterial pressure*. The mean arterial pressure is the average pressure during the cardiac cycle and is usually measured in the aorta or its major branches. To obtain the mean arterial pressure accurately, one must integrate the area under the blood pressure curve and divide this area by the time of integration. An approximation of the

mean arterial pressure can be obtained from the following expression
by knowing only the systolic (P_{as}) and diastolic (P_{ad}) pressures:

$$\overline{P}_a = P_{ad} + \frac{P_{as} - P_{ad}}{3}. \tag{6-7}$$

Fortunately, in most situations today, we can obtain the mean arterial
pressure electronically.

PULSE PRESSURE

The arterial pressure (nonmean) is markedly pulsatile during each
cardiac cycle. This characteristic can be seen in Figure 3–13, or in Figure
6–2, which is an arterial blood pressure tracing recorded from the aorta
of a dog. A sharp, ascending limb is followed by an elongated, descending limb, which usually contains the dicrotic notch (see Chap. 3). The
interval between the dicrotic notch and the beginning of the next ascending limb is referred to as the period of *diastolic run-off*. The zenith
of the ascending limb is the *systolic* pressure whereas the last part of the
diastolic run-off is the *diastolic* pressure. The *pulse* pressure is the difference between the systolic and diastolic pressures.

The pulse pressure is primarily a function of (1) stroke volume (SV),
(2) arterial (largely aortic) compliance (C_a), and (3) arterial resistance
(R_a). At any given level of C_a and R_a, an increase in SV produces an
increase in the ascending limb of the pressure curve, thereby increasing
the pulse pressure. At any given value of R_a and SV, a decrease in C_a
(making the aorta stiffer) results in a larger ascending limb and, there-

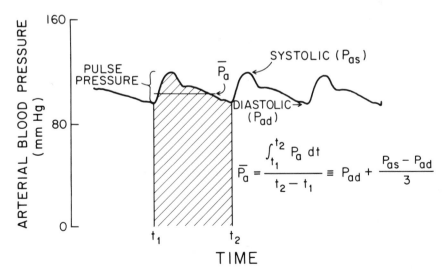

Fig. 6–2. Direct recording of arterial blood pressure from the thoracic aorta of a dog.

fore, a larger pulse pressure. At any given heart rate, SV, and C_a, the level of the diastolic pressure depends purely on the magnitude of the arterial resistance; if R_a falls, the diastolic run-off is greater and, therefore, diastolic pressure is less. Opposite changes in SV, C_a, and R_a, of course, produce opposite changes in pulse pressure. It should be noted that heart rate, per se, has little direct influence on the magnitude of the pulse pressure. At constant cardiac output, C_a and R_a, a change in heart rate changes stroke volume and thus pulse pressure indirectly.

Close inspection of an arterial tracing (Figs. 3–13 and 6–2) reveals an important function of the arterial system. Flow out of the left ventricle ceases at the dicrotic notch. But, flow and pressure throughout the systemic circulation do not drop to zero at this point because of the so-called *windkessel* function of the arterial system. "Windkessel" is a German word for a type of capacitor. The large amount of elastic tissue in the large arteries endows this part of the circulation (aorta and large branch) with the properties of a volume capacitor in series with the arterial resistance. With each beat of the heart, a portion of the left ventricular stroke volume is "stored" during systole. This stored volume then drains through the arterial resistance during the period of diastolic run-off, thus maintaining flow. We should note at this point that, even though the arterial capacitance is important in maintaining flow during diastole, the compliance of the arterial system is still smaller than that of the venous system. Therefore, the total amount of blood "stored" in the arteries during systole is small compared to that held by the small veins and venules.

Transmission of Pulse Pressure

The arterial pulse originates in the ascending aorta (on the side of the aortic valve) and travels in a wavelike fashion down the arterial tree. As the wave travels farther from the heart, a transformation occurs (Fig.

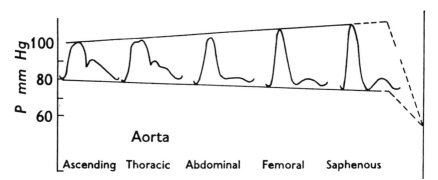

Fig. 6–3. Diagram demonstrating the behavior of the pressure pulse as it travels away from the heart. Mean pressure falls slowly, but the pulsatile pressure variation increases until, in the saphenous artery, it may be double that at the root of the aorta. (From McDonald, D.A.: Blood Flow in Arteries. London, Edward Arnold Ltd., 1974.)

6–3). The systolic pressure increases and the diastolic pressure decreases; the ascending portion of the pulse rises more sharply; the dicrotic notch disappears; and a secondary dip and rise develop in diastole. Two major factors have been identified in this metamorphosis.

1. Damping of the high-frequency waves traveling in a viscous fluid within the visco-elastic arterial system.

2. Reflections of waves that occur whenever the configuration or dimensions of the vessel change (e.g., at branching points). Because of reflections, the pressure at any given point in the arterial tree, at any given time, is the algebraic sum of the antegrade incident waves and the retrograde reflected waves.

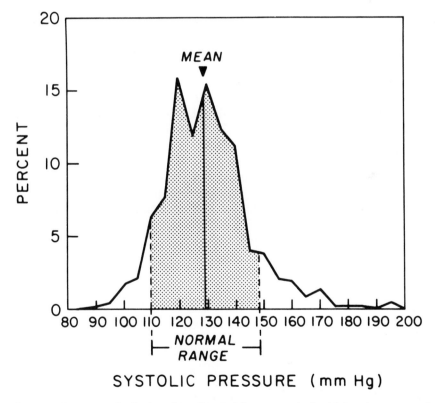

Fig. 6–4. Frequency distribution of systolic arterial pressures obtained from a large group of healthy male industrial workers between the ages of 40 and 44. The abscissa refers to the percent of the total number of individuals having a given value of systolic arterial pressure. (Redrawn from Master, A.M., Garfield, C.I., and Walters, M.B.: Normal Blood Pressure and Hypertension. Philadelphia, Lea & Febiger, 1952.)

Table 6–1.   Normal Range of Arterial Blood Pressure*

	Systolic		Diastolic	
Age	Male	Female	Male	Female
16	105–135	100–130	60–86	60–85
17	105–135	100–130	60–86	60–85
18	105–135	100–130	60–86	60–85
19	105–140	100–130	60–88	60–85
20–24	105–140	100–130	62–88	60–85
25–29	108–140	102–130	65–90	60–86
30–34	110–145	102–135	68–92	60–88
35–39	110–145	105–140	68–92	65–90
40–44	110–150	105–150	70–94	65–92
45–49	110–155	105–155	70–96	65–96
50–54	115–160	110–165	70–98	70–100
55–59	115–165	110–170	70–98	70–100
60–65	115–170	115–175	70–100	70–100

*Data from Master, Garfield, and Walters (1952).

NORMAL VALUES OF ARTERIAL BLOOD PRESSURE IN THE HUMAN

Arterial blood pressure normally varies with sex, age, metabolic rate, emotional state, and various other factors. Thus, normal values of arterial blood pressure can be expressed properly only by specifying a frequency distribution for a given sex, age group, and other conditions. Figure 6–4 presents a frequency distribution of systolic pressures obtained from a large group of "healthy male industrial workers" between the ages of 40 and 44 years (Master, et al., 1952). The distribution falls about a fairly normal distribution curve with a mean value for systolic pressure of 130 mm Hg. Because "physiologic normality" has not been defined, the statistical determination of the normal blood pressure range is thus somewhat subjective. Usually one assumes that any given reading is "normal" if it falls within ±1 standard deviation of the mean from a frequency distribution curve of a given homogeneous group, which includes 80 per cent of the observations under the curve. Table 6–1 presents the normal range of systolic and diastolic pressures obtained for different age groups from frequency distributions similar to that in Figure 6–4. Table 6–1 shows that arterial blood pressure gradually increases with age and that pressures of women are 5 to 10 mm Hg lower, on the average, than those of men until the age of 50; after the age of 50, pressures do not differ.

CONTROL OF THE CARDIOVASCULAR SYSTEM

DETERMINANTS OF VASCULAR TONE

Vascular (or *vasomotor*) tone can be broadly defined as "the state of contraction of the vascular smooth muscle within the walls of blood vessels." The exact amount of tone within any vessel at any time is largely the result of a balance between local control mechanisms, which are independent of nervous influences, and centrally controlled nervous input. We will begin our discussion of the control of circulatory function by first considering briefly the structure and physiological characteristics of vascular smooth muscle. We will then discuss the local and neurogenic mechanisms which control vascular smooth muscle tone.

Vascular Smooth Muscle

The vascular smooth muscle cells are 50 to 60 μ long and about 2 μ wide. They are usually helically arranged although longitudinally arranged smooth muscle fibers can also be found. The distribution of vascular smooth muscle is not uniform within the serial sections of the vasculature.

Unfortunately, the ultrastructure of vascular smooth muscle is not as well understood as that of cardiac and skeletal muscle. The sarcolemma encloses myofilaments, which are about 50 to 80 Å wide; however, the length of the myofilaments is unknown because they twist around each other and are lost when attempts are made to follow them with successive electron microscopic sections. The composition of the myofilaments is also not adequately known. Whereas distinct thin actin filaments and thick myosin filaments are seen in both cardiac and skeletal muscles, only actin filaments have been clearly identified in smooth muscle.

Vascular smooth muscle appears to be functionally differentiated into two basic types: (1) *unitary* smooth muscle and (2) *multiunit* smooth muscle. Unitary smooth muscle is characterized by spontaneous myogenic activity that is initiated in pacemaker areas. The activity then spreads throughout the muscle by some kind of cell-to-cell propagation. The resting membrane potential is only -40 to -50 mV. Rhythmic oscillations are superimposed on this resting potential and build up local potential. The local potential can become large enough to evoke a total depolarization and, through some poorly understood excitation-contraction coupling, a contraction. The spontaneous activity is enhanced by stretching the muscle. The unitary smooth muscle has few or no direct nervous innervations.

The multiunit smooth muscle does not contract spontaneously and is normally activated in more than one region by sympathetic nerves. The multiunit smooth muscle cell usually *does not react* to stretch.

Although some vascular smooth muscle cells clearly exhibit either unitary or multiunit behavior, other vascular smooth muscle cells exhibit both types of activity. Therefore, this classification should be considered as defining two ends of a spectrum. This diversification is one reason why an understanding of the physiology of the smooth muscle cell has taken so long to achieve (Bülbring, et al., 1970; Stephens, 1984).

The various types of vascular smooth muscle cells are not randomly distributed throughout the circulatory system. The unitary type of cell predominates at the site of the precapillary sphincter and probably constitutes the inner sheath of vascular smooth muscle in the small precapillary vessels. The multiunit type of cell appears to dominate the larger arterial vessels, the outer sheath of smooth muscle in the precapillary vessels, the veins, and the AV shunt vessels located in the skin. In general, the closer the vascular smooth muscle cell to the capillaries, the higher the probability that it is the unitary type.

This distribution of cell types has important physiologic significance. As we will see later, there is a considerable level of basal tone throughout the circulation as well as a large degree of local regulation of blood flow. The unitary type of smooth muscle cell, because of its spontaneous myogenic activity that is independent of nervous innervation, is ideally suited to establish local tone and to regulate local blood flow. In response to an increase in transmural pressure, the unitary type of smooth muscle increases its myogenic activity, thereby increasing its tone and the vascular resistance. Similarly, if pressure drops, the resistance drops. Thus, the unitary type of vascular smooth muscle operates to maintain a constant local blood flow despite changing perfusion pressures. On the other hand, the multiunit cell type is situated to produce an override of local mechanisms when, for the good of the organism, a centrally mediated reflex adjustment is necessary. If, for example, a temporary decrease in blood flow is necessary in one area (to increase flow in another parallel area), the multiunit smooth muscle in the outer sheath of the precapillary vessel could be activated, overriding the control of the inner unitary muscle as well as that of the unitary muscle downstream in the precapillary sphincters.

The veins also need predominantly central control (i.e., for reflex adjustment of venous compliance and venous return). Therefore, venous vascular smooth muscle is predominantly the multiunit type. For the same reasons, the AV shunts in the skin, which serve primarily a centrally mediated thermoregulatory function, are composed of multiunit smooth muscle.

The distribution of sympathetic nervous innervation closely follows the distribution of multiunit smooth muscle cells. Thus, arterioles are densely innervated whereas the precapillary sphincters have little or no innervation. On the venous side, the small veins and venules appear to have a greater nerve supply than do the larger drainage veins.

The sympathetic innervation is basically of two types: (1) the sympathetic adrenergic and (2) the sympathetic cholinergic. The adrenergic transmitter (the agent released at the nerve ending) is norepinephrine, which stimulates the alpha-adrenergic receptors (see the following). The cholinergic transmitter is acetylcholine. The sympathetic adrenergic nerves innervate all vascular smooth muscles. Activating the adrenergic nerves produces a constrictor response. The sympathetic cholinergic nerves innervate only the precapillary resistance vessels of the skeletal muscles where they produce, when activated, a dilation response. Sympathetic cholinergic fibers are known to exist in several species including dog, cat and rabbit, but are believed to be absent in primates.

Humoral agents can also act on vascular smooth muscle. They can reach the muscle from both the luminal and interstitial sides of the vessel. Many, although not all, vasoactive agents couple to specific *membrane receptors*. Two important receptors are the alpha- and beta-adrenergic receptors. The alpha-receptors are activated by norepinephrine (as well as other *alpha-adrenergic agonists*) and produce an excitatory response, whereas the beta-receptors are activated by epinephrine and isoproterenol (and other *beta-adrenergic agonists*) and produce an inhibitory response. The distribution of beta-receptors is predominantly (but not solely) located in the smooth muscle of the precapillary vessels, whereas alpha-receptors are fairly evenly distributed.

Certain hormones and drugs can produce contracture changes in vascular smooth muscle without evidence of electrical excitation. This response, known as *pharmacomechanical coupling*, is believed to be mediated by Ca^{++} influx or release. Agents in this category are histamine, acetylcholine, serotonin, angiotensin, adenosine, and the prostaglandins.

Unfortunately, we do not have the necessary knowledge to allow us to discuss in detail the anatomic, physiologic, and biochemical mechanisms that govern the action of vascular smooth muscle. This is an active area of research and we will no doubt know more about this important structure in future years. In the meanwhile, the problems and controversies of smooth muscle, in general, are discussed in an excellent monograph by Stephens (1984).

LOCAL CONTROL OF VASCULAR TONE

The existence of a local control mechanism that is independent of nervous influences is clearly demonstrated in preparations that have no extrinsic nervous influences or blood-borne constrictor agents, such as a surgically isolated and artificially perfused limb. In this preparation, one may observe a precipitous drop in arterial resistance immediately following a period of arrested flow. After a period of a few minutes, the resistance returns to normal. *Reactive hyperemia* is the term given to this phenomenon of active vasodilation. If, in the same preparation, arterial pressure is slowly elevated, flow increases, but in a less-than-proportionate manner. That is, as the driving pressure for flow increases, the vascular bed *autoregulates* in an attempt to maintain a constant flow. Both reactive hyperemia and autoregulation occur without extrinsic nervous influences and blood-borne constrictor agents, thereby indicating these phenomena are controlled by local mechanisms. Hyperemia and autoregulation are widespread throughout the body. For example, autoregulation has been demonstrated in skeletal muscle, in the myocardium, in the brain, and in the kidneys.

The ability of the various regional circuits to respond in the manner discussed indicates that vessels must work from a *basal tone*. If basal tone did not maintain a certain level of arterial resistance, blood flow could not be increased by lowering this resistance. The extent of the basal tone in the various parallel regions may be examined by determining the difference in blood flow (at constant arterial pressure) occurring under normal resting conditions and under maximal vasodilation by a large dose of some suitable drug. This examination reveals that the regions capable of a fairly wide range of metabolic activity, such as skeletal muscles, myocardium, and salivary glands, manifest an especially high level of basal vascular tone, which is primarily myogenic in origin (Fig. 7–1). Tissues with a high degree of innervation exhibit either little basal vascular tone (i.e., the kidney) or a largely neurogenic basal vascular tone (i.e., the skin).

The mechanism by which basal tone is established and maintained has been the subject of many investigations and much debate, and is still unknown. However, two major hypotheses have been advanced (Johnson, 1964). The *myogenic hypothesis* (Johnson, 1980) recognizes the inherent myogenic activity of unitary smooth muscle and attributes basal

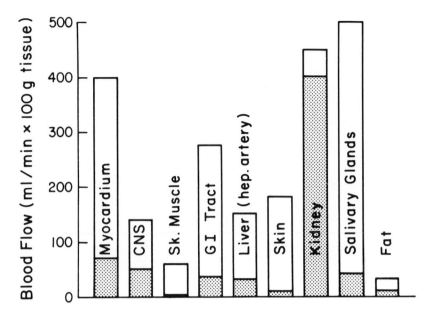

Fig. 7–1. Diagram illustrating regional blood flows at rest (shaded areas) and under conditions of maximal vasodilation. (Redrawn from Mellander, S., and Johansson, B.: Control of resistance, exchange and capacitance function in the peripheral circulation. Pharmacol. Rev., 20(3):117, 1968.)

vascular tone to this property (Fig. 7–2). The myogenic hypothesis also suggests that an increase in arterial distending pressure increases the tone of the unitary smooth muscle, whereas a decrease in pressure has the reverse effect. (Remember that the spontaneous activity of unitary smooth muscle is enhanced by stretching.)

The *metabolic hypothesis* (Sparks, 1980) states that the level of vascular tone is a function of the amount of vasodilator metabolics acting on the

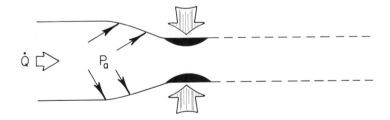

MYOGENIC HYPOTHESIS

Fig. 7–2. Schematic drawing illustrating the hypothesized myogenic mechanism of vascular control. The spontaneous myogenic activity of the unitary type of vascular smooth muscle establishes a basal level of tone. The arterial tone and resistance can then be augmented by the stretch initiated by an increase in the arterial distending pressure.

Cardiovascular Physiology

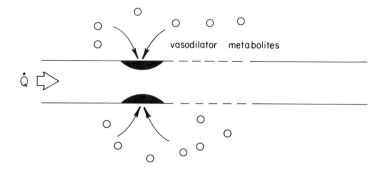

METABOLIC HYPOTHESIS

Fig. 7–3. Schematic drawing illustrating the hypothesized metabolic mechanism of vascular control. Vasodilator metabolites accumulate in the interstitial fluids and act on the vascular smooth muscle to reduce tone and arterial resistance.

vessel at any one moment (Fig. 7–3). There have been attempts to identify a universal vasodilator substance (one that acts equally on all tissues). The candidates for this agent have been low P_{O_2}, high P_{CO_2}, low pH, adenosine, and lactic acid, to mention a few. Apparently, the importance of any individual agent varies from one tissue to another or even within the same tissue from one time to another. Thus, adenosine and low P_{O_2} have powerful effects on the coronary vessels whereas low pH appears to be the main regulator of the cerebral vessels.

Although neither the myogenic nor the metabolic mechanisms can totally and individually account for the establishment of the basal tone, both mechanisms may actually operate together, one complementing the other. The myogenic mechanism would establish a basal level of tone through the inherent properties of unitary smooth muscle. Stretch would provide a positive feedback to augment the tone, and the accumulation of metabolics would provide a negative feedback to reduce the tone. The resulting tone would therefore be the algebraic sum of all factors operating together.

NEUROGENIC CONTROL OF VASCULAR TONE

Vasoconstrictor Innervation

In general, sympathetic adrenergic nerves innervate most vessels of the body, although in varying degrees (Bevan, et al., 1980). The degree of innervation ranges from sparse in the cerebral vessels to heavy in the skin. The density of innervation of the skeletal muscles and the gastrointestinal tract is intermediate between the extremes represented by the cerebral and the skin vessels. As already noted, the density of innervation also varies along the serial sections of the circulation. The large arteries and veins are sparsely supplied whereas the small arterioles are heavily innervated. The precapillary sphincters, composed mostly of unitary smooth muscle, have little or no sympathetic nervous innervation. As a rule of thumb, the vasoconstrictor fibers exert their greatest effect in organs or areas where the intrinsic basal tone of the vessel is small. Thus, the more active the region (i.e., as judged, for example, by the AV oxygen difference), the less the innervation. The kidney is an interesting special case because it is a highly active organ that is also highly innervated. However, under normal conditions, the sympathetic nerves to the kidneys are inactive.

Evidence shows that, in some regions (e.g., skeletal muscles) innervated with sympathetic vasoconstrictor fibers, the tonic activity of these fibers creates an augmentation of the basal tone. Thus, elimination of sympathetic activity to skeletal muscles causes the blood flow to double. Because of the great bulk of skeletal muscles (roughly half of the body mass), the tonic activity of the sympathetic nerves to this tissue has a profound influence on the establishment of central arterial (aortic) blood pressure.

When activated by the sympathetic nerves, the response of the vascular smooth muscle is not an all-or-none reaction, but depends on the frequency of nervous stimulation. When the frequency is increased

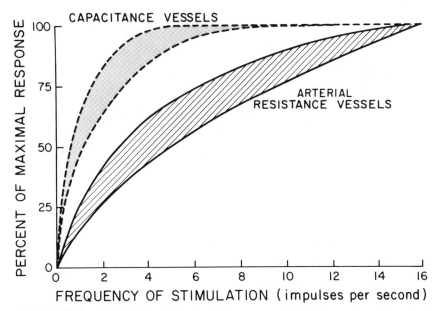

Fig. 7–4. Frequency-response curve for resistance vessels and capacitance vessels in the hindquarters of the cat. (From Mellander, S.: Comparative studies on the adrenergic neurohormonal control of resistance and capacitance blood vessels in the cat. Acta Physiol. Scand., 50[Suppl. 176]:1, 1960.)

slowly from 0 to approximately 20 impulses per second, the elicited response of the vessel increases. Figure 7–4 presents a frequency-response curve for both the resistance and capacitance vessels in the hindquarters (skin and muscle) of a cat. The response is presented as a percentage of the maximal response. It is apparent from Figure 7–4 that the response is a function of frequency and that the responsiveness to stimulation differs between the capacitance and arterial resistance vessels. The capacitance vessels reach their maximal response before the arterial resistance vessels. The physiologic range of stimulation is usually 1 to 10 impulses per second. The veins reach their maximal constriction well within this range, but the arterial resistance vessels only reach 75 percent of their maximal response. This dissociation between the responses of resistance and capacitance vessels suggests an independent control, which would be in keeping with their separate hemodynamic functions.

Vasodilator Innervation

Vasodilator fibers have a limited distribution to the systemic circulation and are not tonically active. They nevertheless have a profound physiologic influence under special circumstances. There are two basic types of vasodilator fibers: (1) *cholinergic sympathetic* nerves found in nonprimates (e.g., dogs, cats, rabbits) and (2) *parasympathetic* nerves (Burnstock, 1980). The cholinergic sympathetic nerves supply only the larger precapillary arterial vessels of skeletal muscles and are activated by a defense-like reaction. They are usually evoked with an intense discharge of other sympathetic nerves, which reduces flow to parallel compartments while increasing flow to the skeletal muscles.

The parasympathetic nerves are of two types: (1) those that produce dilation directly, and (2) those that produce dilation indirectly. The most important direct nerves are those distributed to the external genital erectile tissue through the parasympathetic sacral roots. Some evidence indicates that the pial vessels of the brain are also supplied with parasympathetic vasodilator nerves, but their functional significance is not fully appreciated.

Indirect vasodilation is produced by the parasympathetic nerves distributed to the salivary, sweat, and gastrointestinal glands. These nerves produce their indirect effect by releasing the specific enzyme *kallikrein* from the glands. Kallikrein, in turn, splits off a vasodilator polypeptide, called *kallidin*, from globulin.

Concept of Adrenergic Receptors

Many humoral agents interact with membranes (e.g., vascular smooth muscle or the myocardium) by way of specific membrane receptors. Two adrenergic receptors have been identified by Ahlquist (1948) based on the relative potency of *epinephrine, norepinephrine,* and *isoproterenol* to stimulate the receptors and on the ability of *Dibenzyline* (phenoxyben-zamine hydrochloride) and *dichloroisoproterenol* (DCI) to block their effects. Ahlquist found that epinephrine was the most potent stimulator for one receptor, called the *alpha (α) type*, whereas isoproterenol was the least potent. Isoproterenol was the most potent stimulator for the other receptor, called the *beta (β) type*, and norepinephrine was the least potent. Dibenzyline selectively blocked the action of the alpha-receptors, and DCI selectively blocked the beta-receptors. This differentiation of alpha- and beta-adrenergic receptors is summarized in Table 7–1.

The adrenergic receptors differ in their physical and chemical properties to such an extent that their affinities for various adrenergic agents also differ. In general, the effect of the alpha-adrenergic receptor is excitatory and that of the beta-adrenergic receptor is inhibitory. One important exception to this rule is related to beta-receptors in the myocardium, which are excitatory in nature. Isoproterenol, by activating the myocardial beta-receptors, increases heart rate and force of contraction. (The beta-receptors in the myocardium [heart muscle] should not be confused with possible beta-receptors in the coronary vessels. See Table 7–2.)

In recent years, the myocardial beta-receptors have become known as $beta_1$-receptors and are selectively blocked by such agents as metoprolol. The beta-receptors in the rest of the body (in the systemic vasculature and the bronchial smooth muscle, which responds to beta-stimulation with bronchodilation) are known as $beta_2$-receptors.

The distribution of alpha- and beta-adrenergic receptors in the circulation is not uniform. Some vascular sections may have a preponderance of one type of receptor and a small proportion of the other type. For example, the skeletal muscle vessels have mostly beta-receptors, which produce relaxation when stimulated with epinephrine. These same vessels also have a smaller number of alpha-receptors, which produce vasoconstriction when stimulated with norepinephrine. The predominant type of adrenergic receptors in various vascular areas is presented in Table 7–2. Cholinergic innervation is also listed in this table for comparative purposes.

Review of Factors Acting Directly on Blood Vessels

Table 7–3 summarizes the neurogenic and chemical control mechanisms that exist locally in the major parallel vascular regions. Remember

Table 7–1. Differentiation of Adrenergic Receptors

Type of Receptor	Relative potencies of:			Blocked by:	
	Epinephrine	Norepinephrine	Isoproterenol	Dibenzyline	DCI*
α	500	100	1	+	−
β	20	1	100	−	+

*DCI = dichlorisoproterenol

Table 7–2.   Adrenergic and Cholinergic Response in the Cardiovascular System*

	Adrenergic Responses		
Area	Receptor Type	Response	Cholinergic Responses
Heart:			
SA node	β	increase in heart rate	decrease in heart rate; vagal arrest
Atria	β	increase in contractility and conduction velocity	decrease in contractility and (usually) increase in conduction velocity
AV node and conduction system	β	increase in conduction velocity	decrease in conduction velocity; AV block
Ventricles	β	increase in contractility, conduction velocity, automaticity, and rate of idiopathic pacemakers	—
Blood vessels:			
Coronary	—	dilation[1]	—
Skin	α	constriction	—
Skeletal muscles	α,β	constriction; dilation[2]	dilation
Cerebral	α	constriction (slight)	dilation
Pulmonary	α	constriction	—
Viscera	α,β	constriction; dilation[2]	—
Salivary glands	α	constriction	dilation

*From Gilman, A.G., et al. (eds.): Goodman and Gilman's The Pharmacological Basis of Therapeutics. 7th ed. New York, Macmillan, 1985.
[1]May be largely due to indirect effects.
[2]Over the usual concentration range of physiologically released, circulating epinephrine, β-receptor response (vasodilation) predominates in blood vessels of skeletal muscle and liver; α-receptor response (vasoconstriction), in blood vessels of other abdominal viscera.

that these factors (nervous and chemical) modify the existing basal tone, which is believed to be established by the inherent myogenic properties of the unitary smooth muscle. Several generalities can be made. First, the primary controlling mechanism in those regions that exhibit low resting metabolic activities (i.e., skin, visceral organ, and kidney) is a centrally mediated nervous response; in areas with high resting metabolic activity (i.e., skeletal muscles, heart, and brain), the primary controlling mechanism is local (myogenic modified by chemical metabolites). The resting AV oxygen difference is a good indication of the level of metabolic activity in a given region. Second, although sympathetic cholinergic innervation is present in certain tissues (i.e., skeletal muscle and sweat glands of the skin), these nerves are of secondary importance to the tonically active sympathetic adrenergic system. Finally, alpha- and beta-adrenergic receptors are present throughout the vasculature and can be stimulated by circulating catecholamines or drugs (e.g., epinephrine or isoproterenol). Their effect can be either complementary to the major direct sympathetic innervation (as in skeletal muscle) or opposite (as in the visceral organs). The exact effect elicited by certain agents is also a function of their concentration. For example, epinephrine elicits a constrictor response (α) in the vessels of the heart in a high concentration and a dilation response (β) in a low concentration.

CONTROL OF CARDIAC FUNCTION

The heart's natural properties, such as inherent rhythmicity, excitability, conductivity, and contractility, endow it with certain *intrinsic* control mechanisms. These mechanisms allow the heart to function even when all nervous connections are severed. Today, nothing illustrates this ability more vividly than does a human being who carries out his or her normal routine with a transplanted heart. Nevertheless, much of the heart's activity under normal conditions is governed by *extrinsic* mechanisms, such as nervous and humoral factors (Levy and Martin, 1979; Downing, 1979; Coleridge and Coleridge, 1979).

Nervous Control of Heart Rate and Contractility

Nervous control of the heart comes from the neural innervation received from both the parasympathetic and sympathetic divisions of the autonomic nervous system. Both sets of nerves exhibit tonic activity. Whereas the parasympathetic system inhibits activity, the sympathetic system functions as an excitatory stimulus.

Innervation of the Heart

In addition to playing an important role in the regulation of heart rate, the autonomic nervous system also influences the force of contraction of both the atria and ventricles. This influence probably results from the distribution of the autonomic fibers. The sympathetic nerves supply all areas of the atria and the ventricles. The vagal nerve fibers (parasympathetic) supply the SA node, atrial muscle fibers, AV node, and, according to some recent studies, the ventricles. A schematic drawing representing the efferent autonomic innervation of the heart is presented in Figure 7–5. Afferent (reflex) activity affecting the heart's performance is discussed below.

Effects of Nervous Stimulation

Stimulation of the vagus nerves* results primarily in (1) a diminution in the strength of atrial and ventricular contraction, (2) a reduction in the conduction velocity through the AV node, and (3) a slowing of the heart rate. If the strength of stimulation is increased, a complete atrioventricular dissociation or a temporary cessation of the heartbeat could result.

These effects of vagal stimulation result primarily from a reduction in

---

*Acetylcholine, the chemical mediator liberated at the vagal nerve endings in the heart, mimics the effects of vagal stimulation when applied to the atrial muscle.

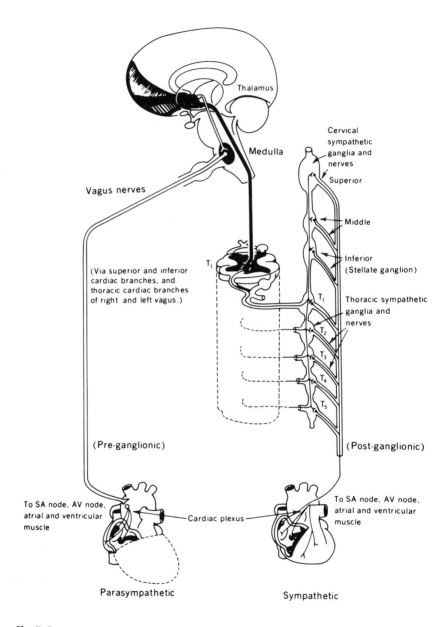

Fig. 7–5.

the slope (phase 4) of the pacemaker potential and from the production of a more negative maximum diastolic potential (see Fig. 2–5). This *hyperpolarization* is believed to be caused by a significant increase in potassium permeability. Although vagal fibers predominantly influence the atrial musculature and the SA and AV nodes, vagal innervation also reaches the ventricles. This may explain why vagal stimulation decreases ventricular contractility.

Stimulation of the sympathetic nerves through the release of norepinephrine at the end of the sympathetic fiber in the heart results primarily in (1) an increase in the strength of myocardial contractions, (2) an increase in conduction velocity through the atria, AV node, and ventricles, and (3) an increase in heart rate.

Sympathetic stimulation results principally from an increase in the slope of the pacemaker potential and possibly from an augmentation of the slow inward currents of sodium and calcium.

The effect of the nervous system on the heart is always the result of the combined effect of both the sympathetic and parasympathetic systems. The vagal parasympathetic system is believed to normally predominate and to maintain the normal resting heart rate of approximately 72 beats per minute.

Effects of Humoral and Chemical (Drug) Agents

Agents that can reach the heart through the blood are forms of extrinsic stimulators. The most obvious of these agents are the normally circulating catecholamines, such as epinephrine and norepinephrine. Such

---

Fig. 7–5. A schematic representation of the efferent autonomic innervation of the heart. The parasympathetic and sympathetic nerves to the heart, many of which closely accompany each other in and through the various cardiac and coronary plexuses, have been separated for illustrative purposes. The parasympathetic innervation of the heart originates in the medulla and passes through the right and left vagus nerves. Two sets of cardiac nerves arise from each vagus nerve: the superior (superior and inferior cervical) cardiac nerves, which arise from the vagi in the neck, and the inferior (thoracic) cardiac nerves, which arise from either the vagus nerves or the recurrent branches of the vagi. The sympathetic innervation of the heart passes from the spinal cord to the upper four or five thoracic ganglions. Some fibers from the upper thoracic ganglions pass up the cervical sympathetic to the superior, middle, or inferior cervical ganglions. The superior (cervical), middle (cervical), and inferior (cervical) cardiac nerves originate from their respective ganglions and pass downward through the deep and superficial parts of the cardiac plexus to the heart. When the inferior cervical and the first thoracic ganglions are fused, the resulting ganglion is known as the stellate ganglion. Additional cardiac branches arise from the upper four or five thoracic ganglions and pass to the cardiac plexuses or to the aorta. The cardiac and coronary plexuses are formed by cardiac branches from both the sympathetic and parasympathetic systems. Both sympathetic and parasympathetic fibers are thought to influence the SA node, the AV node, and both the atrial and ventricular myocardia. (From Silverman, M.E., and Schlant, R.C.: Functional anatomy of the cardiovascular system. *In* The Heart. Edited by J. W. Hurst, and R. B. Logue. New York, McGraw-Hill Book Co., 1966.)

agents tend to mimic the effects of sympathetic stimulation. Epinephrine, when injected into the blood alone, increases the heart rate and improves the efficiency of contraction as exhibited by a decrease in diastolic volume. Carbon dioxide and oxygen can also be considered extrinsic stimulating agents. Excesses of carbon dioxide or lack of oxygen produce dilatation of the heart and increase diastolic volume. Combinations of different agents have different effects on the heart. For example, epinephrine in combination with an increase in partial pressure of carbon dioxide increases the heart rate and prevents the reduction of diastolic volume, a characteristic of epinephrine alone. The numerous agents that are commonly used clinically (e.g., digitalis, calcium, isoproterenol, dopamine, corticosteroids) all function as extrinsic stimulating agents. The specific effect of any given agent is a complex function of not only the physiologic state of the heart, but also of the way the agent is administered, either alone or in combination with other extrinsic agents.

NEURAL CONTROL OF CARDIOVASCULAR FUNCTION

Levels of Neural Control

Until now, our discussion of the neurogenic control of vascular function and of the heart has been limited to a description of the local effects of the vasoconstrictor and vasodilator fibers and the local effects of the various cardiac nerves. These fibers, however, originate in a diffused area of the brain known as the *cardiovascular centers* where all cardiovascular functions (and even pulmonary function) are integrated (Korner, 1979). This integration occurs because the "centers" are not strictly localized, but are rather *a diffused network of interconnected neurons* in the reticular formation, which extends from the lower part of the pons to the obex. The cardiovascular reflexes (discussed later) depend in large part on the neural mechanisms located in the medullary area, which is responsible for the *tonic discharge* sent over the vasoconstrictor fibers. These same mechanisms are excited or inhibited by reflex inputs and by descending influences from higher portions of the brain. Only the sympathetic vasodilator outflow to the skeletal muscle (see the following) seems independent of this part of the medulla.

Electrical stimulation of various sections of the medulla in experimental animals has indicated that two areas regulate the vasculature and two areas appear to have direct control of the heart, although these areas tend to overlap. A *pressor* area in the lateral reticular formation produces a rise in arterial blood pressure when stimulated, and a *depressor* area in the medial reticular formation produces a fall in arterial blood pressure when stimulated. The former area produces its pressor response by evoking excitation of the vasoconstrictor nerves, whereas the depressor

Table 7–3. Summary of Neurogenic and Chemical Control Mechanisms

Region	Special Function	Primary Control	A-VO$_2$ Difference- Rest (Vol %)	Oxygen ml/min	Uptake % total	Neurogenic Control Primary	Response	Secondary	Response	Chemical Control Primary	Response
Skin	Heat exchange	Central	1	5	2	Sympathetic adrenergic (α)	Constriction	Sympathetic cholinergic (to sweat glands)	Dilation	—	—
Visceral organs	Absorption	Central	4.1	57	22	Sympathetic adrenergic (α)	Constriction	β, high [epinephrine]	Dilation	—	—
Kidney	Volume and electrolyte balance	Central and local	1.3	14	5	Sympathetic adrenergic (α)	Constriction			—	—
Skeletal muscles	Metabolic	Local (+ some neurogenic)	8	97	37	Sympathetic adrenergic (α) / Sympathetic cholinergic	Constriction / Dilation	α, high [epinephrine] / β, normal [epinephrine]	Constriction / Dilation	Potassium ions Hyperosmolarity pH low PO$_2$ high PCO$_2$	Dilation
Heart (coronaries)	Metabolic	Local	11.4	26	10	Sympathetic adrenergic	Constriction (functionally insignificant)	α, high [epinephrine] / β, normal [epinephrine]	Constriction / Dilation	Adenosine and its breakdown products low PO$_2$	Dilation
Brain	Metabolic	Local	6.3	48	18	Sympathetic adrenergic	Constriction (functionally insignificant)	Parasympathetic Cholinergic	Dilation	high PCO$_2$	Dilation
Pulmonary	Gas exchange	Local- mechanical	—	—	—	Autonomic innervation present, but of minimal effect, thus the vessels are almost maximally dilated.		—	—	low PO$_2$ (hypoxia)	Constriction
Other	—	—	3	17	6	—	—	—	—	—	—
Cardiac output	—	—	4 (whole body)	254	100	—	—	—	—	—	—

area produces its depressor response by *inhibition* of the vasoconstrictor nerves. Thus, the depressor center should not be considered an active vasodilator center. No vasodilator fibers are activated (by the depressor center) in any depressor reflex; *a fall in pressure is solely caused by release of vasoconstrictor tone and by a slowing of the heart.* Figure 7–6 presents a schematic drawing of the medulla and localizes the pressor and depressor areas.

Closely associated with the pressor area is the *cardioaccelerating center.* Activation of the vascular pressor center also stimulates the cardioaccelerating center and results in tachycardia accompanying the systemic vasoconstriction. The cells from these centers pass their outflow down the spinal cord. This outflow is distributed to the nodal tissue in the heart as well as to the systemic blood vessels by way of the sympathetic nerves. Also closely associated with the vascular depressor areas is the *cardioinhibitory center,* which is a neuronal pool that gives rise to the efferent fibers of the vagus nerves. Stimulation of the cardioinhibitory center leads to bradycardia or even stoppage of the heart.

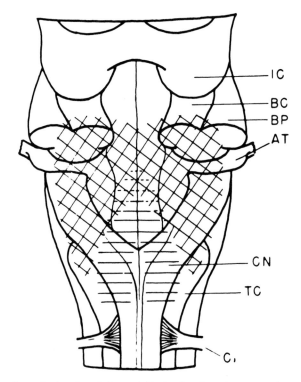

Fig. 7–6. A schematic drawing of the medulla that localizes the pressor (cross-hatched) and depressor (horizontal lines) areas of the cat. IC = inferior colliculus; BC = brachium conjunctivum; BP = brachium pontis; AT = auditory tubercle; CN = caudate nucleus; TC = tuberculum cinereum; C_1 = first cervical nerve. (From Alexander, R.S.: Tonic and reflex functions of medullary sympathetic cardiovascular centers. J. Neurophysiol., 9:205, 1946.)

All the cardiovascular centers receive impulses from the higher areas of the brain and afferent impulses from all parts of the body. Signals received from the cerebral cortex play important roles in the cardiovascular response to exercise, pain, and anxiety. Signals received from the heat-regulating areas of the anterior part of the hypothalamus are another example of a higher center input. Local heating of this area (i.e., by warm blood) causes vasodilation of the skin vessels, resulting from inhibition of the sympathetic constrictor fibers. Examples of afferent input from other parts of the body include those signals carried by the vagus, aortic, and carotid sinus nerves (i.e., from the baroreceptors). The aortic and carotid sinus nerves have inhibitory effects on the cardiovascular centers. We will have more to say about these afferent inputs below.

The sympathetic cholinergic vasodilator nerves have no connection with the various cardiovascular centers. These fibers originate in the motor cortex and move downward to a relay station in the hypothalamus. The efferent fibers from the two sides of the hypothalamus are interconnected and, after passing through another relay station in the collicular region, continue down the ventrolateral parts of the medulla (but do not connect with the pressor or depressor areas). The fibers then move directly to the preganglionic neurons in the lateral horn cells of the spinal cord. These fibers do not participate in carotid or aortic baroreceptor reflexes. A schematic presentation of the central and peripheral extensions of the sympathetic vasodilator pathway is shown in Figure 7–7.

The content of both oxygen and carbon dioxide directly affects the cardiovascular centers. (This effect is independent of their effect on the chemoreceptors—see the following.) If the P_{CO_2} of the arterial blood is low (i.e., by hyperventilation), a marked fall in arterial blood pressure occurs because of the paralysis of the cardiovascular centers in the medulla. On the other hand, hypoxia (a significant decrease in the arterial P_{O_2}) produces a sharp rise in arterial blood pressure because it leads to a stimulation of the cardiovascular centers and an increase in the sympathetic discharge to most organs of the body.

In summary there are four major areas of the central nervous system which play major roles in cardiovascular control: the cortex, hypothalamus, medulla and spinal cord. The functional connections between these areas are shown schematically in Figure 7–8.

Peripheral Receptors

Several areas of the cardiovascular system containing specialized nerve endings evoke profound cardiovascular and pulmonary reflexes when stimulated. These regions are located at the bifurcation of the common carotid artery, at the arch of the aorta, and, to a lesser degree, in the heart, large veins, and pulmonary vasculature. The impulses from these

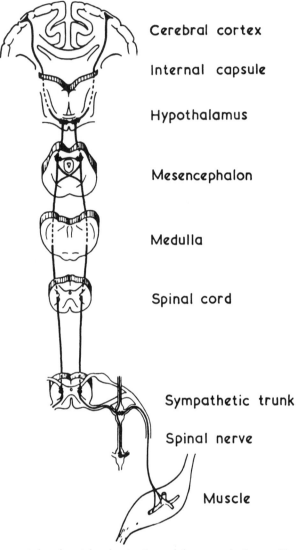

Fig. 7–7. The central and peripheral extensions of the sympathetic vasodilator pathways. (From Lindgren, P.: The mesencephalon and the vasomotor system. Acta Physiol. Scand., *35*[Suppl. 121]:1, 1955.)

specialized regions, known as *baroreceptors* and *chemoreceptors,* travel by afferent nerves to the medullary centers and then through efferent nerves back to the heart and blood vessels where they evoke changes in heart rate, contractility, vascular resistance, and compliance. As their names imply, the baroreceptors respond to changes in arterial pressure, and the chemoreceptors respond to changes in the chemical composition of the blood. Both receptors operate through the principle of *negative*

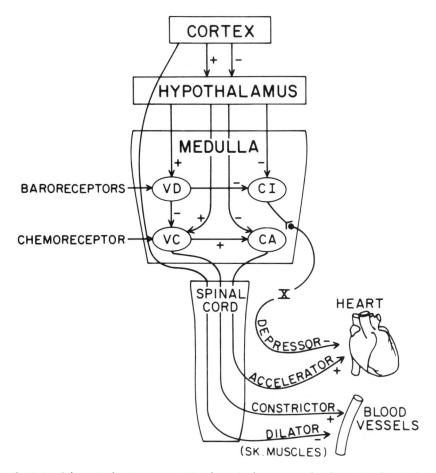

Fig. 7–8. Schematic drawing summarizing the major known neural pathways involved in the central regulation of cardiovascular function. This design is oversimplified to illustrate the major relationships between excitatory (+) and depressor (−) fibers. VD = vasodepressor area; VC = vasoconstrictor area; CA = cardioaccelerator area; CI = cardioinhibitory area.

feedback. Negative feedback mechanisms operate in such a way as to maintain a control variable at a fixed value, often called the *set point.* For example, consider the control of mean systemic arterial blood pressure. Let us assume its normal value (its set point) is 100 mm Hg. If for some reason, say hemorrhage, the mean systemic arterial blood pressure falls to 80 mm Hg, an error signal is created. The error signal is the difference between the set point (100 mm Hg) and its actual value (80 mm Hg). The peripheral receptors sense this error and feed information back to the central nervous system such as to return the mean systemic arterial blood pressure back to its set point. This it does by initiating autonomic adjustments to increase systemic arterial resistance and/or cardiac output. When the error signal is abolished the adjustments stop.

Baroreceptors. In human beings (and other mammals), the common carotid artery divides into the internal and external carotid arteries. At the beginning of the internal carotid is a bulbous enlargement, known as the *carotid sinus,* whose wall contains the arterial baroreceptors. The baroreceptors of the carotid sinus are innervated by the *carotid sinus nerve* (also known as the *nerve of Hering*), which is a branch of the ninth cranial nerve (the *glossopharyngeal*).

In diffuse locations in the wall of the aortic arch, other baroreceptors are innervated by the aortic depressor nerve, which is a branch of the tenth cranial nerve (the *vagus*). The afferent fibers from the carotid and aortic baroreceptors run up their respective nerves and make direct connections with the cardiovascular centers.

The normal stimulus for the baroreceptor is not pressure per se, as its name implies, but rather the deformation in the vessel wall produced by changes in pressure. Thus, these receptors are actually stretch receptors (a better name is *mechanoreceptors*). A schematic representation of the carotid sinus and the carotid body (chemoreceptor) and their innervation in the dog is presented in Figure 7–9.

When the arterial blood pressure (transmural pressure) increases at the baroreceptors (increasing their stretch), the frequency of impulse firing increases, thereby inhibiting the vasoconstrictor center. Consequently, the tonic activity of the medullary centers is diminished. This results in a withdrawal of sympathetic efferent activity reducing systemic arterial resistance and increasing systemic venous compliance. A bradycardia, brought about by stimulation of vagal centers, accompanies the peripheral changes. Lowering the arterial blood pressure reverses this scenario.

Animal experiments have demonstrated that the carotid sinus adapts rapidly to pressure changes and is more responsive to *changing* pressures than to constant pressures. For example, at a mean arterial pressure of 50 mm Hg, an impulse from a single fiber of the sinus nerves is initiated only by the pressure rise in early systole. As the mean pressure increases, the frequency of discharge increases, yet most of the discharges still occur early in systole. Finally, at a high mean arterial pressure (200 mm Hg), a maximal sustained firing is reached.

Chemoreceptors. The chemoreceptors consist primarily of the *carotid* and *aortic bodies.* The carotid body is a small, specialized group of cells situated at the bifurcation of the common carotid artery (see Fig. 7–9). It receives its blood supply from a branch of the occipital or ascending pharyngeal artery. Although it is small, the carotid artery receives the largest blood flow, on a weight basis, of any other organ in the body. The flow is equivalent to about 2000 ml/min/100 gm of carotid body tissue. The carotid body is innervated by the *carotid sinus nerve,* the same nerve that innervates the carotid sinus. The carotid body nerve endings respond to changes in the chemical composition of the blood, most

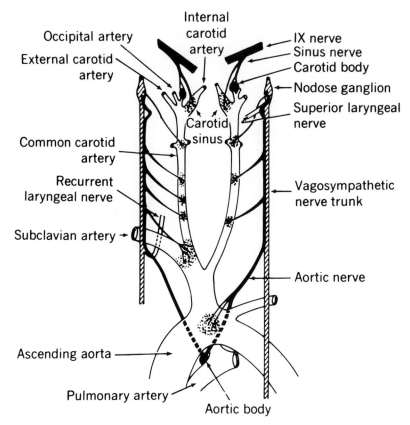

Fig. 7–9. Diagrammatic representation of location and innervation of baroreceptors and chemoreceptors of aortic and carotid regions in cat and dog. (Comroe, 1964; Heymans and Neil, 1958; Kezdi, 1967). Baroreceptor areas are indicated by stippling. Nerves and arteries are labeled. (From Milnor, W.R.: The cardiovascular control system. *In* Medical Physiology. Edition 14. Edited by V. B. Mountcastle. St. Louis, The C.V. Mosby Co., 1980.)

powerfully to a decrease in P_{O_2}, but also to a rise in P_{CO_2} and a fall in pH.

Located in the arch of the aorta is a similar group of chemoreceptors known as the aortic body. Their function is the same as that of the carotid bodies, but they are innervated by the aortic nerve. The chemoreceptors respond mostly to changes in P_{O_2} and P_{CO_2}. The nervous impulse activity from the chemoreceptors increases when the P_{O_2} falls below 150 mm Hg and the P_{CO_2} increases above 35 mm Hg. The most potent stimulus for the peripheral chemoreceptors is hypoxia. The major cardiovascular effects of chemoreceptor stimulation are bradycardia and an increase in arterial resistance. These effects, particularly the vasoconstriction, can be attenuated by the secondary ventilatory reflexes initiated by peripheral chemoreceptors (see Chap. 16).

Vagal Receptors. Although the peripheral baroreceptors and the chemoreceptors are, by far, the most important regulators of cardiopulmonary function, other less understood receptors, whose afferent fibers pass in the vagus nerve, are located in other areas of the vasculature. First, a series of *low pressure baroreceptors* is located in the pulmonary vessels. These receptors are believed to be tonically active and can reflexly alter systemic resistance with changes in pulmonary vascular pressure and blood volume. Second, baroreceptors located in the walls of the ventricles and atria can inhibit sympathetic tone to the systemic vessels, thereby causing dilation. The atria receptors are believed to play a role in urine regulation by controlling the release of antidiuretic hormone (ADH) from the posterior pituitary gland. The exact mechanism for this action has not been fully explained. In recent years, electrophysiologic studies have demonstrated the existence of ventricular receptors that are sensitive to endogenously released substances such as prostaglandins and bradykinin. These substances may be released by the myocardium during ischemia. These receptors may, therefore, play a role under pathologic conditions. Finally, the simple act of lung inflation can bring about a reflex vasodilation. The afferent fibers from these lung stretch receptors also run in the vagus nerves and inhibit the vasomotor center. This lung reflex is closely associated with another pulmonary reflex, the *Hering-Breuer reflex* (discussed later in the pulmonary section).

Sympathetic Receptors. Chemosensitive sympathetic afferent nerve endings in the heart have been shown to respond to algesic agents such as lactic acid and bradykinin. It is believed that the pain of angina results from the stimulation of these sympathetic endings. They may also evoke pressor reflexes, but these mechanisms are poorly understood.

Summary Comments. When one remembers that the cardiovascular system maintains a constant internal environment to all cells of the body, one recognizes that the control system could not have been better designed. The local neurogenic and chemical factors can basically take care of the needs of the tissues without any outside (nervous) help (provided perfusion pressure is adequate). Yet, the nervous control mechanisms can take control when one area of the circulation must cooperate with the other. The integration is excellent. The vasomotor center takes in measurements from the peripheral sensors as to the pressure, volume, and chemical status of the systemic blood vessels. It then integrates this information with "higher order" impulses about such things as body temperature and emotion into a coherent and continuous moment-to-moment control schema.

Consider what happens when, because of hemorrhage, the perfusion pressure is not sufficient to allow local mechanisms to provide adequate nutritional flow. Recall that the arterial and low pressure baroreceptors usually send a steady supply of impulses to the cardiovascular depressor area in the medulla. These impulses inhibit the normally occurring tonic sympathetic vasoconstrictor impulses that are sent to the systemic blood vessels. When the blood pressure is low (because of hemorrhage), the inhibitory effect is reduced and the vasoconstrictor discharge is thereby augmented. In addition, cardiac output is probably low because of blood volume loss. A low cardiac output leads to a large AV oxygen gradient and poor tissue oxygenation. A generalized increase in the discharge to the sympathetic vasoconstrictor and cardiac acceleration fibers decreases the venous compliance, thereby increasing venous return toward normal; increases the heart rate and contractility so that the increase in venous return can be transferred to the arteries; and, finally, increases the arterial resistance so that the elevated cardiac output can support an increase in perfusion pressure to perfuse such important areas as the heart and brain.

As part of this total integration, we would have found that the arterial resistance in the heart muscle and the brain does not increase because such sensitive organs simply cannot tolerate a reduction in blood flow. Therefore, their powerful, active, local control mechanisms maintain their flow at optimal or near optimal levels, even in the face of the generalized sympathetic discharge that occurs following the hemorrhage.

This example has been used to demonstrate how the cardiovascular control mechanisms come together to maintain the homeostatic balance of the organism. By simply understanding the basic principles discussed in this chapter, one can reason through most other circumstances. Try it; it's fun.

8

THE MICROCIRCULATION

The microcirculation—the capillaries and, perhaps, the small veins immediately downstream from the capillaries*—is undoubtedly the "action site" of the circulatory system. At this level, the circulation's primary function of maintaining a constant internal environment (i.e., *le milieu interieur*) is accomplished by the transport of oxygen, carbon dioxide, nutrients, and waste products. We have already briefly considered the structure of the microcirculation (see Chap. 1). This chapter concentrates on its function by considering first the determinants of capillary pressure and, second, the three major types of processes by which transcapillary exchange occurs: (1) filtration-absorption, (2) diffusion, and (3) cytopempsis.

DETERMINANTS OF CAPILLARY PRESSURE

As was discussed in Chapter 4, the pressure at any given point in any flowing system is the product of the flow and resistance downstream from that point plus the effective back pressure (Poiseuille's law). Poiseuille's law can be applied to a capillary as follows:

$$P_c = \dot{Q}R_v + P_v, \qquad (8-1)$$

where P_c is the hydrostatic pressure at the midpoint of the capillary, P_v is the downstream venous pressure (measured either locally or near the right atrium), and R_v is the postcapillary venous resistance, or the resistance to flow between the midpoint of the capillary and the point where venous pressure is measured. Because capillary flow ($\dot{Q}$) is usually a function of arterial pressure (P_a) and the precapillary arterial resistance

---

*Recent studies suggest that the immediate postcapillary segment of veins may be part of the effective exchange vessels because pores appear to be abundant there.

(R_a), capillary pressure is usually expressed as follows (Landis and Pappenheimer, 1963):

$$P_c = \frac{\left(\dfrac{R_v}{R_a} \times P_a\right) + P_v}{1 + \dfrac{R_v}{R_a}}. \tag{8–2}$$

Figure 8–1 shows the derivation of Equation 8–2. Implicit in this expression are the assumptions that the flow into the capillary is equal to the flow out of the capillary and that the overall driving pressure for flow is the arterial and venous pressure differences. Thus, Equation 8–2 shows that, for any given tissue, P_c is determined by the ratio of postcapillary resistance to precapillary resistance and the arterial and venous pressures.

Equation 8–1 is similar in form to Equation 5–2, which defines the mean systemic pressure, P_{MS}, under conditions of flow as:

$$P_{MS} = \dot{Q} R_{VS} + P_{RA}, \tag{5–2}$$

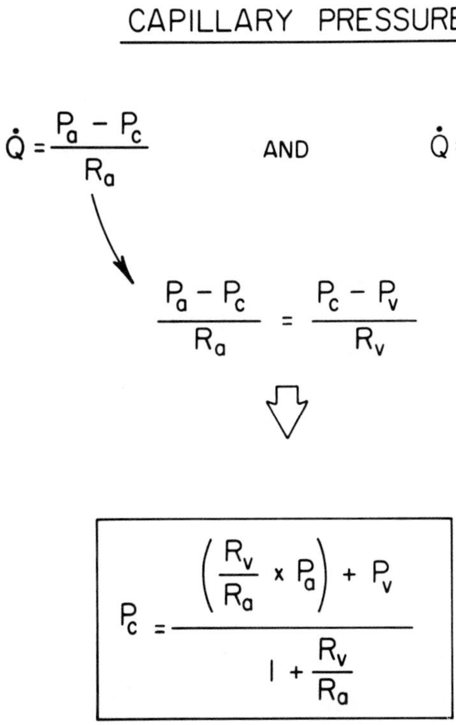

CAPILLARY PRESSURE

$$\dot{Q} = \frac{P_a - P_c}{R_a} \quad \text{AND} \quad \dot{Q} = \frac{P_c - P_v}{R_v}$$

$$\frac{P_a - P_c}{R_a} = \frac{P_c - P_v}{R_v}$$

$$P_c = \frac{\left(\dfrac{R_v}{R_a} \times P_a\right) + P_v}{1 + \dfrac{R_v}{R_a}}$$

Fig. 8–1. Derivation of Equation 8–2, expressing capillary pressure (P_c) as a function of arterial resistance (R_a), venous resistance (R_v), arterial pressure (P_a), and venous pressure (P_v). Flow equations from capillary inflow and outflow are set equal and solved for P_c.

where $\dot{Q}$ is the venous return, P_{RA} is the right atrial pressure, and R_{VS} is the hydraulic resistance between the small veins and venules and the right atrium. The significance of the similarity between these two equations is interesting. Recall that P_{MS} is the upstream driving pressure for venous return to the heart and is believed to be the pressure in the capacitance areas of the systemic circulation (i.e., the small veins and venules immediately downstream from the capillaries). In the form of Equation 5–2, P_{MS} represents an average of all the pressures in the small veins and venules in all the various parallel vascular areas (weighted by their compliances), and R_{VS} represents an average resistance to blood flow between these small veins and venules and the right atrium. Because any given tissue must have its own P_{MS} as well as its own P_c, the individual venous resistances for that tissue, R_v and R_{VS}, must overlap and, thus, link the control of venous return from that segment to the control of capillary pressure. The extent to which these two *functionally different* hydraulic resistances overlap has yet to be adequately determined. But, for any given tissue, the closer the capillary pressure to the mean systemic pressure, the closer the magnitudes of R_v and R_{VS}.

FILTRATION-ABSORPTION

The Starling Principle. One of the most important aspects of the circulation is the process by which plasma is held in the circulatory system. The principle of fluid balance was first formulated by Starling (1896) and now bears his name (the *Starling Principle* of fluid balance). The five primary factors that determine whether fluid moves into or out of the capillary, according to the Starling principle, are the capillary and interstitial hydrostatic pressures, the capillary and interstitial colloid osmotic pressures, and the hydraulic conductivity of the capillary wall. The hydrostatic pressures may be thought of as forces that tend to push fluid across the capillary membrane, whereas the colloid osmotic pressures may be thought of as forces that tend to retard this flow. Because hydrostatic and colloid osmotic pressures are on both sides of the capillary membrane, the difference in these pressures is important. Thus, the Starling principle describes the flow of fluid across the capillary, $\dot{Q}_c$, as:

$$\dot{Q}_c = CFC[(P_c - P_i) - (\pi_p - \pi_i)], \tag{8–3}$$

where P_c and P_i are the capillary and interstitial hydrostatic pressures; π_p and π_i are the plasma and interstitial colloid osmotic pressures; and CFC, the capillary filtration coefficient, is the filtration "constant" for the capillary membrane and expresses the resistance of the capillary wall to fluid flow. When Equation 8–3 is expressed as $\dot{Q}_c = CFC \times \Delta P$, it becomes quite apparent that the Starling principle is a similar expression to Poiseuille's law for flow across the capillary wall.

Colloid Osmotic Pressures

The capillary and interstitial colloid osmotic pressures (also referred to as *oncotic pressures*) occur because the capillary wall is not freely permeable to the plasma proteins. The plasma contains about 300 milliosmoles/L of crystalloids that pass freely across the capillary wall; thus, their concentration is equal on both sides of the capillary. The concentration of plasma protein is about 7 gm/100 ml of plasma, exerting a plasma colloid osmotic pressure of around 28 mm Hg. The plasma protein concentration is considerably less in the interstitium and differs in various regions. In skeletal muscle, this concentration is about 20 percent of that in plasma and exerts a colloid osmotic pressure of around 5 mm Hg. The interstitial protein concentration in the intestine varies between 40 to 60 percent of that of the plasma, whereas the liver interstitium contains up to 80 percent of the protein content of plasma.

The Conventional Starling Balance

Equation 8–3 illustrates that, when there is no net flow across the capillary wall, i.e., $\dot{Q}_c$ equals zero, the difference in hydrostatic pressures across the capillary wall just balances the differences in colloid osmotic pressures, or

$$(P_c - P_i) = (\pi_p - \pi_i). \tag{8–4}$$

Thus, by knowing these four pressures, one can predict the conditions under which there is no net fluid movement. The conventional appli-

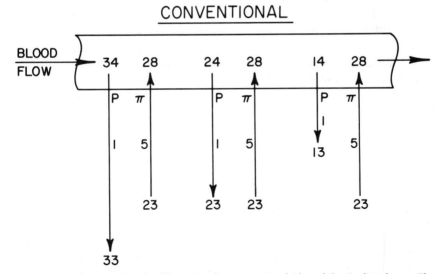

Fig. 8–2. Schematic drawing illustrating the conventional idea of the Starling forces. The arrows indicate the direction and magnitude of the pressure gradients for both hydrostatic and osmotic pressures. P = hydrostatic pressure and π = colloid osmotic pressure.

cation of this relationship made use of direct measurements of capillary pressure with micropipets (Fig. 8–2), which ranged from around 34 mm Hg at the arterial end of the capillary to around 14 mm Hg at the venous end. Also of use was the knowledge that plasma colloid osmotic pressure was 28 mm Hg, whereas interstitial osmotic pressure was approximately 5 mm Hg (at least for skeletal muscle). Thus, assuming a mean capillary hydrostatic pressure of 24 mm Hg and an interstitial hydrostatic pressure of 1 mm Hg, one could obtain a reasonable value of 23 mm Hg of hydrostatic pressure difference, which was believed to balance 23 mm Hg of osmotic pressure difference (see Fig. 8–2). The high hydrostatic pressure at the arterial end of the capillary produced a net filtration force at the arterial end of 10 mm Hg whereas, at the venous end, a net absorption force was 10 mm Hg.

A More Probable Starling Balance

In recent years, new considerations have come to light that suggest that the Starling forces may be different from those considered in Figure 8–2. Recent measurements of functional (mean) capillary pressure (Intaglietta et al., 1970; Wiederhielm, et al., 1964) have yielded results from 10 to 15 mm Hg lower than 24 mm Hg. In addition, Guyton and colleagues (1975) used a newly developed technique for measuring interstitial hydrostatic pressures and found them to average about 8 mm Hg *subatmospheric.*

The concept of a negative interstitial hydrostatic pressure is of such significance that it requires brief consideration. Guyton and colleagues measure interstitial hydrostatic pressure by chronically implanting into tissues small hollow plastic spheres perforated by several hundred small holes. At the end of a few weeks, tissues grow inward through the holes to line the inner surface of the sphere. The remainder of the cavity fills with fluid. Guyton reasons that this pressure is in equilibrium with the interstitial hydrostatic pressure. When he measures this pressure, he finds it is around 8 mm Hg negative in most tissues of the body, except in the kidney where the pressure ranges from -1 to $+8$ mm Hg and in the lung where the pressure is around -18 mm Hg.

If P_i is truly -8 mm Hg, then P_i is not set by any close relationship to atmospheric pressure (as previously assumed) and other factors must be important. Furthermore, if P_i is 9 mm Hg lower than previously thought (-8 instead of $+1$), the mean capillary pressure must also be 9 mm Hg lower. These relationships are shown in Figure 8–3. To balance the Starling equation, capillary pressure must be 15 mm Hg. Because it is difficult to imagine a high pressure gradient for flow down the capillaries, this figure has been adjusted to show a pressure drop of only 2 mm Hg. The magnitude of the hydrostatic pressures presented in Figure 8–3 is consistent with the more recent measurements of capillary pressure.

MORE PROBABLE

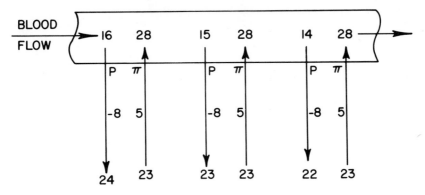

Fig. 8–3.   Schematic drawing illustrating the more probable values of the Starling forces based on recent measurements of capillary pressure and interstitial hydrostatic pressures. This figure is interpreted in the same manner as Figure 8–2.

Now that we have seen that the mean capillary pressures in most tissues may be a lot closer in magnitude to the mean systemic pressure (7 to 10 mm Hg) than previously recognized, we are in the position to appreciate the significance of the overlapping venous resistances (previously discussed). If P_c is close to P_{MS}, R_V and R_{VS} may not be too dissimilar in magnitude. This possibility implies that the control of capillary pressure is inescapably linked to the control of venous return, at least on a region-by-region basis, and that P_c and P_{MS} should change together by the same or similar magnitudes.

A comment is needed at this point concerning the various values for hydrostatic and colloid osmotic pressure used in the preceding examples. The only principal pressure in the Starling balance of which we can be certain is the plasma colloid osmotic pressure. This pressure can be measured directly from a small blood sample. As we have seen, the other values are, at best, estimates that are changing as research continues in this field. The absolute values used in the preceding examples are not important; however, the principles they were used to illustrate, i.e., the Starling balance, are important. Furthermore, these values are constantly changing in a dynamic organism. Thus, as arterial tone increases, a capillary that may have been filtering at its arterial end and absorbing at its venous end suddenly absorbs along its entire length as capillary hydrostatic pressures fall along its entire length. Thus, one must realize that the establishment of a Starling equilibrium must not necessarily be conceived as a balance between filtration at the arterial end of the capillary and absorption at the venous end. Periods of predominate filtration may alter with periods of absorption.

Capillary Filtration Coefficient

Thus far, this discussion has been primarily limited to the condition where there is no net transfer of fluid across the capillary membrane. Thus, the constant of proportionality (the capillary filtration coefficient) in Equation 8–3 (CFC) was not of concern. However, when fluid does move across the capillaries, its rate of movement not only depends on the algebraic sum of the hydrostatic and osmotic forces, but also on the area of the capillary wall available for filtration, A_c; the distance across the capillary wall, ΔX; the viscosity of the filtrate, η; and the filtration constant of the capillary membrane, k. Thus, the capillary filtration coefficient is actually a complicated factor, where

$$CFC = \frac{k \, A_c}{\eta \, \Delta X}. \qquad (8\text{–}5)$$

CFC is said to express the "hydraulic conductivity" of the capillary wall. Its units are usually expressed as ml/min per 100 gm of tissue per mm Hg. Because the thickness of the capillary wall and the viscosity of the filtrate are relatively constant under any given set of circumstances, the CFC can be used as a measure of the capillary permeability *and* the area available for diffusion. Changes in permeability alone or surface area alone cannot be distinguished by the CFC.

Filtration-Absorption Process

Thus, the net transport of fluid across the capillary wall is a function of the difference in hydrostatic and colloid osmotic pressures across the capillary wall as well as of the hydraulic conductivity of the wall itself. If we knew, or could at least qualitatively assess, the various parameters and variables occurring in Equations 8–3 and 8–5, we could then predict the magnitude and direction of the fluid flow. Fortunately, transient changes in arterial pressure produce little direct effect on capillary pressure because these changes are usually countered by the automatic adjustment of arteriolar tone by one or more of the mechanisms discussed in Chapter 7. However, prolonged reductions in arterial pressure, such as occur with a severe hemorrhage, initiate reflex constriction of the arterial vessels (in an attempt to maintain arterial pressure). The arterial vessels produce reductions in capillary hydrostatic pressure. The result is absorption of fluid from the interstitial spaces. Of course, as this absorption continues, both the interstitial hydrostatic pressure and the plasma colloid osmotic pressure fall; therefore, the process tends to be self-limiting. During hemorrhage, such absorption of fluid acts as an internal transfusion for the vascular system, increasing the mean systemic pressure (see Chap. 5) and helping to bring venous return, cardiac output, and arterial pressure to normal.

Essentially the opposite scenario occurs during right heart failure. The elevated right atrial pressure (essentially P_v in Eqs. 8–1 and 8–2) causes capillary hydrostatic pressures to rise and filtration to occur. With prolonged elevation of venous pressure (severe heart failure), the filtration exceeds the capacity of the lymphatic system to remove the excess interstitial fluid and edema occurs (see the following). In fact, systemic vascular edema is like the *sine qua non* of congestive right heart failure.

When crystalloids (isotonic solutions without proteins) are administered to patients as volume therapy (for whatever reason), the plasma colloid osmotic pressure drops. The Starling balance is thus upset and filtration occurs. If crystalloid therapy continues edema develops.

In addition to upsetting the pressure gradients, the capillary filtration coefficient can be changed, altering the magnitude of the fluid shift that occurs for any given pressure gradient. Bradykinin and histamine, which can be released locally, increase capillary permeability probably by widening the membrane pores. This contributes to inflammatory edema and to the increased interstitial protein concentration that occurs during inflammation.

In normal humans, the cardiac output approaches 7200 L per day, yet only about 20 L per day are filtered from the capillaries (excluding the kidney glomeruli). This suggests that under normal conditions our capillaries are in a near perfect Starling balance. Although these 20 L appear almost insignificant when compared to the total circulating blood volume, they are, nevertheless, extremely significant because they carry all the 100 to 200 gm of proteins that escape from the capillaries each day. The amount of protein lost from any given system depends on the size of the pores which, in turn, depends on the type of capillary, e.g., "continuous" or "fenestrated" (see Fig. 1–8). This "leaked" protein not only serves as an important determinant of the fluid transport process itself (by establishing the interstitial colloid osmotic pressure), but also serves as a substrate for various chemical and hormonal reactions and takes an important role in the body's immune system.

Formation of Edema

Edema is defined as the occurrence of an abnormal amount of interstitial fluid. The amount of edema that accumulates depends not only on the amount of fluid filtered, but also to a large extent on the pressure-volume characteristics of the interstitial spaces. Guyton and colleagues (1975) have determined experimentally the pressure-volume curve of the interstitium and have devised a model that helps us to understand these characteristics (Fig. 8–4). Small water-filled balloons (the tissue cells) are placed inside a plastic envelope (the skin), which is also filled with water (the interstitial fluid). As the interstitial fluid is sucked away, the cells, which are spheres when floating free, become packed together in a flat-sided geometric configuration. Finally, interstitial fluid is almost eliminated, except at the angles where the cells meet. Interstitial hydrostatic

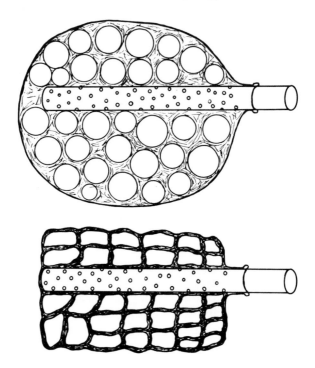

Fig. 8–4. Guyton's physical model of the tissue spaces. See text for details. (Reproduced by permission of the American Heart Association from Guyton, A.C.: Interstitial fluid pressure. II. Pressure-volume curves of interstitial space. Circ. Res., *16*:452, 1965.)

pressure is now below atmospheric pressure while cellular pressure is only slightly positive. We will discuss the mechanism that is believed to keep the interstitial spaces "dry" and the interstitial hydrostatic pressure negative in the section on lymphatics (see below).

Pressure-volume curves of the interstitial spaces of the model and of the hindlimb of the dog are shown in Figure 8–5 (Guyton, 1975). When the interstitial hydrostatic pressure, P_i (referred to as a fluid pressure in this figure) is negative, the interstitial fluid volume is minimal and changes little as P_i is raised. However, when P_i is positive, a large increase in interstitial fluid volume causes only a small increment in P_i because the cells are now separated, and P_i increases only as the tissue septa or skin is stretched. As P_i rises, the accumulation of interstitial fluid is not appreciable until P_i has risen by about 9 mm Hg. Only then is the fluid clinically identifiable as edema. If, as conventionally believed, P_i were zero, large amounts of fluid would begin to accumulate with the first rise in P_i, and edema would therefore be a frequent occurrence. With P_i normally negative, the system is protected against edema formation following mild changes in the Starling balance. This phenomenon has been referred to as the *safety factor against edema.*

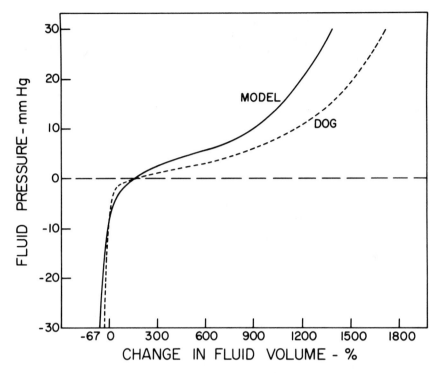

Fig. 8–5. Pressure-volume relationship of the interstitial spaces of Guyton's model and the hindlimb of a dog. (Redrawn by permission of the American Heart Association from data of Guyton, A.C.: Interstitial fluid pressure. II. Pressure-volume curves of interstitial space. Circ. Res., 16:452, 1965.)

Role of the Lymphatic System

So far, our discussion of filtration and absorption has referred several times to the amount of fluid (about 20 L) and protein (about 200 gm) that is filtered during a 24-hour period. We have ignored what happens to this fluid and protein when it leaves the circulation, saving this important topic for last. Actually, approximately 16 of the 20 L of filtered fluid are reabsorbed by the systemic capillaries, either at their downstream end or through parallel capillaries that absorb along their entire length. Consequently, only about 4 L of interstitial fluid per day return to the circulation by way of the lymph vessels under normal conditions (see Chap. 1). However, nearly all the protein must be returned to the circulation by the lymph vessels because protein cannot diffuse back into the capillaries against the large protein gradient that exists. Thus, the plasma capillary filtrate is returned to the circulation by finding its way into the terminal lymphatic capillaries and then through the lymph vessels. This movement is facilitated by compression external to these vessels (e.g., skeletal muscle contractions and arterial pulsations) and by the actual contraction of the lymph vessels themselves. The one-way valve system of the lymphatic vessels prevents backflow. If the lymphatic vessels did not continually remove filtered fluid and, especially, proteins, edema would develop rapidly because the accumulating proteins would increase the interstitial colloid osmotic pressure.

The lymphatic vessels are also believed to be responsible in large part for the development of the negative interstitial hydrostatic pressure. Although the following explanation is a hypothesis, it is consistent with the available evidence. By continually removing proteins, the lymphatic system keeps the colloid osmotic pressure low (approximately 5 mm Hg) relative to that of plasma (28 mm Hg). This allows the venous ends of the capillaries to reabsorb tremendous quantities of fluid (80 per cent or more of that which is filtered), thus creating (when the rest of the filtered fluid is removed from the interstitial space by the "lymphatic pump") the negative interstitial hydrostatic pressure (for further details of this hypothesis see Guyton et al., 1975).

Diffusion

The process of filtration-absorption is important for the net movement of water across the capillary wall; however, diffusion is the most important process by which nutrients (e.g., glucose and O_2) and waste products (e.g., lactate and CO_2) cross the capillary wall. Diffusion occurs down a concentration gradient and Fick's law of diffusion describes this process as it occurs across a capillary wall as:

$$J_s = \frac{DA}{X} (C_1 - C_2), \tag{8-6}$$

where J_s is the flux (or flow) of a given solute particle (moles/sec), D is the diffusion coefficient (cm^2/sec) measuring the "resistance to diffusion" through a capillary wall of area (cm^2), A, and thickness (cm^2), X. $C_1 - C_2$ is the concentration difference (mole/cm^3) of the solute particle across the capillary wall.

Diffusion can occur across a capillary wall by basically two routes: (1) through the entire wall or (2) through restrictive pores within the wall. Solutes that tend to pass through the entire wall are usually lipid-soluble substances, such as oxygen and carbon dioxide. Solutes that are water-soluble and cannot pass through the endothelial cell membranes diffuse through pores.

Lipid-soluble molecules, because they are not restricted by pores, move quickly across the capillary wall. Because oxygen and carbon dioxide are both lipid-soluble, the oxygen supply (and CO_2 transport out of the tissues) is not limited by the membrane. (This fact is extremely important to the discussion of pulmonary gas exchange in Chapter 14.)

Diffusion of water-soluble solutes, on the other hand, is restricted by the pores. For small molecules and ions, such as glucose, Na^+, and Cl^-, there is little restriction to diffusion because the capillary pores are so large relative to the size of the solute. However, as molecule size increases relative to pore size, diffusion becomes progressively more restrictive. As molecules approach the size of albumin, with a molecular weight of about 70,000, diffusion becomes minimal at best, thus accounting for the semipermeable nature of the capillary membrane to large plasma proteins.

Cytopempsis

The third and last major process of transcapillary exchange is known as *cytopempsis* (sometimes referred to as *micropinocytosis*). Whereas filtration and diffusion are passive processes, cytopempsis involves active transport and is a much slower process. Essentially, a small part of one side of the capillary endothelium pinches off, enclosing the substance to be transported into a small vesicle. The vesicle then moves across the capillary membrane, depositing its substance on the other side. Cytopempsis is probably of minor importance except for the transport of large lipid-insoluble molecules, such as gamma globulins.

9

THE PULMONARY CIRCULATION

MECHANICAL DETERMINANTS OF PULMONARY BLOOD FLOW

The most important determinants of pulmonary blood flow are the mechanical determinants. We will, therefore, begin this chapter with a discussion of the basic mechanical determinants of blood flow through the lung. We will then discuss how neurogenic and chemical determinants influence the pulmonary circulation. For a more comprehensive review of this most interesting of circulations, see Fishman (1986).

Starling Resistor Concept Applied to the Pulmonary Circulation

The most important feature of the pulmonary circulation is the collapsible nature of the pulmonary capillaries. Thin-walled and surrounded by alveolar pressure, these capillaries can function as Starling resistors. In fact, the pulmonary circulation is the classic example of the physiologic importance of collapsible tubes (see Chap. 4).

In Chapter 4, we summarized the pressure-flow relationships through an ideal Starling resistor by the following three succinct statements: (1) Whenever the pressure surrounding a collapsible tube is greater than the inflow pressure which, in turn, is greater than the outflow pressure, no flow occurs through the tube. (2) Whenever surrounding pressure is greater than outflow pressure, flow is proportional to the difference between inflow pressure and surrounding pressure; changes in outflow pressure have no influence on flow, (3) Whenever outflow pressure is greater than surrounding pressure, flow is proportional to the difference between inflow pressure and outflow pressure; changes in surrounding pressure have no influence on flow. The three possible conditions of a Starling resistor were depicted as hydraulic models in Figure 4–9.

Because the pulmonary capillaries are collapsible tubes, the pressure-flow relationships through pulmonary capillaries can be described by the preceding three statements when the following substitutions are made: pulmonary arterial pressure for inflow pressure, pulmonary venous pressure for outflow pressure, and alveolar pressure for surrounding pressure. Thus, (1) Whenever the alveolar pressure surrounding a pulmonary capillary is greater than the pulmonary artery pressure which, in turn, is greater than the pulmonary venous pressure, no flow occurs through the capillary. (2) Whenever alveolar pressure is greater than pulmonary venous pressure, but is less than pulmonary arterial pressure, flow is proportional to the difference between pulmonary arterial pressure and alveolar pressure; changes in pulmonary venous pressure have no influence on flow. (3) Whenever pulmonary venous pressure is greater than alveolar pressure, flow is proportional to the difference between pulmonary arterial pressure and pulmonary venous pressure; changes in alveolar pressure have no influence on flow.

Studies demonstrating that the pressure-flow relationships of the pulmonary circulation are analogous to those of a Starling resistor were done originally in dog lungs. Figure 9–1 presents the pressure-flow

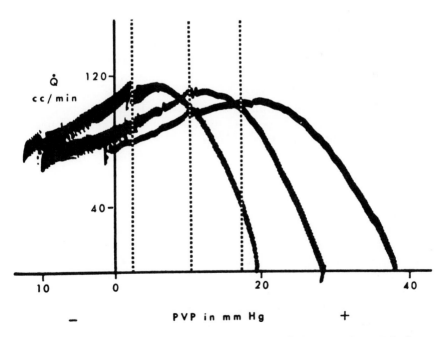

Fig. 9–1. Pressure-flow relationships of the pulmonary capillaries. (From Permutt, S., Bromberger-Barnea, B., and Bane, H.N.: Alveolar pressure, pulmonary venous pressure and the vascular waterfall. Medicina Thoracilis, *19*:239, 1962.)

relationships obtained by Permutt, Bromberger-Barnea, and Bane (1962). They cannulated the pulmonary veins of the left lower lobe of a lung in an anesthetized dog with the chest open and recorded changes in flow as the venous pressure was slowly changed. Venous return from the lobe is plotted on the ordinate, and pulmonary venous pressure is plotted on the abscissa. Three curves are shown. The left-hand curve was obtained at an alveolar pressure of 3 mm Hg and a pulmonary artery pressure of 19 mm Hg. The middle curve was obtained at an alveolar pressure of 10 mm Hg and a pulmonary artery pressure of 29 mm Hg. The right-hand curve was obtained at an alveolar pressure of 18 mm Hg and a pulmonary artery pressure of 38 mm Hg. In general, flow increased as outflow pressure (pulmonary venous pressure) was lowered and inflow pressure (pulmonary arterial pressure) was kept constant until outflow pressure was lowered below the pressure surrounding the pulmonary capillaries (alveolar pressure). As outflow pressure was lowered further, flow decreased slightly, but this decrease is not the significant feature of these curves. These curves have the same general shape as the curve presented in Figure 4–10, which considered a theoretic Starling resistor. They are also similar to a systemic venous return curve in which the inflection can be accounted for in terms of veins collapsing as they enter the chest.

Evidence that the Starling resistor concept can be used to interpret the pressure-flow relationships of the pulmonary circulation in normal humans has been provided by West and Dollery (1965). These investigators used radioactive isotopes to measure ventilation and blood flow in different regions from top to bottom of the upright human lung. Both pulmonary arterial and venous pressures increase from superior to dependent regions of the lung because of the hydrostatic effect resulting from gravity.* In a typical human lung 30 cm in height, the pulmonary artery pressure may be 20 cm H_2O and the pulmonary venous pressure may be 10 cm H_2O at the most dependent portion of the lung (the diaphragmatic surface). Thus, 10 cm from the bottom of the lung the pulmonary venous pressure falls to atmospheric pressure; 20 cm from the bottom of the lung, the pulmonary artery pressure falls to atmospheric pressure. The alveolar pressure, however, remains essentially constant throughout the lung.

This distribution of pressures results in the distribution of blood flow within the lungs to essentially three major zones, depending on the magnitudes of the pressures. In the upper third of the lung (zone I),

---

*The increase in blood pressure caused by gravity is equal to ρgh, where ρ is density of blood (1.05 gm/cm^3), g is gravity acceleration constant (980 cm/sec^2), and h is vertical distance down the lung. Because ρ and g are constants and the density of blood is approximately that of water, the blood pressure increases approximately 1 cm H_2O for each cm distance moved down the lung.

the alveolar pressure is greater than or equal to pulmonary artery pressure, and there is no flow. In the middle zone (zone II, the Starling resistor zone), pulmonary arterial pressure is greater than alveolar pressure, which is greater than pulmonary venous pressure. In zone II, flow through the pulmonary capillaries is proportional to the difference between pulmonary arterial and alveolar pressure. In zone III, the dependent region, pulmonary arterial pressure is greater than pulmonary venous pressure, which is also greater than alveolar pressure. Alveolar pressure has no influence on flow. Thus, three major blood flow zones correspond roughly to the three possible pressure-flow conditions of a collapsible tube, as previously discussed. Note that in the normal upright human lung there is no zone I, although this condition can develop if pulmonary arterial pressure falls or alveolar pressure rises. Figure 9–2 is a schematic drawing of the three zones of West; compare each zone with its hydrodynamic equivalent depicted in Figure 4–9.

Blood flow increases toward the dependent regions of both zones II and III (see Fig. 9–2). The mechanism for this increase is currently not completely understood. A major cause for the increase in blood flow down zone II must be related to the increase in the pressure gradient for flow toward the dependent regions of zone II. The pressure gradient for flow in zone II is the pulmonary arterial pressure minus the alveolar

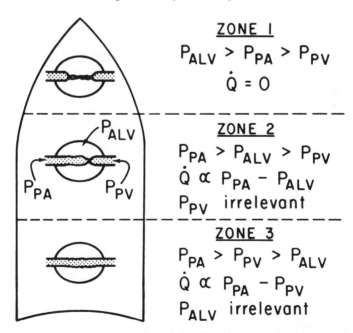

ZONE I

$$P_{ALV} > P_{PA} > P_{PV}$$

$$\dot{Q} = 0$$

ZONE 2

$$P_{PA} > P_{ALV} > P_{PV}$$

$$\dot{Q} \propto P_{PA} - P_{ALV}$$

$$P_{PV} \text{ irrelevant}$$

ZONE 3

$$P_{PA} > P_{PV} > P_{ALV}$$

$$\dot{Q} \propto P_{PA} - P_{PV}$$

$$P_{ALV} \text{ irrelevant}$$

Fig. 9–2. Schematic drawing of the three zones of West. P_{pa} = pulmonary arterial pressure; P_{ALV} = alveolar pressure; P_{pv} = pulmonary venous pressure; and $\dot{Q}$ = regional pulmonary blood flow. (Reproduced by permission from Green, J.F.: The pulmonary circulation. *In* The Peripheral Circulations. Edited by R. Zelis. New York, Grune & Stratton, 1975.)

pressure. Alveolar pressure is constant throughout the zone, but pulmonary arterial pressure increases toward the dependent regions of the lung because of the hydrostatic effects. Thus, the pressure gradient increases down zone II.

This mechanism cannot account for the increase in blood flow down zone III. The pressure gradient for flow in this zone is the pulmonary arterial pressure minus the pulmonary venous pressure, and both pulmonary arterial and venous pressures increase by the same amount toward the dependent regions of zone III (1 cm H_2O per cm distance down the lung). Thus, the pressure gradient ($P_{PA} - P_{PV}$) remains constant in zone III. The increase in blood flow toward the dependent regions of zone III is attributed to a constantly decreasing pulmonary vascular resistance. The mechanism for this decrease in resistance is still unsettled. Two hypotheses have been proposed (Fig. 9–3): distension of existing flow channels (West, 1965) and recruitment of additional channels (Maseri, et al., 1972).

The *distension hypothesis* uses the fact that, although the pressure gradient does not change in zone III, the transmural pressure increases toward the dependent regions of this zone. An increase in transmural

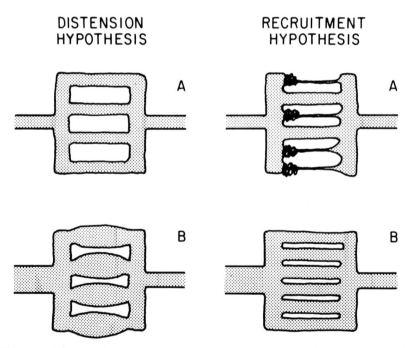

DISTENSION HYPOTHESIS   **RECRUITMENT HYPOTHESIS**

Fig. 9–3. Schematic drawing representing the two proposed mechanisms for the decreasing vascular resistance down zone III. *A:* A portion of the pulmonary vasculature toward the top of zone III. *B:* A portion of the pulmonary vasculature toward the dependent region of zone III. (Reproduced by permission from Green, J.F.: The pulmonary circulation. *In* The Peripheral Circulations. Edited by R. Zelis. New York, Grune & Stratton, 1975.)

pressure should cause an increase in the radius of the pulmonary capillaries, thereby decreasing their resistance. The *recruitment hypothesis* suggests that there is a spectrum of critical opening pressures within the pulmonary vasculature and implies that the pulmonary arterial pressure must rise above the opening pressure of an individual vessel to allow its perfusion. The pulmonary artery pressure is higher at the more dependent regions of the lung; therefore, a greater number of vessels are perfused. This reduces the pulmonary vascular resistance. Some evidence (Glazier, et al., 1969) suggests that recruitment predominantly occurs when pulmonary venous pressure is less than alveolar pressure, and distension predominantly occurs when pulmonary venous pressure is greater than alveolar pressure. Thus, recruitment and the increasing pressure gradient may account for the increase in blood flow down zone II, whereas distension may account for the increase in blood flow down zone III. Undoubtedly, we have not heard the last about why blood flow increases toward the dependent regions of the lung.

Pulmonary Vascular Resistance

The resistance of the pulmonary vasculature is conventionally calculated as the difference between pulmonary arterial pressure and left atrial pressure divided by the cardiac output. This calculation implicitly assumes that left atrial pressure is the effective back pressure for blood flow through the lungs. With the recognition that, under zone II conditions, alveolar pressure, and not pulmonary venous pressure, is the back pressure, some investigators have questioned the meaning of pulmonary vascular resistance as conventionally calculated (Permutt, et al., 1962). An increase in the ratio of driving pressure to flow merely indicates that something has happened within the vascular bed somewhere between the points where the pressures were measured to cause an increase in the amount of potential energy dissipated. Given laminar flow and constant blood viscosity and vessel lengths, a change in pulmonary vascular resistance, calculated using left atrial pressure as back pressure, can only be interpreted as evidence of a change in total vascular cross-section somewhere in the pulmonary vascular bed. Poiseuille's law (see App. 2) implies this change, but the cause and site of the change cannot be determined from such a measurement (Milnor, 1972). However, under zone II conditions (see Fig. 9–2), inferences can be drawn concerning arterial diameter and some undetermined proximal part of the capillary bed if alveolar pressure is substituted for left atrial pressure in the resistance formula. Thus, to interpret measurements of pulmonary vascular resistance correctly, one must know the zonal conditions under which the measurements were made and must also use the appropriate back pressure in the resistance formula.

Effect of Lung Inflation on Pulmonary Pressure-Flow Relationships

Lung inflation affects the pressure-flow relationships of the pulmonary vasculature both directly, by compressing the small vessels, and indirectly, through the effect of pleural pressure on venous return and pulmonary blood flow. We shall first consider the direct effect of lung inflation per se by considering the pulmonary blood flow constant.

An increase in lung volume necessitates an increase in transpulmonary pressure (the difference between alveolar pressure and pleural pressure, see Chap. 13). This increase may be accomplished by either a decrease in pleural pressure relative to atmospheric pressure (spontaneous respiration) or an increase in alveolar pressure relative to atmospheric pressure (positive pressure respiration). Left atrial pressure relative to pleural pressure tends to remain constant at constant cardiac output (see Chap. 3). Thus, an increase in lung volume, which necessitates an increase in alveolar pressure relative to pleural pressure, results in an increase in alveolar pressure relative to left atrial pressure. This increase occurs regardless of whether the lung is inflated by spontaneous respiration or by positive pressure ventilation. Lung inflation, therefore, causes compression of the small alveolar vessels (those directly exposed to alveolar pressure). The end result is an increase in that portion of the lung in zone II and an increase in the resistance of flow in all vessels exposed to alveolar pressure.

Pulmonary vascular resistance increases not only at high states of lung inflation, but also at low levels of inflation (Howell, et al., 1961; Hughes, et al., 1968). Consequently, the curve of pulmonary vascular resistance versus lung inflation is U-shaped. The high vascular resistance at low states of lung inflation is probably caused by a narrowing of extra-alveolar vessels (those arteries and veins that are not directly exposed to alveolar pressure and that run through the lung parenchyma). The caliber of extra-alveolar vessels is affected by lung volume; decreasing lung volume decreases the radius of extra-alveolar vessels, thereby increasing the pulmonary vascular resistance.

The pulmonary vasculature is also influenced by lung inflation's effect on venous return. During a spontaneous respiration, right atrial pressure falls with pleural pressure. The fall in right atrial pressure increases venous return which, when passed to the lungs, causes a fall in pulmonary vascular resistance by one of the possible mechanisms previously discussed. With positive pressure ventilation, right atrial pressure rises, venous return falls, and pulmonary vascular resistances increase. Thus, the rise in pulmonary vascular resistance by compression of the small alveolar vessels with spontaneous inspiration tends to be negated by the increases in venous return. However, with positive pressure ventilation, resistance tends to be accentuated by the fall in venous return. Overdistension of the lungs during positive pressure breathing therefore results in an increase in the amount of work required from the right ventricle to pump the same amount of blood. Thus, this overdistension can be associated with harmful consequences, particularly for patients with pre-existing impairment of right ventricular function.

Pulmonary Venous Return

In Chapter 5, the pressure-flow relationship through the systemic venous system was described by the following expression:

$$\dot{Q}_s = \frac{P_{MS} - P_{RA}}{R_{VS}}, \qquad (5\text{-}2)$$

where $\dot{Q}_s$ is systemic venous return, P_{MS} is mean systemic pressure (pressure within the compliant area of the systemic circulation), P_{RA} is right atrial pressure, and R_{VS} is resistance of the veins between the compliant areas and the right atrium, i.e., the systemic venous resistance. This pressure-flow relationship is the inevitable consequence of the structure of the systemic venous system in which the major compliant areas are upstream from the small but significant resistance to venous return. Evidence also suggests that the same condition exists in the pulmonary circulation. Engelberg and Du Bois (1959) have shown that approximately 45 per cent of the total pulmonary vascular compliance is located at the level of the small pulmonary veins, whereas the compliance of the large pulmonary veins accounts for only 15 percent of the distribution of the total pulmonary vascular compliance. The remaining compliance is divided about equally among large arteries, small arteries, and capillaries. This division allows us to consider pulmonary venous return ($\dot{Q}_p$) with the aid of the same kind of conceptual model used with systemic venous return:

$$\dot{Q}_p = \frac{P_{MP} - P_{LA}}{R_{VP}}, \qquad (9\text{-}1)$$

where P_{MP} is mean pulmonary pressure (pressure within the compliant areas of the pulmonary circulation), P_{LA} is left atrial pressure, and R_{VP} is the resistance of the veins between the compliant areas of the pulmonary vascular bed and the left atrium, i.e., the pulmonary venous resistance.

The important parameters for the systemic and pulmonary venous systems are compared in Table 9–1. The gross disparity between the compliances is immediately apparent. The systemic compliance is approximately 12 times greater than the pulmonary compliance. The significance of this difference was discussed briefly in Chapter 4; the pulmonary vessels cannot be a significant vascular reservoir. The next most obvious dissimilarity between the greater and lesser circulations is the venous resistances. The pulmonary venous resistance is only one seventh that of the systemic venous resistance, which suggests (as is the

Table 9–1. Comparison of the Circulatory Parameters for the Systemic and Pulmonary Vascular Beds*

C_s	C_p	P_{ms}	P_{mp}	P_{ra}	P_{la}	R_{vs}	R_{vp}	$\dot{Q}_s$	$\dot{Q}_p$
(ml·mm Hg^{-1}·kg^{-1})		(mm Mg)				(mm Hg·L^{-1}·min)		(L/min)	
2.6	0.2	7.0	5.0	0	4.0	4.4	0.6	1.6	1.6

*Parameters listed are mean values.

case) a small pressure drop (1 mm Hg) between the primary capacitance areas, immediately downstream from the capillaries and the left atrium.

NEUROGENIC DETERMINANTS OF PULMONARY BLOOD FLOW

The pulmonary vasculature is innervated with both sympathetic adrenergic vasoconstrictor fibers from the stellate ganglion and parasympathetic cholinergic vasodilator fibers from the vagus nerve. Alpha-adrenergic receptors also appear present. Yet, it has been difficult to unequivocally demonstrate the extent to which vasomotor control operates in vivo. This hardship stems partially from the difficulty of excluding the bronchial circulation, which provides the arterial blood supply to the lung tissue itself, from experimental preparations. But, more importantly, demonstrating neurogenic control has been difficult because, under normal conditions, this control is probably slight. Even in experiments during which the bronchial circulation was controlled, maximum stimulation of the stellate ganglion increased pulmonary vascular resistance by no more than 30 percent (Daly and Hebb, 1967). Weak responses are also induced in the pulmonary vasculature by both baroreceptor and chemoreceptor stimulation. Thus, even though the pulmonary vessels are subjected to autonomic control, the control apparently is normally minimal.

From the neurogenic point of view, the pulmonary circulation is probably more important for the origination of controlling impulses. In the walls of the pulmonary trunk and in the walls of both the right and left pulmonary arteries are mechanoreceptors innervated from the vagus nerve. When pulmonary artery pressure rises, these receptors can reflexly initiate bradycardia and hypotension in a similar manner to the carotid and aortic mechanoreceptors (Coleridge and Kidd, 1960).

LOCAL DETERMINANTS OF PULMONARY BLOOD FLOW

The pulmonary vessels apparently have little or no resting basal tone; it is nearly impossible to *reduce* pulmonary vascular resistance under normal conditions. The pulmonary vessels are unique in their response to local chemical and blood-borne humoral agents because, in nearly every case, their response is opposite that of the systemic vasculature.

An entire series of substances that produces vasodilation in the systemic circulation also produces pulmonary vasoconstriction. These include norepinephrine, serotonin, histamine, hypercapnia, acidosis, and hypoxia. Unfortunately, the mechanisms for these responses are not adequately understood.

By far, the most important of these agents are hypoxia and hypercapnia because their responses represent an important mechanism for matching regional pulmonary blood flow to regional changes in ventilation. If, for example, a lobe of lung is underventilated, the alveolar oxygen tension falls and the carbon dioxide tension rises, bringing about a local increase in pulmonary vascular resistance. This rise in pulmonary vascular resistance shunts flow away from the region of poor ventilation to other areas more adequately ventilated. Similarly, if a lobe becomes underperfused, alveolar hypocapnia occurs. Low carbon dioxide tension increases bronchial smooth muscle tone. The end result is a decrease in ventilation that readjusts the ventilation-perfusion relationship to a more appropriate level (see Chap. 14).

OTHER REGIONAL CIRCULATIONS

CORONARY CIRCULATION

Distribution of Coronary Blood Flow

The blood supply to the myocardium arises from the right and left coronary arteries, which begin at the root of the aorta immediately behind the cusps of the aortic valve. The vascular channels in the heart are numerous and complex, and the normal distribution of blood flow within the coronary vessels can vary greatly. Usually, the left coronary artery supplies most of the left ventricle, whereas the right coronary artery supplies most of the right ventricle and some of the left. In about 50 percent of all humans, blood flow through the right coronary artery exceeds that through the left; however, this flow pattern is reversed in about 20 percent of all individuals. In the remaining 30 percent of all humans, blood flow is about equal between right and left coronaries. Blood is returned from the coronary arteries through both a superficial and a deep system of veins. The main source of venous drainage from the subepicardial (superficial) veins is the coronary veins that drain into the right atrium through the *coronary sinus.* Another system of superficial coronary veins, the *anterior cardiac veins,* drains directly into the right atrium. Blood drains from the deep aspects of the myocardium through (1) the *thebesian veins* directly into the heart chambers; (2) the *arterioluminal vessels,* which connect small coronary arterial branches directly to the cardiac chambers; and (3) the *arteriosinusoidal vessels,* which originate as arterioles and rapidly lose their arterial structure as they divide into anastomosing sinuses before draining into the cardiac chambers. The

complexity of the coronary circulation is demonstrated by flow measurements in the veins that have revealed that, although nearly all the
coronary sinus outflow comes from the left coronary artery, this outflow
constitutes only about 75 percent of the left coronary artery inflow. The
remaining fraction of the left coronary artery inflow and the right coronary artery inflow drains through the anterior cardiac veins and the
other drainage systems. The exact distribution is, as one might imagine,
difficult to determine.

Mechanical Determinants of Coronary Blood Flow

The most important determinant of coronary blood flow is aortic pressure. Changes in aortic pressure (increased or decreased) produce parallel changes in coronary blood flow, whose magnitude is proportional
to the change in aortic pressure. Another important physical determinant
of *mean* coronary blood flow is the direct external compression of the
coronary vessels produced by the contracting myocardium. During systole, the contracting heart muscle actually squeezes the coronary vessels
sufficiently to stop briefly or to even reverse the direction of blood flow.
Because of this rhythmic systolic compression and varying aortic blood
pressure (from systolic to diastolic), the coronary blood flow is markedly
phasic. The maximum flow occurs early in diastole when the compression has subsided and the aortic pressure is greatest (see Fig. 3–13). As
diastole progresses, coronary flow decreases as aortic pressure falls.

The external compression to which the coronary vessels are subjected
makes separating the effects of other determinants of coronary blood
flow difficult. For instance, an increase in heart rate increases the length
of time spent in systole (and subjected to external compression) thereby
decreasing coronary blood flow; however, this decrease in blood flow
tends to be counteracted by the release of vasodilator metabolites, which
accumulate as a result of increased activity of the myocadium.

Neurohumoral Determinants of Coronary Blood Flow

The coronary vasculature is innervated with sympathetic adrenergic
and parasympathetic cholinergic (vagal) fibers, but not with sympathetic
cholinergic fibers. Stimulation of the cardiac sympathetic fibers increases
coronary blood flow; however, because stimulation of these nerves also
increases myocardial metabolism, the increase in blood flow results
chiefly from the accumulation of metabolic dilators. This possibility was
suggested in studies where the increase in myocardial activity was experimentally prevented by inducing fibrillation in the isolated perfused
heart and by using Practolol* to block the metabolic effects in the intact

---

*A beta-adrenergic blocking agent that selectively blocks the excitatory beta receptors of
the myocardium, but does not block the inhibitory beta receptors in the coronary vessels
(see Chap. 7).

beating heart. In these studies (Mark and Abboud, 1975), sympathetic nerve stimulation produced direct constrictor responses in coronary vessels. This constriction was reduced by phentolamine, an alpha-adrenergic blocking agent, suggesting that stimulation of the cardiac sympathetic nerve elicits the response of alpha-adrenergic receptors in the coronary vasculature.

Beta-adrenergic receptors are also present in the coronary vasculature; they can be demonstrated by the fact that coronary vasodilation is elicited by isoproterenol, a beta-adrenergic stimulator. However, these receptors apparently do not play a significant role in the response of the coronary vessels to sympathetic nerve stimulation because blocking these receptors with propranolol does not augment the constrictor response that occurs with sympathetic nerve stimulation in the absence of metabolic changes.

Stimulation of the vagus nerve in the beating heart produces an increase in coronary blood flow (Feigl, 1969). These responses were blocked by atropine, a cholinergic blocking agent. Thus, parasympathetic cholinergic nerves are also active in the coronary vessels.

Both carotid chemoreceptor and baroreceptor reflexes effectively alter coronary blood flow. Stimulation of the carotid chemoreceptors with such agents as nicotine or cyanide produces coronary vasodilation that is blocked by atropine and vagotomy, thereby suggesting that this coronary vasodilation results from direct neurogenic influences mediated through the vagus nerve (Hackett, et al., 1972). Two types of responses have been elicited from the carotid baroreceptors. When direct carotid sinus hypotension occurs, reflex coronary vasodilation occurs presumably by the indirect effects of metabolites because carotid sinus hypotension also activates adrenergic-constrictor nerves to the coronary vessels (Feigl, 1968). When the carotid sinus nerve is directly stimulated (a situation analogous to carotid sinus hypertension), a decrease in mean arterial blood pressure occurs. However, the coronary blood flow does not fall proportionately, indicating reflex vasodilation that must be of direct neurogenic origin because slowing of the heart also occurs. Under these conditions, metabolic vasodilation would not be expected. This decrease in coronary resistance is believed to be the result of withdrawal of adrenergic constrictor tone and stimulation of vagal dilator fibers (Hackett, et al., 1972). Although questions of coronary vascular control are far from answered, these observations suggest that neurogenic control of coronary vessels may predominate over metabolic influences in the reflex control of coronary vessels (Mark and Abboud, 1975; Berne, 1975). However, metabolites are still believed to be the most important determinants of coronary blood flow under normal nonreflex conditions.

Metabolic Determinants of Coronary Blood Flow

By far the most important determinant of coronary blood flow (secondary to aortic pressure) is the metabolic activity of the heart itself.

This is not surprising when we realize that, under resting conditions, the oxygen content of coronary sinus blood flow is only about 5 vol % (maximum content is about 20 vol %). Thus, little reserve oxygen is available for extraction by the myocardium; the heart can get more oxygen only by increasing its blood flow. A close correlation between myocardial oxygen consumption and coronary blood flow exists in a number of situations. By and large, whenever the amount of work done by the heart muscle increases, which requires an increase in the oxygen consumption (e.g., an increase in heart rate, an elevation of aortic blood pressure, or aortic valve stenosis), coronary blood flow also increases. This relationship is true despite the increase in extravascular compression. The reverse occurs when the work load of the heart decreases. This relationship between coronary blood flow and oxygen requirement is found in the denervated heart, the completely isolated heart, and in the fibrillating heart in addition to its normal occurrence in the innervated beating heart. Thus, this relationship appears to be a generalized phenomenon of the myocardium.

The actual mechanism for the metabolic control of coronary blood flow has been unsettled since the relationship was first observed in 1879 (Roy and Brown). Numerous metabolic agents have been suggested as the mediator of this vasodilation. These agents include hypoxia (low partial pressure of oxygen), carbon dioxide, lactic acid, hydrogen ions, potassium ions, increased osmolarity, histamine, and adenosine. Any one of these agents alone or in combination with any other agent may eventually prove to account for the metabolic determinants of coronary blood flow. Whatever the actual mechanism, the rate of myocardial metabolism is undoubtedly the most important determinant of coronary blood flow.

SKELETAL MUSCLE CIRCULATION

Neurohumoral Determinants of Skeletal Muscle Blood Flow

The blood vessels of skeletal muscles are innervated by sympathetic adrenergic vasoconstrictor fibers, and in certain species (but not primates), by sympathetic cholinergic vasodilator fibers. Both sympathetic nerve stimulation and infusion of exogenous norepinephrine cause constriction of the arterial resistance vessels of skeletal muscles. Because this response can be blocked by an alpha-adrenergic blocking agent, such as *phenoxybenzamine hydrochloride* or *phentolamine*, it is believed to be mediated through alpha-adrenergic receptors. Beta-adrenergic receptors are also found in skeletal muscle vessels, but probably respond only to circulating humoral agents. Isoproterenol infusion produces a marked vasodilation of skeletal muscle resistance vessels. This response can be prevented with the beta-adrenergic blocking agent propranolol (Mellander and Johansson, 1968; Shepherd and Vanhoutte, 1975).

Although the arterial resistance vessels of skeletal muscles normally possess a high degree of basal tone (see Chap. 7), an additional amount of resting tone can be attributed to a continuous low frequency discharge of the sympathetic vasoconstrictor fibers. Elimination of this resting neurogenic tone approximately doubles skeletal muscle blood flow in humans.* In animal experiments, stimulation of the sympathetic nerves at frequencies of about 2 impulses per second causes 75 percent of the response (decrease in flow) obtained at frequencies 5 to 10 times as great. During maximal vasodilation, such as can occur during exercise, skeletal muscle blood flow can increase to 70 ml/min per 100 gm tissue! These observations suggest that the resting tone in skeletal muscles is high, that the resting tone is determined predominantly by elements other than neurogenic factors, and that sympathetic adrenergic nerves control a small fraction of the overall maximal flow capacity in skeletal muscles.

In certain species, including dog, cat, and rabbit (but not human), stimulation of the sympathetic nerves after the alpha receptors have been blocked produces a vasodilation that can be prevented with atropine. These sympathetic cholinergic dilator fibers begin in the hypothalamus and pass down the spinal cord, bypassing the vasoactive areas in the medulla. They apparently innervate only the precapillary resistance vessels of skeletal muscles and are usually activated in anticipation of exercise. Although the cholinergic fibers increase blood flow to skeletal muscles, they apparently do not recruit additional capillary beds; therefore, these fibers are said to increase flow through *thoroughfare* or *nonnutrient* channels. Thus, the sympathetic cholinergic fibers may serve to redistribute cardiac output preferentially to skeletal muscles during exercise. Once contraction starts, metabolic vasodilation of the precapillary sphincters increases the flow to nutritional areas. In humans, a similar response is believed to occur by withdrawal of sympathetic constrictor tone to the precapillary resistance vessels.

The tonic activity of the sympathetic nerves to skeletal muscles is greatly influenced by reflexes from the baroreceptors and chemoreceptors. Thus, an increase in carotid sinus pressure results in dilation of the skeletal muscle vasculature and in constriction when carotid sinus pressure falls. Because about 40 percent of the mass of the entire body is skeletal muscle, this tissue has a profound effect in controlling arterial blood pressure.

Local Determinants of Skeletal Muscle Blood Flow

Based on the general principles discussed in Chapter 7, one should not be surprised to find that metabolic factors influence skeletal muscle

---

*In resting humans, skeletal muscle blood flow is about 5 ml/min per 100 gm tissue.

blood flow. First, there is a considerable degree of basal vascular tone in the arterial vessels of skeletal muscles even after all neurogenic influences have been eliminated. Second, skeletal muscle is usually a metabolically active tissue. Despite these factors, separating metabolic factors from myogenic factors is difficult. This problem is best illustrated by the phenomenon of *reactive hyperemia*. If we were to stop arterial inflow to a skeletal muscle by clamping an inflow artery for a few moments, we would find, upon unclamping the artery, that flow would be considerably augmented over what it had been before the clamp was initiated. Flow would then slowly return to normal. Considering that most, if not all, of the basal tone in skeletal muscle is produced by a myogenic-like response (Chap. 7), the drop in arterial pressure that occurs during the stop-flow period may remove the facilitation of myogenic tone in the precapillary resistance vessels, thus allowing for greater flow immediately after pressure is restored. However, more happens during the stop-flow period; tissue oxygen concentration is also reduced and vasodilator metabolites are accumulated. Thus, both mechanical and chemical influences contribute to this response. With prolonged periods of occlusion, the recovery time is lengthened considerably, suggesting that the myogenic mechanism becomes involved when abrupt changes in blood pressure occur. However, metabolic mechanisms also contribute significantly to reactive hyperemia as well as to the local control of skeletal muscle blood flow in general. Numerous metabolic agents have been suggested as the mediator of this vasodilation. These agents have also been attributed to producing metabolic vasodilation in the coronary vasculature. Like the coronary vasculature, no single metabolite has been identified as the most important causative agent.

CEREBRAL CIRCULATION

The blood flow to the brain is the best regulated. In the human, the cerebral blood flow is maintained within a narrow range of around 55 ml/min per 100 gm of brain tissue. The brain is also the organ that can least tolerate hypoxia. Interruption of cerebral blood flow for as little as 5 seconds leads to blackout (loss of consciousness). No one knows this better than the aviator subjected to acceleration stress.

The cerebral vessels are innervated from the cervical sympathetic nerves; however, the exact role played by these sympathetic nerves is currently a controversial question. The evidence is conflicting, but most physiologists feel that sympathetic neurogenic control of cerebral blood flow is probably minimal, at best, and that metabolic factors play the major role in the control of cerebral blood flow (Scheinberg, 1975).

Unlike other tissue where metabolic control of blood flow is important, the cerebral vasculature is influenced strongly by a single metabolite—carbon dioxide. Increases in the arterial CO_2 tension produce profound cerebral vasodilation, and decreases in arterial CO_2 tension produce the opposite effect, profoundly. Carbon dioxide is not the only metabolite that influences cerebral blood flow, but it appears to be the most important.

SPLANCHNIC CIRCULATION

The splanchnic circulation can be defined as all vascular beds that drain through the hepatic veins. Organs included in the splanchnic circulation are the liver, pancreas, spleen, and gastrointestinal tract. We treat these organis together because their anatomic arrangement allows them to function hemodynamically as a single vascular channel. Furthermore, when the venous compliance of this channel (the splanchnic circulation) is measured and compared with that of the rest of the body, we find that approximately one half or more of the venous compliance of the entire systemic circulation is located in the splanchnic circulation (Green, 1977). Thus, the splanchnic circulation serves as the most important site of the vascular reservoir and, as such, as a major influence on venous return (see Chap. 5).

Neurohumoral Determinants of Splanchnic Blood Flow

The splanchnic circulation is richly supplied with sympathetic vasoconstrictor nerves from the *splanchnic nerve;* however, sympathetic cholinergic vasodilator innervation of the splanchnic circulation is not apparent. Electrical stimulation of the splanchnic nerves causes both a marked decrease in splanchnic blood flow as splanchnic arterial resistance* rises and large decreases in splanchnic blood volume (Rowell, 1975). In the dog, about 48 percent of the total splanchnic blood volume can be expelled by stimulating the splanchnic nerves at relatively low frequencies (2 cps). At higher stimulation frequencies (15 cps), as much as 90 percent of the dog's splanchnic blood volume can be expelled. The main effect of splanchnic sympathetic stimulation on the rest of the circulation is thus a redistribution of blood volume to other areas. This redistribution increases venous return, cardiac output, and arterial blood pressure (Green, 1979).

The splanchnic circulation participates in both baroreceptor and chemoreceptor reflexes. A fall in carotid sinus pressure results in increased vasoconstrictor nerve activity, and a rise in carotid sinus pressure has the opposite effect. Stimulation of the chemoreceptors, such as occurs with hypoxia, also leads to vasoconstriction. Considering the important

---

*The splanchnic arterial resistance is a conceptual resistance determined by lumping together all the arterial inflow resistance from all the various splanchnic organs. The splanchnic venous resistance is more easily identified both anatomically and functionally as the common venous outflow path of the splanchnic circulation, i.e., the hepatic veins.

effect of the splanchnic circulation on venous return, it must be considered a major "target" area for the reflex control of circulatory function.

The splanchnic vasculature has both alpha- and beta-adrenergic receptors. Both epinephrine and norepinephrine can cause marked changes in splanchnic blood flow. In humans, physiologic concentrations of epinephrine cause splanchnic vasodilation whereas physiologic concentrations of norepinephrine cause vasoconstriction (Rowell, 1975).

For years, beta-adrenergic stimulation with isoproterenol was recognized for its ability to increase venous return in the dog despite its vasodilation effect. The actual mechanism remained in question, however, until isoproterenol was found to dilate the hepatic outflow vessels, thereby reducing splanchnic venous resistance and increasing venous return from the splanchnic circulation (Green, 1977).

Local Determinants of Splanchnic Blood Flow

Following section of the splanchnic nerves, a high degree of basal tone remains in the arterial vessels of the intestinal and hepatic regions of the splanchnic circulation, thereby suggesting a degree of local regulation. An interesting phenomenon in the cat further points to local mechanisms operating in the splanchnic circulation. Stimulation of the splanchnic nerves for several consecutive minutes initially reduces blood flow, but blood flow then returns to control levels. This phenomenon, known as *autoregulatory escape*, is associated with a redistribution of intestinal blood flow from the outer mucosal region to the submucosa and suggests a local action of vasodilator metabolites that overrides the neural vasoconstriction.

CUTANEOUS CIRCULATION

The blood flow to the skin usually far exceeds its metabolic needs because the primary function of the cutaneous circulation is temperature regulation. Thus, the skin can accommodate a wide range of blood flows depending on the body's need to lose or to conserve heat. The blood flow to the skin must be integrated with other bodily functions; therefore, it is primarily under the control of nervous elements and, in large part, controlled directly from a temperature-regulating center in the anterior hypothalamus.

The arteries carrying blood to the skin pass through the underlying muscles and are accompanied by the veins that drain the skin (called *venae comitantes arteriae femoralis*). Thus, *countercurrent heat* exchange is possible. For instance, under cold conditions, blood returning from the skin can be warmed by the deep, warmer blood going to the skin.

Once blood reaches the skin it can return by two alternative routes. First, it may pass through a superficial network of venules that have thin walls and through which heat can be lost. Second, it may pass through communicating veins directly to the deep veins where countercurrent heat exchange can occur. In certain areas of the body, most notably in the skin of the fingertips, toes, hands, and feet, *arteriovenous anastomoses* can shunt blood directly to the superficial venous networks.

Nervous control of the skin vasculature is mediated almost exclusively through the sympathetic vasoconstrictor system. There is no evidence for parasympathetic vasodilator fibers; however, the skin (at least the sweat glands of the skin) is innervated with sympathetic cholinergic fibers which, under certain circumstances, can cause indirect vasodilation (see Chap. 7). The arteriovenous anastomoses are heavily innervated with sympathetic vasoconstrictor fibers and become maximally dilated when these fibers are cut and maximally constricted when these nerves are stimulated (to the point where their lumens close). The arteriovenous anastomosis has no nonneurogenic basal tone and is sensitive to vasoconstrictor agents. The rest of the skin arterial vessels exhibit some degree of nonneurogenic basal tone, but neurogenic factors are still more important in regulating flow in these vessels.

When exposed to cold, the cutaneous vessels constrict, thereby diverting blood flow away from the body's surface and conserving heat. Whenever the body temperature is elevated, such as by exposure to a warm environment or by internal increases in metabolism (e.g., during exercise), the cutaneous vessels, especially the arteriovenous anastomoses, dilate and consequently divert blood to the superficial venous plexus where heat is lost.

In addition to the basic heat-regulating mechanism just described, there are a few interesting phenomena of the skin vasculature. When the hand is immersed in a bucket of ice, vasoconstriction and pain develop. If the cold exposure is prolonged, the skin begins to dilate and becomes red. With continued exposure, periods of alternating vasoconstriction followed by vasodilation occur. The cause of this *cold-induced vasodilation* is unknown, but may be the result of direct inhibition of the vascular smooth muscle. The pink faces and hands of snow skiers are an example of cold-induced vasodilation.

Other examples of cutaneous vasoconstriction phenomena are the *white reaction* and *triple response* of *Lewis* (1930). If one lightly strokes the skin with a thin, blunted object, a pallored appearance develops along the line of stroking after a latent period of about 20 seconds. This color change is believed to be the result of localized venoconstriction. It disappears in about 5 minutes. If the blunted instrument is drawn more forcefully across the skin, a red line soon appears. This *red reaction* is probably caused by dilation of the cutaneous venules. If the stimulus is repeated still more forcefully, a *red flare* develops for some distance around the line of stroking. This flare is most likely caused by dilation of cutaneous arterioles.* and venules. Finally, when the stimulus is still

---

*This dilation is attributed to an *axon reflex* that originates at the site of injury. A nerve impulse travels up the sensory nerves and then down their branching collaterals, thereby evoking dilation of the arterioles.

more intense, the skin along the line of stimulation becomes blanched and a *wheal* is raised. This swelling is the result of transudation of fluid from the injured vessels. The triple response, especially the wheal, has been attributed to the release of histamine from the injured cells, but this mechanism is not certain (Hsieh, 1975).

11

THE BLOOD

As was stated in Chapter 1, the primary function of the cardiovascular system is to maintain a constant internal environment for the body. To do so, the circulation participates in the transport of nutrients and waste products. It also distributes various hormones that regulate and coordinate the body's activities and participates in the regulation of fluid balance and body temperature. Several of the most important transport processes performed by the circulation (e.g., the transport of oxygen and carbon dioxide and the maintenance of acid-base balance) are accomplished by passing the blood through the gas exchange environment of the lungs.

COMPOSITION

The fluid part of the blood is the *plasma,* which accounts for about 60 percent of the blood by volume. The blood plasma is an extremely complex liquid. About 90 percent of the plasma consists of water. The major solute in plasma is a group of proteins that constitute between 7 to 9 percent of the plasma by weight. *Albumin* is the most abundant *plasma protein* and is an extremely important determinant of fluid balance because of the semipermeable property of the capillaries and its resulting osmotic activity (see Chap. 8). Less than 1 percent of plasma consists of inorganic salts and small amounts of urea, uric acid, creatine, amino acids, sugar, fats, and various hormones.

The *formed elements* of the blood account for approximately 40 percent of the blood by volume (Figs. 11–1 and 11–2). The most numerous formed element is the *red blood cell* or *erythrocyte.* There are about 4.5 to 5.0 million erythrocytes per cubic mm of blood. They are nonmotile, highly differentiated cells that have lost their nuclei and most of their cytoplasmic organelles. Erythrocytes are soft and flexible and can pass through the smallest capillaries. An important constituent of erythro-

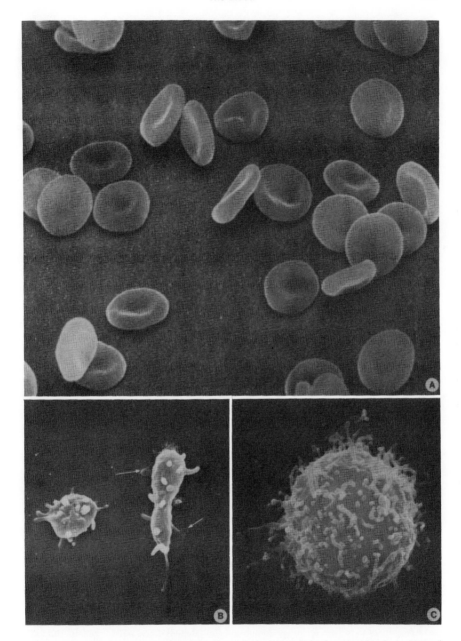

Fig. 11–1. Electron micrographs of the formed elements of the human blood. *A:* Normal human erythrocytes. Note the characteristic biconcave appearance of these anucleated cells (×5000); *B:* Two human blood platelets. The filamentous extensions of the platelet's surface continuously change in form and direction in the living state. When one of these extensions contacts a glass slide it adheres and spreads out (arrows) (×8000); *C:* A lymphocyte exhibiting many long microvilli. Isolated from the blood of a patient with chronic lymphocytic leukemia (×9000). (From Motta, P., et al.: Microanatomy of Cell and Tissue Surfaces: An Atlas of Scanning Electron Microscopy. Philadelphia, Lea & Febiger, 1977.)

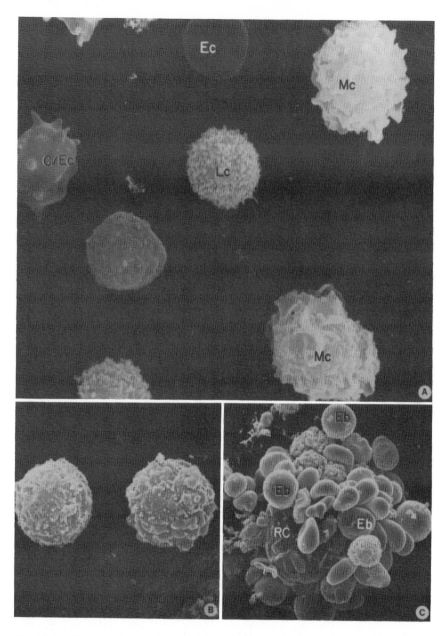

Fig. 11–2. Electron micrographs of the formed elements of the human blood. *A:* Human monocytes (Mc), lymphocytes (Lc), and normal (Ec) and created (C/Ec) erythrocytes. Note that some lymphocytes possess relatively smooth surfaces whereas others possess variable numbers of microvilli. The ruffles or folds that characterize the monocyte free surface represent potential pseudopodia. Isolated from normal human blood (×6500). *B:* Two neutrophilic leukocytes. Neutrophilic leukocytes possess variable rough free surfaces. From a patient with acute granulocytic leukemia (×6500). *C:* Erythroblastic islet. In the bone marrow, erythroblasts (precursors to erythrocytes) are arranged in small islets composed of a central reticulation (RC) surrounded by maturing erythroblasts (Eb). From cultured human bone marrow (×3000). (From Motta, P., et al.: Microanatomy of Cells and Tissue Surfaces: An Atlas of Scanning Electron Microscopy. Philadelphia, Lea & Febiger, 1977.)

cytes is *hemoglobin*, which accounts for about 33 percent of the weight of the cell. Hemoglobin is a conjugated protein composed of a *heme*, a porphyrin ring to which iron is linked, and *globin*, a protein. Hemoglobin is the chemical that permits these cells to bind and to transport oxygen. Figure 11–1 presents a scanning electron micrograph of several erythrocytes. The individual erythrocyte is a biconcave disk about 8 μm in diameter and 2μm thick at its margins. The thinner concave region in the center represents the space the nucleus had occupied before it was expelled.

Another major type of formed element of the blood is the *leukocyte.* These cells are less numerous than the erythrocytes; there are only about 6000 to 10,000 per cubic mm of blood. Leukocytes primarily defend the body against invasion by infectious agents, repair damaged tissues, and participate in immune reactions. There are several types of leukocytes; all retain their nuclei. The *nongranular leukocytes* are composed of *lymphocytes* and *monocytes.* Lymphocytes make up about 25 percent of the leukocyte population (Figs. 11–1C and 11–2A). They are spheric cells, are 6 to 10 μm in diameter, and have a relatively large nucleus surrounded by a thin layer of cytoplasm. They may have a smooth surface or may possess variable numbers of long or short microvilli. The lymphocytes are concerned with cellular immunity, hypersensitivity, and the production of antibodies.

The monocytes comprise about 3 to 8 percent of the total leukocyte population (Fig. 11–2A). They are approximately 12 to 18 μm in diameter and possess considerably more cytoplasm than do lymphocytes. The free surface of monocytes is characterized by thin folds that can be modified into pseudopodia when the cells engulf material by endocytosis.

Granular leukocytes are characterized by heavily granulated cytoplasm and are named according to the staining characteristics of their cytoplasmic granules: *neutrophils, eosinophils,* and *basophils.* Granular leukocytes are also known as *polymorphonuclear* leukocytes because of the lobulated nature of their nuclei.

Neutrophils are approximately 12 to 15 μm in diameter (Fig. 11–2B). They comprise about 60 to 70 percent of the leukocyte population and are chemotactically attracted to damaged tissue and other foreign bodies (i.e., bacteria), which they engulf and phagocytize. They also release enzymes that can initiate lysis of the surrounding tissues.

Eosinophils account for about 3 percent of the leukocyte population. They have an abundance of large refractile granules. In allergic reactions, eosinophils increase in number and can phagocytize antigen-antibody complexes.

Basophils comprise less than 1 percent of the leukocyte population. They range in size from 10 to 20 μm and are important because they manufacture heparin and histamine.

Blood platelets are the smallest formed elements (Fig. 11–1B). They are approximately 2 to 5 μm in diameter and often exhibit filamentous projections of various lengths. There are about 250,000 platelets per cubic mm of blood. Platelets are believed to be fragments of cytoplasm of larger cells, the *megakaryocytes,* which reside in the bone marrow. They are a source of *thromboplastin,* an important factor needed for the coagulation of blood.

NORMAL VALUES OF BLOOD VOLUME IN THE HUMAN

Like arterial blood pressure (see Chap. 6), blood volume varies with sex, age, and various other factors. Weight is one of the most important factors to consider when determining a person's normal blood volume. Thus, blood volume is usually expressed as ml per kg of body weight. "Normal" values of blood volumes for young healthy men are presented in Table 11–1. Although these are mean values, it should be emphasized that there is considerable individual variation. Thus, an individual's blood volume that ranges by as much as plus or minus 20 percent from the mean is not uncommon. One reason for the difference in blood volume is the amount of an individual's body fat. As a rule, obese people have less blood volume per kg of body weight than do thin individuals. It has been estimated that the lean mass of the body has a blood content of about 93 ml/kg, whereas adipose tissue has a blood content of only 18 ml/kg (Alexander, et al., 1962). This could account for the lower blood volumes per kg of body weight in women. Blood volume appears to be best correlated with lean body mass (Fig. 11–3).

REGULATION OF BLOOD VOLUME

Important factors in determining blood volume are (1) the acute exchange of fluid between plasma and the interstitium; (2) the long-term regulation of plasma volume by the kidneys; and (3) the regulation of erythrocyte volume. We will consider each of these factors in turn.

Filtration-Absorption

In Chapter 8 we considered the process by which plasma is held in the circulatory system. The five primary factors that determine whether

Table 11–1. Average Blood Volumes Determined in Normal Young Man*

Plasma volume (ml/kg)	46
Cell volume (ml/kg)	31
Blood volume (ml/kg)	77
Hematocrit (%)	44.5
Plasma protein concentration (gm %)	6.86

*Data from Gregersen, M.I., and Nickerson, J.L.: Relation of blood volume and cardiac output to body type. J. Appl. Physiol., 3:329, 1950.

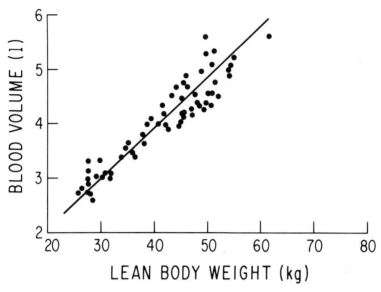

Fig. 11–3. Relationship of blood volume to lean body mass. (Data from Allen, T.H., et al.: Prediction of blood volume and adiposity in man from body weight and cube of height. Metabolism, 5:328, 1956.)

fluid moves into or out of the circulation, according to the Starling hypothesis, are the capillary and interstitial hydrostatic pressures, the capillary and interstitial colloid osmotic pressures, and the hydraulic conductivity of the capillary wall. The most important of these factors in determining acute changes in blood volume is the capillary hydrostatic pressure. The ways in which changes in capillary pressure can alter blood volume may be illustrated by discussing the sequence of events that follows an acute hemorrhage. An acute loss of blood volume results in an immediate reduction in venous return, cardiac output, arterial blood pressure, and perfusion to many vascular beds (e.g., skeletal muscles). This reduction in tissue perfusion results in a decrease in the capillary hydrostatic pressure and upsets the Starling balance, causing an immediate absorption in extravascular fluid that continues until a new balance of forces is achieved (see Chap. 8). Consequently, plasma volume increases toward normal. The baroreceptors play an important role in this reabsorption following hemorrhage because, in an attempt to keep arterial pressure elevated (to maintain perfusion of the vital coronary and cerebral circulations), the reflexes produce strong constriction of the skeletal muscle arterioles, which further accentuates the fall in skeletal muscle capillary pressure.

Capillary pressure also helps to bring blood volume back toward normal when the circulatory system has too much blood volume. Under these conditions, capillary pressure rises and fluid is lost into the interstitial spaces.

Regulation of Plasma Volume by the Kidney

Although the Starling balance is important in helping to bring about acute changes in plasma volume, the long range, steady-state regulation of plasma volume is accomplished by a balance of fluid intake and urinary output. The mechanisms responsible for the kidney's role in the regulation of blood volume are complex and linked to the kidney's role in the regulation of fluid osmolality.

One major factor responsible for the renal regulation of plasma volume is the extremely sensitive effect arterial blood pressure has on urinary output. For each 1 mm Hg change in arterial blood pressure (increase or decrease), there is approximately a onefold change in urinary output. Thus, an increase in blood volume (e.g., by an overinfusion of intravenous fluid) rapidly results in an increase in urine; a decrease in blood volume (e.g., by hemorrhage) results in a reduction in urine formation.

Another mechanism for the control of plasma volume is linked to the body's osmolality regulatory system. Located in the anterior hypothalamus near the supraoptic and paraventricular nuclei are so-called *osmoreceptors,* which can sense the osmolality of the tissue fluids (normally around 300 mOsm/kg). The osmoreceptors somehow know when the osmolality changes from normal. They transmit a signal through nerve connections to the neurohypophyseal cells of the posterior lobe of the pituitary where *antidiuretic hormone* (ADH) is produced and secreted. ADH has its main effect on the distal tubules of the nephron where it increases the permeability to water. When the osmolality increases, ADH is released and water reabsorption *(antidiuresis)* increases. The result is a decrease in urine formation and an increase in blood volume. Some evidence (Gupta, et al., 1966) suggests that low-pressure mechanoreceptors located in the atria and heart chambers may also affect ADH release. Thus, in addition to initiating pressor reflexes, these receptors also are believed to relay ascending fibers to the hypothalamus and to influence the osmoreceptors. Thus, an increase in circulating blood volume would stretch these low pressure (volume) receptors and inhibit ADH secretion, resulting in greater fluid loss through the kidneys. One might suspect that if blood volume affects ADH secretion through a mechanoreceptor system it should also affect *aldosterone* release through a similar mechanism. Aldosterone is the salt-retaining corticosteroid from the adrenal cortex that acts on the kidney to exchange hydrogen and potassium for sodium ions. There is little evidence for release of aldosterone through mechanorceptor stimulation, but some linkage between ADH and aldosterone no doubt exists because osmolality (salt content) is generally regulated with plasma water.

Although aldosterone has not been shown to be released through mechanoreceptor stimulation, it has been shown to affect blood volume through the renin-angiotensin system. When arterial blood pressure falls (such as occurs during hemorrhage) renin is released by the juxtaglomerular apparatus (Bunag, et al., 1966). Renin leads to the formation of angiotensin II, which not only is a powerful vasopressor, but also stimulates the release of aldosterone from the zona glomerulosa of the adrenal cortex. Consequently, the amount of sodium retained by the kidney increases. Because salt cannot be retained without an osmotic equivalent of water, this renin-angiotensin-aldosterone system increases plasma volume. This mechanism may, indeed, prove to be one of the most important mechanisms for plasma volume regulation.

Regulation of Erythrocyte Volume

In the adult human, the production of red cells, or *erythropoiesis*, occurs in the bone marrow. The erythrocyte evolves from a stem cell of uncertain identity. Early in development, the cell contains a nucleus that becomes progressively smaller as maturation proceeds. Hemoglobin slowly appears in the cytoplasm as the cell decreases in size. By the time the cell enters the circulation, its nucleus has disappeared.

The rate of erythrocyte production is controlled by the hormone, *erythropoietin*. Erythropoietin is a glycoprotein produced in the kidney and possibly elsewhere. It probably exerts its effect on the stem cells causing them to differentiate into the early erythroblasts. When the volume of red blood cells decreases, a receptor somewhere in the body appears to sense the decrease and the output of erythropoietin increases. Hypoxia also appears to stimulate erythropoietin and, thus, red blood cell production.

PHYSICAL CHEMISTRY OF BLOOD

Partial Pressures and Solubility of Gases in Blood

According to Henry's law (Perry and Chilton, 1973), the amount of a gas in physical solution in a liquid (including blood) at constant temperature is directly proportional to its partial pressure.* To determine the partial pressure of a gas in a liquid, one must determine its partial pressure in an equilibrated gas phase because, under equilibrium conditions, the partial pressures of the gas in the gas phase and in the liquid

---

Dalton's law (Perry and Chilton, 1973) states that each gas in a gas mixture acts as if it alone occupied the total volume of its container and, therefore, exerts a pressure independent of other pressures (its *partial pressure*). The sum of all partial pressures is equal to the total pressure. The partial pressure of a gas in a mixture is equal to the product of its mole fraction and the total pressure. For example, the partial pressure of oxygen in dry air (in mm Hg) when the total pressure is 760 mm Hg is equal to 0.21×760 or 160 mm Hg.

phase are equal. This is because the number of gas molecules leaving the liquid per unit time is equal to the number entering the liquid.

The partial pressure of a gas in solution is not the same as the amount of gas dissolved in physical solution. For example, at the partial pressures normally found in arterial blood, the blood contains, in physical solution, the following amounts of gas per 100 ml of blood: 0.25 ml of O_2, 2.69 ml of CO_2 and 1.04 ml of N_2. The units used to express the amount of a gas in blood are usually ml per 100 ml of blood. These units for convenience are referred to as volume percent (vol %); therefore, 2.69 ml of CO_2 per 100 ml of blood is usually referred to as simply 2.69 vol %. The total amount of oxygen and carbon dioxide found in each 100 ml of blood is considerably greater than that held in physical solution because of the amount held in chemical combination. The total amount of oxygen found in arterial blood is around 20 vol %, whereas that held in physical solution amounts to only 0.25 vol %. If it were not for the oxygen and carbon dioxide held in chemical combination, a circulating blood volume of about 75 times larger than normal would be needed to satisfy the metabolic requirements of the body!

Oxygen Transport

As we discussed earlier, a major constituent of the erythrocyte is the conjugated protein hemoglobin (HHb), which can combine reversibly with O_2 and CO_2. In blood, hemoglobin's reaction with oxygen proceeds as follows:

$$HHb + O_2 \rightleftharpoons HHbO_2. \tag{11-1}$$

The rate of formation of *oxyhemoglobin* ($HHbO_2$) is governed by the partial pressure of oxygen. At a P_{O_2} of 100 mm Hg, about 97 percent of the available HHb has been converted to $HHbO_2$. Under normal conditions, blood contains about 15 gm of HHb per 100 ml and each gm of HHb can combine with 1.36 ml of O_2; therefore, *fully* oxygenated blood contains 20 vol % of O_2 (100 percent saturated). Normally, arterial blood leaving a well-ventilated pulmonary capillary is about 98 percent saturated because the process is not complete until the P_{O_2} reaches 150 mm Hg (the alveolar P_{O_2} is normally around 100 mm Hg.).

When the amount of oxygen held by the blood (mostly by hemoglobin) is plotted against the partial pressure of oxygen in the blood, the resulting curve is known as the *oxygen dissociation curve* (Fig. 11-4). The amount of oxygen held in the blood can be plotted either as content (vol %) or as percent saturation (where 20 vol % equals 100 percent saturation). As the oxygen dissociation curves graphically show, the amount of oxygen in the blood is not directly proportional to the partial pressure. The dissociation curve is markedly S-shaped. The steep portion of the curve (between 20 to 60 mm Hg) means that large amounts of oxygen can be delivered to the tissues at relatively small partial pressure gra-

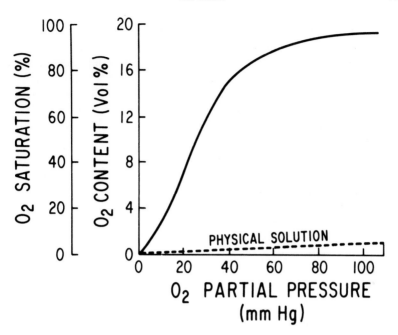

Fig. 11–4. The oxygen dissociation curve. Oxygen content (and saturation) plotted against the partial pressure of oxygen in the blood. The dashed line represents the oxygen held in plasma by physical solution.

dients; the flat upper portion of the curve means that the composition of arterial blood will remain relatively constant despite possibly wide fluctuations in P_{O_2}.

Various factors affect the shape and position of the oxygen dissociation curve. A decrease in temperature shifts the curve to the left so that more oxygen is held by the hemoglobin at any P_{O_2} (Fig. 11–5A). This shift is physiologically significant because as body temperature rises (i.e., with an increase in metabolism), more O_2 is released to the tissues at any given driving pressure.

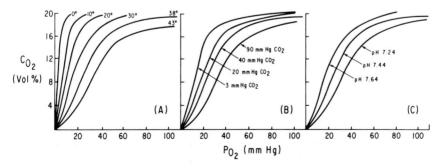

Fig. 11–5. Examples of the effects of (A) temperature (°C), (B) CO_2 tension, and (C) pH on the oxygen dissociation curve.

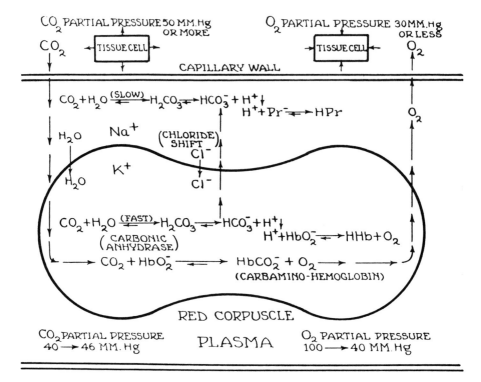

Fig. 11–6. Summary of the transport processes for carbon dioxide. As CO_2 diffuses from the tissues into the plasma, it slowly reacts with water to form H_2CO_3 and then HCO_3^- and H^+. The hydrogen ions that are formed by this reaction immediately combine with the plasma proteins, which act as buffers. Most of the CO_2 diffuses into the erythrocytes where the carbonic anhydrase catalyzes the formation of H_2CO_3, which ionizes to HCO_3^- and H^+. The H^+ reacts with HbO_3^- to form HHb and thus releases O_2 to the tissues. The HCO_3^- that is formed diffuses into the plasma. To keep the ionic charges in balance, Cl^- ions diffuse into the cells. This diffusion is known as the *chloride shift* and allows large amounts of HCO_3^- to be carried in the plasma. The rest of the CO_2 combines directly with HbO_2^- to form $HbCO_2^-$ and free O_2. (From Riley, R.L.: Gas exchange and transportation. *In* Physiology and Biophysics. 9th Edition. Edited by T. C. Ruch, and H. D. Patton. Philadelphia, W. B. Saunders, 1965.)

Increasing the P_{CO_2} or decreasing the pH also shifts the oxygen dissociation curve to favor the dissociation of $HHbO_2$ (Figs. 11–5B and 11–5C). The physiologic significance of this reaction is that the production of CO_2 by the metabolizing tissues themselves facilitates the release of O_2. The effect of CO_2 and pH on the oxygen dissociation curve is known as the *Bohr effect*.

Carbon Dioxide Transport

Carbon dioxide is transported in blood in three forms: (1) as carbonic acid (H_2CO_3), (2) as the bicarbonate ion (HCO_3^-) and (3) in combination

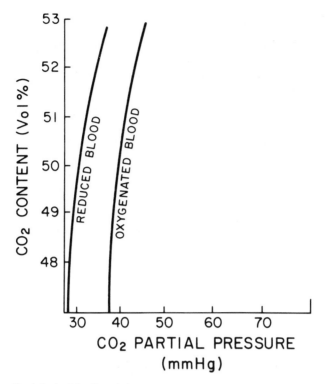

Fig. 11–7. Physiologic CO$_2$ dissociation curve.

with hemoglobin (carbamino hemoglobin, HHbCO$_2$). HHbCO$_2$ is found only in the erythrocyte whereas H$_2$CO$_3$ and HCO$_3^-$ are found in both the erythrocyte and the plasma. An enzyme within the erythrocyte, *carbonic anhydrase*, speeds up the reaction between CO$_2$ and H$_2$CO$_3$. The processes by which carbon dioxide is transported in the blood are summarized in Figure 11–6.

As with oxygen, a *physiologic carbon dioxide dissociation* curve can be constructed by plotting the CO$_2$ content against P$_{CO_2}$. This is done in Figure 11–7 for the range of P$_{CO_2}$ values normally found in human blood. As can be seen from this figure, the CO$_2$ dissociation curve is nearly a straight line over the physiologic range of P$_{CO_2}$. This result has extremely important and practical advantages that will be discussed in detail in this section on pulmonary gas exchange (see Chap. 14). Figure 11–5 also illustrates that the position of the CO$_2$ dissociation curve depends on whether hemoglobin is in its oxygenated or its reduced forms. Thus, picking up O$_2$ by hemoglobin aids in the unloading of CO$_2$ in the lung, and the absorption of CO$_2$ in the tissues aids in the unloading of O$_2$. This phenomenon is known as the *Haldane effect*.

PULMONARY PHYSIOLOGY

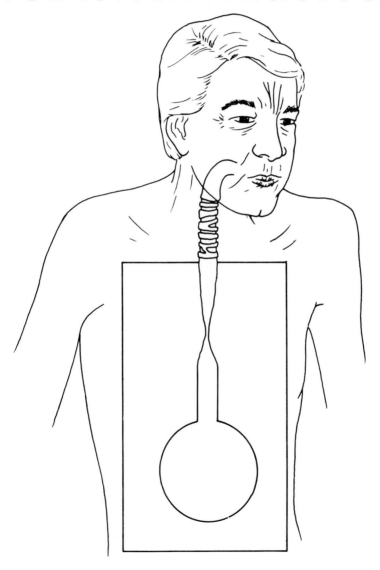

12

THE PULMONARY SYSTEM—A BRIEF OVERVIEW

FUNCTION

The pulmonary system has several functions; however, its primary function is *respiration*. When our muscles of respiration contract, our lungs expand. By so doing, the lungs move air from the ambient environment through a series of smaller and smaller conducting passages until it reaches the millions of minute air sacs, the *alveoli*. Here, *gas exchange* occurs. Oxygen is taken up by the body by diffusion across the thin walls of the alveolar air sacs into the blood, which literally bathes the alveolar sac. Similarly, carbon dioxide is given off and finds its way to the outside air as the muscles of respiration relax, allowing the lung-chest wall system to recoil to its initial lung volume.

In addition to gas exchange, the pulmonary system performs a number of accessory functions. One such function, which is often overlooked, is *vocalization*. During this process, the expired air passes over the vocal cords in the *larynx*, which then vibrates. The sound that results is the voice. The lungs also filter toxic material from the blood and metabolize many endogenous as well as exogenous materials. Because the pulmonary vessels are compliant structures, the lungs also serve as a reservoir of blood, although this reservoir is not as great as that found in the systemic veins.

To begin our study of the pulmonary system we will briefly discuss its anatomy, starting at the macroscopic level and proceeding in stepwise

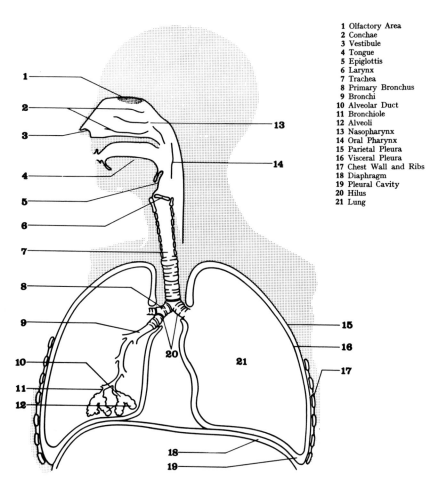

1 Olfactory Area
2 Conchae
3 Vestibule
4 Tongue
5 Epiglottis
6 Larynx
7 Trachea
8 Primary Bronchus
9 Bronchi
10 Alveolar Duct
11 Bronchiole
12 Alveoli
13 Nasopharynx
14 Oral Pharynx
15 Parietal Pleura
16 Visceral Pleura
17 Chest Wall and Ribs
18 Diaphragm
19 Pleural Cavity
20 Hilus
21 Lung

Fig. 12–1. Schematic representation of the respiratory airways.. (From Motta, P., et al.: Microanatomy of Cell and Tissue Surfaces: An Atlas of Scanning Electron Microscopy. Philadelphia, Lea & Febiger, 1977.)

fashion to the microscopic level. We will then define the basic pulmonary air volumes that result when the system functions as a whole.

BASIC ANATOMY

The pulmonary airways are composed of a series of conducting tubules followed by the respiratory portions of the lung, where gas exchange occurs. Figure 12–1 is a schematic respresentation of the respiratory airways.

The conducting airways begin with the nose (and mouth) and are followed by the *pharynx, larynx, trachea,* and varying sizes of *bronchi.* The nose consists of two cavities separated by the *nasal septum*. The opening of the nose is called the *naris,* which widens into the *vestibule.* Behind the vestibule is the *nasopharynx.* Above the vestibule is the *olfactory region,* lined with *olfactory cells,* which are bipolar neurons whose proximal end becomes the *olfactory nerve.* These cells are specialized and react to airborne scents. Openings from spaces of bones, called the *paranasal sinuses,* reach into the nasal cavities. The nasal cavities, nasal pharynx, and paranasal sinuses are lined with ciliated cells, which are interspersed with cells bearing only microvilli and with goblet cells. The goblet cells and the glands in the underlying lamina provide a secretion of mucus that coats the nasal airways.

In addition to conducting air, the upper part of the airway system has other physiologic functions. The hair found in the naris filters out gross objects, and the mucous membranes that line the nasal cavities warm and humidify the inspired air. This viscous fluid also carries particles of dust and dirt through the nasopharynx to the oral pharynx by the beating of the cilia. When the mucous membrane becomes infected or inflamed (e.g., by the common cold or rhinitis), it swells and increases the resistance to breathing.

Below the pharynx is the *larynx,* which is the opening to the airways leading to the lungs. The position of the larynx in the neck is made obvious by the *laryngeal prominence* or *Adam's apple.* The entrance to the *laryngeal cavity* is bound anteriorly by the *epiglottis,* which serves as a valve to prevent the passage of solids and liquids into the conducting airways below. Located in the inferior part of the laryngeal cavity are the *vocal folds* and the slit between them, the *glottis.* The vocal folds and glottis comprise the apparatus for vocalization. All parts of the laryngeal cavity are lined with a mucous membrane similar to that found in the trachea.

The major *windpipe* or *trachea* is about 11 cm long and extends from the larynx to the level of the fifth thoracic vertebra. At this level, it divides into right and left *main bronchi.* The trachea is supported by a C-shaped *hyaline cartilage,* which prevents it from collapsing. The bronchi are constructed much like the trachea. The mucous membranes of the trachea and bronchi are lined with *pseudostratified columnar ciliated epithelium.* The cilia of this epithelium beat in an upward direction to carry foreign material along a mucous blanket.

The main bronchi conduct the air into the *lungs,* which are paired structures occupying most of the thoracic cavity (see Fig. 12–1). The right lung is composed of three lobes, whereas the left lung has only two lobes. Each lobe, in turn, can be subdivided into smaller sections called *lobules.* When the main bronchi enter the lungs they begin to divide into smaller and smaller branches. The branches of the *bronchial tree* that finally enter the lobules are usually less than 1 mm in diameter and are called *bronchioles.* The nature of the bronchial tree can be seen in Figure 12–2, which presents a bronchogram of a left lung. As the bronchial divisions take place, the cartilaginous supports within their wall decrease as the amount of *bronchial smooth muscle* increases. In general, cartilage is not found in bronchioles that are less than 1 mm in size. The bronchioles continue to divide, forming *terminal bronchioles* which lead to *respiratory bronchioles*. The respiratory bronchioles break up into alveolar ducts, alveolar sacs, and finally, the alveoli (Fig. 12–3). The alveolus is the smallest unit of the respiratory tree. Only the thin epithelium of the alveolus and the endothelium of the pulmonary capillaries separate the air from the blood. It has been estimated that approximately 150 million alveoli are in each lung and have a surface area

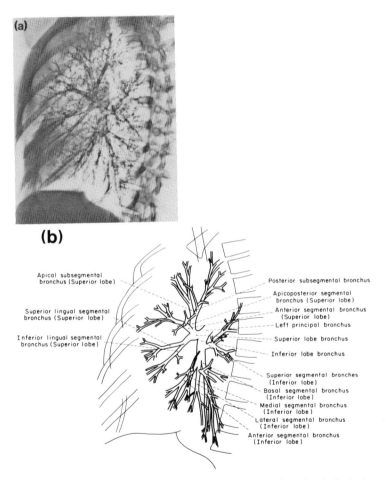

Fig. 12–2. Bronchogram from a left lung. (From Wicke, L.: Atlas of Radiologic Anatomy. Baltimore, Urban & Schwarzenberg, 1979.)

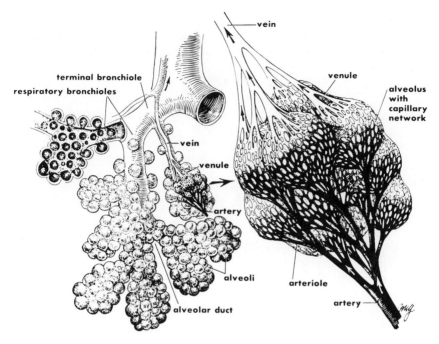

Fig. 12–3. Schematic representation of the respiratory units of the lung. The left side of the figure illustrates the system of air passages. The right side of the figure illustrates how the pulmonary capillaries envelop the air sacs to form the gas exchange units of the lung. (From Crouch, J.E.: Functional Human Anatomy. 4th Edition. Philadelphia, Lea & Febiger, 1985.)

of between 50 and 100 square meters. Diffusion of oxygen and carbon dioxide between air and blood takes place within the alveolar units.

The structure of the alveoli can be seen in the scanning electron micrograph presented in Figure 12–4. The alveoli are separated by an *interalveolar septum.* Small openings called *pores* are found in the thin walls separating adjacent alveoli. These pores provide *collateral ventilation,* which helps to prevent *atelectasis* (alveolar collapse) when the bronchi become obstructed. Each alveolus is lined by *squamous pulmonary epithelial cells* as well as by *septal cells.* These later cells occur singly or in groups of two or three and possess microprojections on their free surface (see Fig. 12–4). They are believed to secrete a *surfactant* material that reduces the surface tension of the alveoli and thereby helps to prevent alveolar collapse. A third type of alveolar cell can often be found moving about the surface of the squamous alveolar cells. These cells are *alveolar phagocytes,* which remove various particles, such as bacteria, from the alveolus (see Fig. 12–4).

Pulmonary Physiology

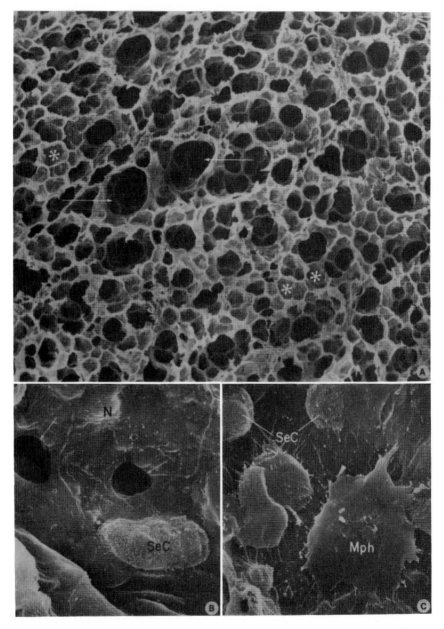

Fig. 12–4. Scanning electron micrograph. *A:* Low magnification view of a sectioned lung. Many alveolar ducts (arrows), alveolar sacs and alveoli (*) can be distinguished (× 75; hamster). *B:* Luminal surface of an alveolus. A protruding septal cell (SeC) covered with microvilli and two alveolar pores (arrows) are depicted. The protruding nuclear regions (N) and cell borders of the squamous epithelial cells can also be distinguished (× 2900; hamster). *C:* Luminal surface of an alveolus. Several alveolar macrophages (Mph) are seen attached to the pulmonary epithelium. Two protruding septal cells (SeC) are also present (× 2900; hamster). (From Motta, P., et al.: Microanatomy of Cell and Tissue Surfaces: An Atlas of Scanning Electron Microscopy. Philadelphia, Lea & Febiger, 1977.)

LUNG VOLUMES

Air volume is to the pulmonary airways what blood volume is to the circulatory system. Therefore, it is appropriate as part of our overview of the pulmonary system to define the various lung volumes that can be measured from any individual. Figure 12–5 depicts the relationship between the various volumes. We can define four primary volumes that do not overlap and, from these volumes, can further define four lung capacities that include two or more of the primary volumes.

The primary lung volumes are defined as follows:

1. *Tidal volume* is the volume of gas inspired (and expired) during each breath.

2. *Inspiratory reserve volume* is the maximal amount of gas that can be inspired above the tidal volume.

3. *Expiratory reserve volume* is the maximal amount of gas that can be expired below tidal volume.

4. *Residual volume* is the volume of gas remaining in the lung at the end of a maximal expiration.

The lung capacities are as follows:

1. *Total lung capacity* is the total amount of gas in the lung at the end of a maximal inspiration.

2. *Vital capacity* is the maximal amount of volume that can be expelled from the lungs during a forced expiration from maximal inspiration.

3. *Inspiratory capacity* is the maximal amount of gas that can be inspired from the resting expiratory level.

4. *Functional residual capacity* is the volume of gas remaining in the lung at the end of a normal expiration.

These volumes and capacities are important not only because they are

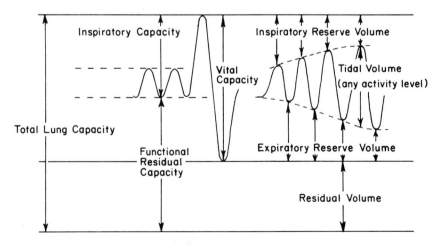

Fig. 12–5. Schematic representation of lung volumes and lung capacities. (From Breazile, J.E.: Textbook of Veterinary Physiology. Philadelphia, Lea & Febiger, 1971.)

Table 12–1.   Lung Volume (in ml) in Healthy Recumbent Subjects*

	Male age 20–30 years (1.7 M²)	Male age 50–60 years (1.7 M²)	Female age 20–30 years (1.6 M²)
Inspiratory capacity	3,600	2,600	2,400
Expiratory reserve capacity	1,200	1,000	800
Vital capacity	4,800	3,600	3,200
Residual volume	1,200	2,400	3,200
Functional residual capacity	2,400	3,400	1,800
Total lung capacity	6,000	6,000	4,200

*Data from Comroe, 1965.
†These are typical values for only healthy subjects at the sex, age, and body surface area specified.

the physiologic manifestation of the anatomic system, but also because they can and do change as a result of the physiologic process (e.g., by age or disease). Therefore, they form the basis for the measurement of pulmonary function. A listing of "normal" values of lung volumes is presented in Table 12–1.

13

PULMONARY MECHANICS

VOLUME-PRESSURE RELATIONSHIPS OF THE LUNG

We begin our discussion of pulmonary mechanics by discussing the elastic nature of the lung.

Volume-Pressure Hysteresis

If an isolated, degassed lung is inflated and then deflated by changing the tracheal pressure relative to that at the surface of the lung, a marked volume-pressure hysteresis loop is obtained (Fig. 13–1A). During inflation, a tracheal pressure of between 8 and 12 cm H_2O is needed before the lung begins to inflate (point a, Fig. 13–1A). This pressure is necessary because the small airways and alveoli are held closed by surface forces, and at least 8 cm H_2O are needed to overcome these forces. As additional pressure is applied, the remaining alveoli are opened (recruited) as lung volume sharply increases (point b). At high pressures, the increase in volume per unit change in pressure decreases because most all alveoli are recruited, and the elastic fibers within the lung are stretched to nearly their elastic limit (point c). As tracheal pressure is lowered, deflation occurs as all the alveoli uniformly decrease in size; that is, there is no initial derecruitment of alveoli. However, upon further deflation (below point d), small alveolar units begin to collapse, and the rate of volume decrease is accelerated. Finally, when tracheal pressure is reduced to zero, additional airways collapse, trapping volume in the lungs (point e). If the lung is reinflated from this point, a different inflation curve is obtained, but the same deflation curve is followed. If the lung is reinflated from a point on the deflation curve (Fig. 13–1B), two important observations are made. First, the size of the hysteresis loop is greatly reduced. Second, the marked nonlinear volume-pressure curve of the lung becomes essentially linear over a small region of the "deflation

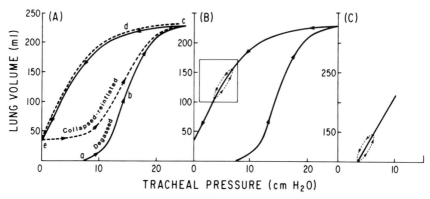

Fig. 13–1. Volume-pressure curves of a normal, excised cat lung. *(A):* The degassed lung requires an opening pressure of between 8 and 12 cm H₂O. At the start of deflation, volume drops are small. Volume drops then increase as tracheal pressure approaches zero. When tracheal pressure returns to zero, some gas remains trapped in the lung. If the lung is reinflated from this point, the hysteresis is less. *(B):* Reinflation over a small portion in the mid-range of the deflation curve. Hysteresis is small as the volume-pressure curve approximates a linear relationship. *(C):* A linearized volume-pressure curve obtained by fitting a straight line to the portion of the deflation curve marked in *(B)* by the box. (Adapted from Hildebrandt, J., and Young, A.C.: Anatomy and physics of respiration. *In* Physiology and Biophysics. 19th Edition. Edited by T. C. Ruch, and H. D. Patton. Philadelphia, W. B. Saunders, 1965.)

curve." This last type of hysteresis curve (Fig. 13–1B) is similar to the curve the lung actually exhibits in the intact person whose lung is prevented from completely collapsing by its interaction with the chest wall (see the following).

Before characterizing the elastic behavior of the lung as it exists in the intact person, we must consider the reasons for this distinct volume-pressure hysteresis found in the excised lung.

Alveolar Surface Forces

The experiment depicted in Figure 13–2 illustrates that alveolar surface forces contribute significantly to alveolar recruitment (and derecruitment). The volume-pressure hysteresis of the lung is also illustrated. Because the alveolar wall is moist, the air-liquid interface produces a surface tension that can be abolished when the interface is eliminated.* This can be done by filling a degassed lung with an isosmotic fluid, such as saline (von Neergaard, 1929). The saline-inflated lung has essentially no hysteresis and has a lower tracheal pressure at any given lung volume than does the air-filled lung. This result suggests that the recoil force decreases when the surface tension is eliminated. It further suggests that, because the air-filled lung has a greater inflation pressure than

---

*Surface tension develops between an air-liquid interface because the attractive forces between liquid molecules are stronger than the forces between the molecules of the liquid and gas. Consequently, the liquid surface areas tend to become as small as possible.

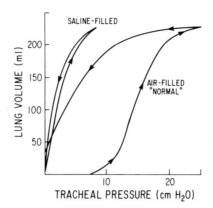

LUNG VOLUME (ml)

SALINE-FILLED

AIR-FILLED "NORMAL"

200

150

100

50

10   20

TRACHEAL PRESSURE (cm H₂0)

Fig. 13–2. Volume-pressure curves of normal and saline-filled excised cat lungs. The curve for the normal, air-filled lung shown here is the same as that presented in Figure 13–1B. Inflation of the saline-filled lung produced lower inflation pressures at any lung volume, showed negligible hysteresis, and emptied nearly completely. (Adapted from Hildebrandt, J., and Young, A.C.: Anatomy and physics of respiration. *In* Physiology and Biophysics. 19th Edition. Edited by T. C. Ruch, and H. D. Patton. Philadelphia, W. B. Saunders, 1965.)

deflation pressure at any given lung volume, fewer surface forces act on the alveoli during deflation than during inflation in the "normal" lung. This characteristic becomes extremely important when one realizes that, if the alveolar surface tension were constant, a lowering of the tracheal pressure below some critical value should collapse all alveoli. Happily, this does not occur because of the nature of the surface active material that lines the alveolar walls. This material is known as *pulmonary surfactant.*

Pulmonary surfactant is believed to be produced by the septal cells, which line the alveolar wall (see Fig. 13–4). This cell's exact composition has not yet been determined, but it does contain phospholipids, polysaccharides, and proteins. Surfactant can alter its surface tension as the areas of the surface film are changed, i.e., as the lung volume changes (Fig. 13–3). As the lung inflates, the surface tension of the pulmonary surfactant increases; as the lung deflates, the surface tension decreases. Lowering the surface tension in the alveoli as deflation occurs prevents collapse of the alveoli (until low pressures and volumes occur), thus bestowing a good deal of stability on the volume-pressure characteristics of the lung (particularly the deflation curve where our lungs usually "operate"). If this were not the case, we would continually need to do more "work of breathing" to overcome collapse. In addition, gas exchange would be severely affected because of the collapsed alveoli.

Pulmonary (Alveolar) Compliance

To characterize the elastic nature of the lung, one must study the volume-pressure relationship of the lung in much the same way as was

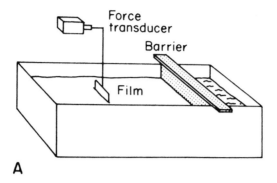

A

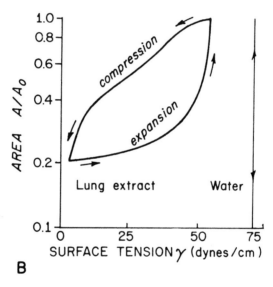

B

Fig. 13–3. Surface tension as a function of film area. *A:* A surface balance instrument is used to measure the surface tension of a lung extract containing surfactant. It consists of a tray filled to the top with fluid. A film of the material to be studied is spread on the surface. A barrier then compresses the film as a hanging plate continuously records the surface tension. *B:* Lung extracts from healthy mammals show extensive hysteresis and a minimum tension of 0 to 5 dynes per cm. For comparison, the surface tension of water is shown to be constant at about 70 dynes per cm. (From Hildebrandt, J., and Young, A.C.: Anatomy and physics of respiration. *In* Physiology and Biophysics. 19th Edition. Edited by T.C. Ruch, and H. D. Patton. Philadelphia, W. B. Saunders, 1965.)

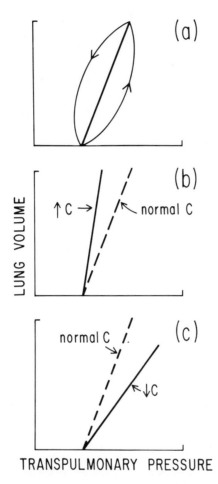

TRANSPULMONARY PRESSURE

Fig. 13–4. *(a):* Hypothetic pressure-volume curves of the normal lung. The straight line represents the static pressure-volume relationship. The curved lines represent the pressure-volume relationships obtained under dynamic conditions. *(b):* Hypothetic pressure-volume curve of a lung with increased compliance. A lesser pressure change is required to achieve a unit change in volume. *(c):* Hypothetic pressure-volume curve of a lung with decreased compliance. A greater pressure change is required to achieve a unit change in volume. (From Green, J.F.: Mechanical Concepts in Cardiovascular and Pulmonary Physiology. Philadelphia, Lea & Febiger, 1977.)

done with the circulatory system (see Chap. 4). This study is greatly facilitated when the volume-pressure relationship is linear. As we saw previously, the volume-pressure relationship of the lung over its entire range is markedly nonlinear in the intact person, following a characteristic "deflation" kind of curve. Fortunately, over the range of normally occurring lung volume (over the range of a normal tidal volume that begins at the functional residual capacity), the volume-pressure characteristics of the lung are essentially linear. This lucky circumstance allows us to "linearize" our discussion of pulmonary compliance, thereby facilitating our understanding of the elastic characteristics of the intact lung.

The relationship of a change in lung volume to a change in distending pressure of the lungs is the compliance of the lungs, which is determined by their elastic properties. The elasticity of the lungs is derived essentially from two sources: elastic elements within the lungs and the alveolar surface tension. Abnormalities in either of these elastic sources can alter pulmonary compliance and interfere with normal functioning of the lungs.

Because the lungs are elastic, an increase in their volume depends on an increase in their transmural pressure (distending pressure). The transmural pressure of the lungs is called the *transpulmonary pressure* and is the difference between the pressure inside the lungs (the alveolar pressure, P_A) and the pressure at the outer surface of the lungs. Under normal conditions, when the lungs are within the chest cavity, the pressure at the outer surface of the lungs is the pleural pressure (P_{PL}); however, when the chest is open, the pressure at the outer surface of the lungs is atmospheric pressure (P_{ATM}, considered zero).* The transpulmonary pressure (P_{TP}) may be summarized as:

$$P_{TP} = P_A - P_{PL}, \text{ normal conditions.} \qquad (13\text{--}1)$$

$$P_{TP} = P_A - P_{ATM} = P_A, \text{ chest open.}$$

Because there are two determinants of the transpulmonary pressure under normal conditions, there are two ways of increasing the lung volume: either by increasing the pressure inside the lung relative to that at the surface (increasing P_A relative to P_{PL}) or by decreasing the pressure at the surface relative to that inside (decreasing P_{PL} relative to P_A). The former situation occurs during positive pressure respiration and is used by the anesthesiologist to ventilate a paralyzed patient. The latter circumstance occurs during normal spontaneous breathing. With an open chest, lung volume can be increased only by positive pressure ventilation. Thus, a patient undergoing thoracic surgery is ventilated in this manner.

Regardless of how the transpulmonary pressure is increased (by positive pressure ventilation or spontaneous inspiration), the increase in lung volume divided by the increased transpulmonary pressure ($\Delta V/ \Delta P_{TP}$) defines the compliance. A plot of ΔV against ΔP_{TP} is known as the compliance curve of the lungs, the slope of which is equal to the compliance.

---

*For convenience, the atmospheric pressure is always considered to be zero. The measured values for P_A and P_{PL} under different circumstances thus denote the change (increase or decrease) in pressure (ΔP) from P_{ATM}.

Introduced here is one of the most potentially confusing issues in this book. In Chapter 4, which discussed the basics of the volume-pressure relationship, a figure was presented of volume plotted on the abscissa and pressure on the ordinate (see Fig. 4–4). Figure 13–4 presents a plot of pressure on the abscissa and volume on the ordinate and is called a pressure-volume relationship. The important question here is whether to plot volume or pressure on the abscissa. By convention, the independent variable is usually thus plotted. To change lung volume, transpulmonary pressure is changed independently, and the resultant change in lung volume is observed. The final volume depends on the magnitude of the change in transpulmonary pressure. Thus, the transpulmonary pressure is plotted on the abscissa and lung vlume on the ordinate. In Chapter 4, we talked about changing the volume in hypothetic balloons and observing the resulting change in pressure. Here volume (the independent variable) was plotted on the abscissa and pressure on the ordinate. We also discussed compliance curves of the circulatory system. These curves are obtained by changing the blood volume and observing the resulting change in blood pressure. Again, volume was plotted on the abscissa. If two important facts are remembered, confusion over this convention can be avoided: (1) the independent variable (that which is initially altered) is plotted on the abscissa and (2) the ratio of change in volume over change in pressure is always called the compliance, i.e., $\Delta V/\Delta P = C$. The ratio of the change in pressure over the change in volume is equal to the reciprocal of compliance, i.e., $\Delta P/\Delta V = 1/C$. If one wishes to apply a name to $\Delta P/\Delta V$, it can be called the elastance; however, this term is seldom used.

Figure 13–4 illustrates hypothetic compliance curves of a lung, assuming linear compliance. Figure 13–1C shows how this curve (and all subsequent compliance curves) represents a small portion of the volume-pressure relationship of the lung taken over the mid-range of normally occurring lung volumes. The straight line represents the pressure-volume relationships that would be obtained under static conditions, that is, if P_{TP} were increased and held constant until volume stopped changing. The static pressure-volume curve would be the same regardless of whether P_{TP} was increased by increasing P_A relative to P_{PL} or by decreasing P_{PL} relative to P_A. This relationship represents the true compliance curve of the lung. The curved lines represent the pressure-volume relationships that would be obtained during a dynamic inspiration and expiration. The horizontal distance at any volume between the dynamic and static curves represents the pressure needed to overcome the resistance to air flow through the lungs. The effect of airway resistance on the pressure-volume curves of the lung is introduced here only to demonstrate that lung compliance curves must be obtained under static conditions (when no flow is occurring). For this reason, the rest of the discussion of lung compliance assumes static measurements. An increase in lung compliance (a flabby lung) would be evident as an increase in the slope of the pressure-volume relationship, whereas a decrease in lung compliance (a stiff lung) would be indicated by a decrease in the slope of the pressure-volume relationship. Hypothetic compliance curves representing increased and decreased lung compliances, respectively, are presented in Figures 13–4b and c.

Chest Wall Compliance

The chest wall is also an elastic structure. Although the chest wall is nonlinear over its entire range of volumes, it, like the lung, can be considered linear over its middle range of volumes (see Fig. 13–10). In a manner analogous to that of the lung, the compliance of the chest wall (see Fig. 13–6) is defined as the change in thoracic volume divided by the distending pressure on the thorax, P_{CW}. P_{CW} is the difference between the pressure at the inside surface of the chest wall (the pleural pressure) and the pressure at the outside surface of the chest wall (the atmospheric pressure). Thus,

$$P_{CW} = P_{PL} - P_{ATM}. \qquad (13–2)$$

Unlike the lung, which recoils only inward, the chest wall recoils either inward or outward, depending on the volume of the chest.

For the purposes of discussing the elastic properties of the chest wall, consider the hypothetic thought experiment illustrated by Figure 13–5. Assume that the thoracic contents (heart, lungs, etc.) have been removed and that the chest wall has been sewn up to be air tight. The pressure throughout the empty cavity is still the pressure at the inner surface of the chest wall and, as such, can be called the pleural pressure. If, under conditions of relaxed respiratory muscles, the volume of the thorax is now adjusted so that the pleural pressure is zero, the thorax is at its *unstressed volume* (V_0), in which case the chest wall will not recoil in either direction (see Fig. 13–5a). That is, when the thorax is at its unstressed volume (V equals V_0), the compliant parts of the chest wall are placed under no tension, thus P_{PL} equals 0. If, while the muscles are still relaxed, air is removed from the thorax so that the thoracic volume is less than the unstressed volume (V is less than V_0), the compliant elements of the chest wall are placed under tension and recoil in the outward direction (indicated by the arrows, see Fig. 13–5b). The outward recoil creates a negative pleural pressure. If volume is now added to the thorax (muscles relaxed) until the thoracic volume is greater than the unstressed volume (V is greater than V_0), the compliant elements of the chest wall are again placed under tension and recoil in the inward direction (see Fig. 13–5c). This inward recoil creates a positive pleural pressure.

The pressure-volume relationship obtained in this manner represents the compliance curve of the chest wall, and the change in volume divided

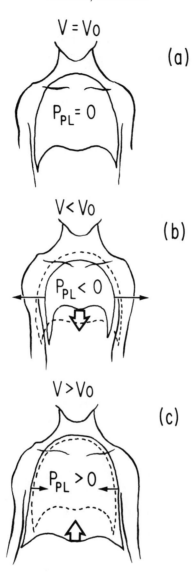

Fig. 13–5. Chest wall recoil illustrated for three hypothetic situations in which the lungs are absent. *(a):* The intrathoracic pressure is atmospheric so that the thoracic volume equals the unstressed thoracic volume ($V = V_0$), i.e., there is no deformation of the chest wall so pleural pressure (P_{PL}) equals ambient pressure (0). *(b):* Air is removed from the thorax so that thoracic volume is less than the unstressed thoracic volume ($V < V_0$). When $V < V_0$, the chest wall recoils in the outward direction and P_{PL} (intrathoracic pressure) becomes subatmospheric. *(c):* Air is forced into the thorax so that thoracic volume is greater than the unstressed thoracic volume ($V > V_0$). When $V > V_0$, the chest wall recoils in the inward direction, and pleural pressure becomes greater than atmospheric pressure. The dashed lines represent V_0. (From Green, J.F.: Mechanical Concepts in Cardiovascular and Pulmonary Physiology. Philadelphia, Lea & Febiger, 1977.)

by the change in pleural pressure defines the compliance of the chest wall. If the thorax were stiffer than normal (less compliant), the same volume added to or removed from the thorax would create a greater change in pleural pressure. If the thorax were flabbier than normal (more compliant), the same volume change would create a smaller change in pleural pressure.

A hypothetic compliance curve of a normal chest wall is plotted in Figure 13–6. Figures 13–6b and c represent the volume-pressure relationships that would be obtained from chest walls of increased and decreased compliances, respectively. Although the thorax was considered as having no contents, the analysis would be identical if the heart and lungs were in the thorax because thoracic contents merely represent volume. Thus, if we take a deep breath (so that thoracic volume is greater than V_0) and relax our muscles of respiration against a closed airway,

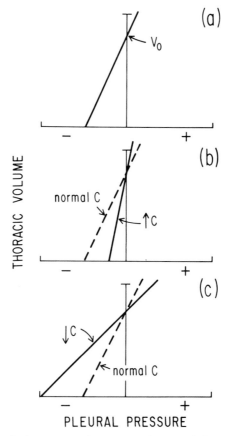

Fig. 13–6. *(a):* Hypothetic pressure-volume curve of a normal chest wall. V_0 = unstressed volume. *(b):* Hypothetic pressure-volume curve of a chest wall with increased compliance and *(c)* with decreased compliance. (From Green, J.F.: Mechanical Concepts in Cardiovascular and Pulmonary Physiology. Philadelphia, Lea & Febiger, 1977.)

pleural pressure becomes positive because of the inward recoil of the chest wall. Similarly, if we exhale to a low volume (so that thoracic volume is less than V_0) and relax our muscles of respiration against a closed airway, pleural pressure becomes negative because of the outward recoil of the chest wall. Try it, and feel the direction the chest wall wants to move.

In the preceding example, the respiratory muscles were considered relaxed. This is essential for the analysis because when the muscles are contracted (against a closed glottis) pressure swings are superimposed on the purely elastic pressure-volume relationship. Consider what happens at any given but constant thoracic volume. Contraction of the expiratory muscles causes an increase in pleural pressure, whereas contraction of the inspiratory muscles causes a decrease in pleural pressure. The magnitude of the change in pleural pressure caused by contraction of the respiratory muscles at constant volume is related to the contractile properties of the muscles, but provides no information about the elastic properties of the lung or chest wall.

Thus, the ratio of the change in lung volume to change in transthoracic pressure under conditions of relaxed respiratory muscles is, by definition, the compliance of the chest wall and is an index of chest wall elasticity. An important fact arising from this relationship is that the pleural pressure under relaxed conditions with glottis closed is determined only by the elastic properties of the chest wall and the volume of the thorax. If the respiratory muscles are contracted at constant volume, the pleural pressure is further determined by the magnitude of contraction—more positive (less negative) if the expiratory muscles are contracted and less positive (more negative) if the inspiratory muscles are contracted. The presence (or absence) of the heart and lung has no effect on pleural pressure except that the volume of the thorax is usually determined by the volume of the lungs.

Functional Residual Capacity

At the end of a normal expiration, when the muscles of respiration are relaxed, the lung-chest wall system comes to rest at a volume known as the functional residual capacity (FRC). What determines FRC? The lung is anatomically independent of but functionally linked to the chest wall by a thin layer of fluid that lines the visceral and parietal pleurae. The thin layer of pleural fluid actually holds the visceral and parietal pleurae together in much the same way that a thin layer of water between two sheets of glass holds the sheets together. Thus, the elastic recoil characteristics of the lung can influence the chest wall and vice versa. FRC is determined when the inward-acting recoil of the lung just balances the outward-acting recoil of the chest wall (Fig. 13–7). The pressure-volume curves of both the lung and the chest wall are plotted on the same coordinates in Figure 13–8. FRC occurs when the transmural

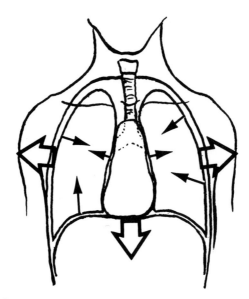

Fig. 13–7. Lung-chest wall system illustrated at functional residual capacity (FRC). The elastic recoil of the lung tends to pull the chest wall in, and the elastic recoil of the chest wall tends to pull the lung out. FRC occurs when the inward elastic recoil of the lung just balances the outward elastic recoil of the chest wall. (From Green, J.F.: Mechanical Concepts in Cardiovascular and Pulmonary Physiology. Philadelphia, Lea & Febiger, 1977.)

pressure of the lungs (the transpulmonary pressure) is equal but opposite to the transmural pressure of the chest wall (the pleural pressure).

Compliance of the Lung Plus Chest Wall

The relationship of thoracic volume to distending pressure of the lung-chest wall system, known as the *transthoracic pressure,* is the total compliance of the lungs plus chest wall. The transthoracic pressure (P_{TT}) is the sum of the transpulmonary pressure plus the distending pressure of the chest wall:

$$P_{TT} = P_{TP} + P_{CW,}$$

or

$$P_{TT} = (P_A - P_{PL}) + (P_{PL} - P_{ATM}).$$

Because all pressures are referred to atmospheric pressure and because these measurements are usually made under static conditions, where alveolar pressure is equal to tracheal pressure (P_T),

$$P_{TT} = P_T. \tag{13–3}$$

Thus, under static conditions, when the muscles of respiration are relaxed (or paralyzed), a pressure applied to the trachea opposes the elastic recoil of the lung plus the elastic recoil of the chest wall. The lung always

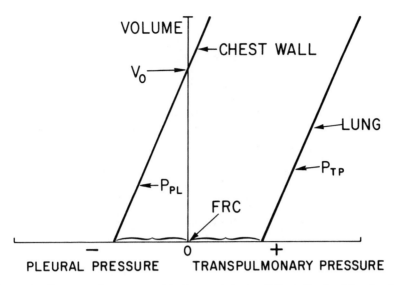

Fig. 13–8. Pressure-volume curves of the lung and chest wall illustrating the determinants of functional residual capacity (FRC). FRC occurs when the elastic recoil of the lung is equal but opposite to that of the chest wall. These lines represent relaxation curves. They are applicable only to relaxed expiration from TLC to FRC point. The actual pleural pressure is different from this during normal inspiration. P_{TP} = transpulmonary pressure and P_{PL} = pleural pressure. (From Green, J.F.: Mechanical Concepts in Cardiovascular and Pulmonary Physiology. Philadelphia, Lea & Febiger, 1977.)

recoils in an inward direction; however, the direction of the chest wall recoil depends on the thoracic (lung) volume. When the thorax is at its unstressed volume (V_0), the chest wall recoils in neither direction and a pressure applied at the trachea at this volume opposes only lung recoil. It is, therefore, equal to the transpulmonary pressure. When the thorax is at a volume greater than V_0, both the lung and chest wall recoil inward, and a pressure applied at the trachea at this volume opposes the inward recoil of both the lung and chest wall. When the thorax is at a volume less than V_0, the chest wall recoil is opposite to that of the lung, and a pressure applied to the trachea at this volume is less than the transpulmonary pressure because of the "help" provided by the outward-recoiling chest wall. At FRC, when the inward recoil of the lung is just balanced by the outward recoil of the chest wall, no pressure need be applied at the trachea to oppose the elastic recoil of the lung plus chest wall. The compliance curves of the lung and chest wall, plus the series compliance curve (marked total) of the lung plus chest wall, are plotted in Figure 13–9. The total curve represents the force that must be applied at the trachea to oppose the elastic recoil of the lung plus chest wall.

Until now, we have assumed linear static compliance for the lung, chest wall, and total respiratory system. As we discussed earlier, this assumption is correct over the middle range of lung volume, immediately

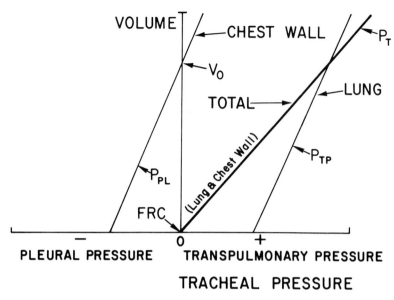

Fig. 13–9. Compliance curves of the lung and chest wall and the series compliance curve (marked total) of the lung plus chest wall. P_T = tracheal pressure, P_{TP} = transpulmonary pressure, and P_{PL} = pleural pressure. (From Green, J.F.: Mechanical Concepts in Cardiovascular and Pulmonary Physiology. Philadelphia, Lea & Febiger, 1977.)

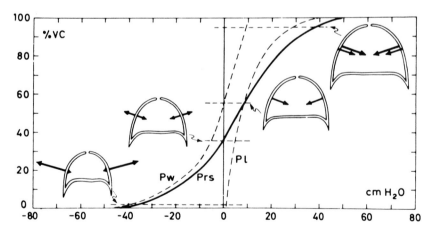

Fig. 13–10. Static pressure-volume curves of the lung, chest wall, and total respiratory system during relaxation in the upright posture. The static forces of the lung and chest wall are pictured by the arrows in the drawings. The volume corresponding to each drawing is indicated by the horizontal broken lines. (From Agostoni, and Mead: Statics of the respiratory system. In Handbook of Physiology. Bethesda, American Physiological Society, 1963.)

above FRC; however, these compliances become alinear at high and low lung volumes. The static pressure-volume curves of the intact lung, chest wall, and total respiratory system over the entire range of vital capacity are presented in Figure 13–10.

PRESSURE-FLOW RELATIONSHIPS OF PULMONARY AIRWAYS

Spontaneous Ventilation

The pressure-flow relationships of the pulmonary airways are not unlike those of the circulatory system. The pressures and resistances must be considered. Also, the pressure-volume relationships of the lung must be taken into account because the elasticity of the lung is, in large part, responsible for the driving pressure for air flow in much the same way that the elasticity of the systemic veins determines to a large extent the upstream driving pressure for venous return.

A basic schematic drawing of the pulmonary airways is presented in Figure 13–11, which is another lumped parameter model. All alveoli are lumped together and represented by a spherical elastic element. Similarly, all airways between the mouth and the alveoli are lumped into a single equivalent airway. The box surrounding the lung represents the thorax.

There is one major difference in the pressure-flow relationships of the pulmonary airways compared with those of the circulation. In the circulation, the direction of flow is always the same, i.e., from arteries to veins. In the pulmonary airways, the direction of flow reverses periodically. Air moves in and out, in and out, and so forth. Thus, our discussion of air flow in the lungs should be broken into two categories: inspiration and expiration.

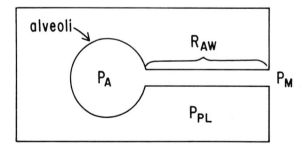

Fig. 13–11. Lumped parameter model of the pulmonary airways. P_A = alveolar pressure, P_M = mouth pressure, P_{PL} = pleural pressure, and R_{AW} = airway resistance. (From Green, J.F.: Mechanical Concepts in Cardiovascular and Pulmonary Physiology. Philadelphia, Lea & Febiger, 1977.)

The pressure-flow relationships of the pulmonary airways during inspiration may be described by the following expression:

$$\dot{V}_I = \frac{P_M - P_A}{R_{AW}}, \tag{13–4}$$

where $\dot{V}$ is inspiratory flow,[*] P_M is pressure at the mouth, P_A is pressure in the alveoli, and R_{AW} is airway resistance. The pressure-flow relationships of the pulmonary airways during expiration are similarly described by

$$\dot{V}_E = \frac{P_A - P_M}{R_{AW}}, \tag{13–5}$$

where $\dot{V}_E$ is expiratory air flow. To draw air into the lungs, the mouth pressure (upstream pressure) must be greater than the alveolar pressure (downstream pressure). To expire air from the lungs, the alveolar pressure (now the upstream pressure) must be greater than the downstream mouth pressure. The pressure at the mouth is atmospheric pressure, except during periods of positive pressure ventilation (see the following). It remains constant over any given respiratory cycle. Therefore, the determinants of alveolar pressure become important because they determine the magnitude of the pressure drop down the airways.

To consider alveolar pressure, we must also consider the pressure-volume characteristics of the lungs, a subject previously discussed in terms of pulmonary compliance. At FRC (functional residual capacity), the elastic recoil of the lung is equal to and opposite that of the chest wall, and the lung-chest wall system is stationary. Being stationary, the alveolar pressure is equal to mouth pressure. There is no pressure gradient and, therefore, no flow. The lungs nevertheless are inflated, which necessitates a positive transpulmonary pressure. This inflation is accomplished by the subatmospheric pleural pressure, which is generated by the outward recoil of the chest wall. As inspiration commences, the muscles of inspiration contract, causing pleural pressure to fall. The drop in pleural pressure is transmitted to the alveoli, and alveolar pressure falls relative to mouth pressure.[†] Figure 13–12a illustrates the temporal changes in pleural and alveolar pressures that occur during inspiration and expiration.

The drop in alveolar pressure with inspiration establishes a pressure gradient, and air rushes in to expand the lungs. The lung volume is greater at end-inspiration (TV, Fig. 13–12) than at FRC. Therefore, the

---

[*]When speaking of air, the symbol V is used to represent air volume and $\dot{V}$ to represent air volume per unit time or air flow. The symbolic language used in cardiovascular and pulmonary physiology is summarized and defined in Appendix 1.
[†]All pressures are measured relative to atmospheric pressure. Because mouth pressure is equal to atmospheric pressure, alveolar pressure falls to a subatmospheric pressure.

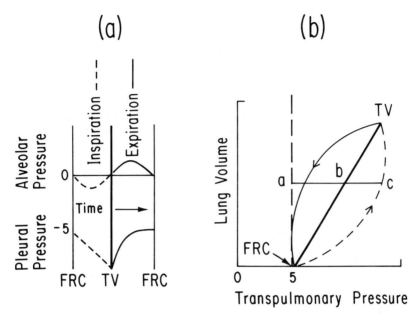

Fig. 13–12. *(a):* Respiratory pressures as a function of time throughout the respiratory cycle. FRC = functional residual capacity and TV = tidal volume. *(b):* Pressure-volume diagram of the lung illustrating the difference between the static and the dynamic transpulmonary pressure. Line segment a—b represents the static component of transpulmonary pressure; line segment b—c represents the dynamic component. (From Green, J.F.: Mechanical Concepts in Cardiovascular and Pulmonary Physiology. Philadelphia, Lea & Febiger, 1977.)

elastic recoil of the lung is greater. (The increase in lung volume during a normal inspiration is called a tidal volume, TV.) As the muscles of inspiration relax, the lung is allowed to recoil inward. This inward recoil at this higher lung volume is unopposed by the chest wall; therefore, the inward recoil elevates alveolar pressure relative to mouth pressure, thereby establishing a pressure gradient for expiration. Expiration continues until the elastic recoil of the lung directed inward is again equal to the outward recoil of the chest wall. When this occurs, the lung-chest wall system has returned to FRC, alveolar pressure is equal to mouth pressure, and expiration has ended (FRC, see Fig. 13–12).

During inspiration, the dynamic transpulmonary pressure increases (i.e., the transpulmonary pressure measured during the period when air rushes in). There are basically two components to this increase: (1) the increase in transpulmonary pressure necessary to overcome the elastic properties of the lung, the so-called static transpulmonary pressure, and (2) the further increase in dynamic transpulmonary pressure needed to overcome resistance forces, mostly resistance to air flow.

Figure 13–12b illustrates a hypothetic pressure-volume diagram of the lung. Initially, the lung is at FRC with a transmural pressure of about 5 cm H_2O. The transpulmonary pressure is then increased to 10 cm H_2O, and the lung inflates to TV. Therefore, line segment FRC-TV represents the static compliance curve of the lung. At any volume between the two static points, the dynamic transpulmonary pressure is greater than the static transpulmonary pressure by an amount proportional to the amount of air moving into the lung per unit time (the air flow) and the resistance to air flow. In Figure 13–12b line segment a-b represents the static transpulmonary pressure, and line segment b-c represents the added component necessary to overcome the resistance to air flow.* Equation 13–4 shows that segment b-c is equal to $\dot{V}_I R_{AW}$ or to alveolar pressure (mouth pressure remaining at atmospheric pressure). In a similar manner, the dynamic transpulmonary pressure during expiration is less than the static transpulmonary pressure by an amount proportional to the air flow and to the resistance to air flow.

Forced Expiration

During spontaneous breathing, expiration is passive because of the elastic recoil of the lung. The muscles of expiration are brought into play during a forced expiration. Such an expiration becomes active. Recall that, at any given lung volume, the transpulmonary pressure is a function of the elastic property of the lungs. Thus, the transpulmonary pressure can be thought of as an elastic recoil pressure, P_{EL}, such that P_{EL} equals P_A minus P_{PL}, where P_A and P_{PL} are alveolar and pleural pressures, respectively. This expression can be rearranged as:

$$P_A = P_{EL} + P_{PL}. \tag{13–6}$$

During a forced expiration, the contraction of the expiratory muscles causes the pleural pressure to rise to a positive pressure. Equation 13–6 demonstrates that this pressure is transmitted directly to the alveoli. The large rise in alveolar pressure that results during an active respiratory effort produces tremendous expiratory flow. This flow, however, becomes limited at some point, and greater expiratory efforts do not increase flow. This maximum expiratory flow ($\dot{V}_{E\ MAX}$) that is effort independent can be accounted for on the basis of the pressure-flow relationship of Starling resistors. The pleural pressure is the effective surrounding pressure of the large, extrapulmonary, intrathoracic air-

---

*A small component of segment b-c would be elastic resistance created by movement or distortions of lung tissue and chest wall. Fortunately, this is normally small enough to be ignored. Another component of segment b-c, which at times can be significant, is pressure drops in the airways caused by convection acceleration as defined by the Bernoulli equation:

$$P_{TP} = \frac{\rho}{2} \left(\frac{1}{A_2^2} \frac{1}{A_1^2} \right) \dot{V}_I,$$

where ρ is density of the air and A is area of the airway at two different points.

ways. As pleural pressure rises with increasing expiratory effort, it reaches a point where it equals the pressure within these large airways. When this occurs, the airways collapse and begin to function as Starling resistors. Recall that the driving pressure for flow through a Starling resistor is the upstream pressure (in this case, the alveolar pressure) minus the surrounding pressure (here, the pleural pressure, see Chap. 4). Thus, one can apply the pressure-flow relationships of a Starling resistor to the pulmonary airway:

$$\dot{V}_{E\ MAX} = \frac{P_A - P_{PL}}{R_{AW}}. \tag{13–7}$$

Substituting Equation 13–6 into this expression yields:

$$\dot{V}_{E\ MAX} = \frac{P_{EL}}{R_{AW}}. \tag{13–8}$$

Thus, under conditions of large airway collapse, the pleural pressure acts both as part of the upstream pressure (P_A) and as back pressure. Consequently, when collapse occurs, the driving pressure for flow is generated simply from the inward elastic recoil of the lung. A greater muscular effort, which increases pleural pressure, has no effect on flow because the effect of pleural pressure on alveolar pressure is exactly counterbalanced by the back-pressure effect of pleural pressure. A convenient way of demonstrating maximum effort-independent flow caused by airway collapse is the *expiratory volume-flow curve*. (From convention, volume is plotted on the ordinate and flow on the abscissa.)

Figure 13–13 shows a series of expiratory volume-flow curves obtained from a normal healthy individual. In traces A, B, and C, expiration starts

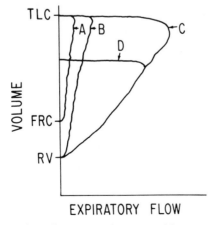

Fig. 13–13. Expiratory volume-flow curves. TLC = total lung capacity, FRC = functional residual capacity, and RV = residual volume. (From Green, J.F.: Mechanical Concepts in Cardiovascular and Pulmonary Physiology. Philadelphia, Lea & Febiger, 1977.)

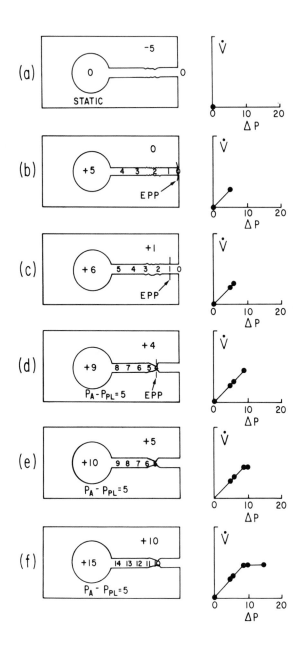

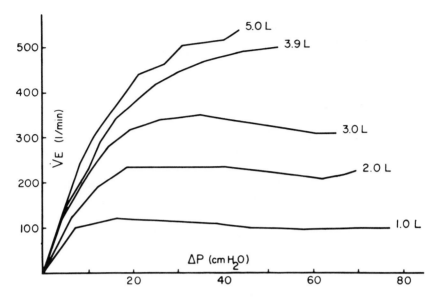

Fig. 13–15. A family of isovolume pressure-flow curves at different lung volumes above residual volume in a normal man. Note that the greater the lung volume, the greater the flow when airway collapse occurs (plateau). Contrast these isovolume pressure-flow curves with the expiratory volume-flow curves presented in Figure 13–10. (From Pride, N.B., et al.: Determinants of maximal expiratory flow from the lungs. J. Appl. Physiol., *23*(5):646, 1967.)

Fig. 13–14. Schematic drawing of the airway dynamics responsible for the isovolume pressure-flow curve. The collapsible portion of the airway is represented in the model by wavy lines. Panel (a) illustrates a static condition. Pleural pressure is −5 units, and alveolar pressure is atmospheric. Because the pressure drop down the airways is zero, flow is zero. Transpulmonary pressure is 5 units and remains 5 in all panels because the lung volume remains the same (isovolume). As expiratory effort begins (panel b) and pleural pressure rises from −5 to 0 to +1 (panel c), alveolar pressure rises from 0 to +5 to +6. As a pressure gradient between alveoli and mouth (ΔP) is now established, flow begins and increases. As flow increases, the equal pressure point (EPP), or the point where airway pressure equals pleural pressure, moves back toward the alveoli. In panel (d), pleural pressure has risen sufficiently to cause the equal pressure point to reach the collapsible segment of airway. When this occurs, the airway collapses and begins to function as a Starling resistor, i.e., the pleural pressure becomes the back pressure. Once collapse occurs, any further rise in pleural pressure (panels e and f) results in an equal rise in alveolar pressure and back pressure; therefore, the pressure gradient for flow ($P_A = P_{PL}$) remains constant and flow remains constant despite an increasing ΔP ($P_A - P_M$). (From Green, J.F.: Mechanical Concepts in Cardiovascular and Pulmonary Physiology. Philadelphia, Lea & Febiger, 1977.)

at total lung capacity (TLC). Trace A shows the flow with decreasing volume to FRC during a relaxed expiration, and trace B shows the volume-flow changes during some submaximal expiratory effort to residual volume (RV). Trace C is a maximal expiratory flow curve. Increasing the expiratory effort from TLC neither increases the flow nor moves the curve farther to the right of trace C. In addition, any expiratory effort at any other lung volume does not increase the maximum expiratory flow. Trace D shows the expiratory flow during a forced expiration starting at 75 percent TLC. Note that the flow follows the maximal expiratory flow curve (trace C). If a maximal expiratory effort is started at any lung volume, the maximal flow never exceeds that of trace C, but follows C to RV. Airway collapse occurs along the descending portion of curve C. Flow decreases when collapse occurs because the lung volume decreases as expiration continues. A lower lung volume means a lower elastic recoil (P_{EL}) and, therefore, from Equation 13–8, a lower flow. Thus, Equation 13–8 can represent an infinite number of points along the descending limb of the expiratory volume-flow curve depending on lung volume, which is constantly changing.

Effort-independent expiratory flow caused by large airway collapse can also be viewed through the *isovolume pressure-flow relationship.* By drawing a horizontal line at any volume in Figure 13–13, one can see that flow increases with increasing effort (we go from trace A to trace B to trace C); thereafter, flow shows no further increase despite increasing effort (there is no curve to the right of C). Expiratory effort may be measured as the difference between the pressure within the alveoli (P_A) and mouth pressure (P_M), ΔP. Figure 13–14 illustrates schematically the airway dynamics responsible for the isovolume pressure-flow curve. Figure 13–15 shows a series of isovolume pressure-flow curves obtained in the human at different lung volumes. The expiratory air flow of the human subject was interrupted at a selected lung volume; the subject then increased expiratory effort against a closed valve until the mouth pressure (which was equal to alveolar pressure because flow was zero) reached a preset value at which the valve opened. Expiratory flow immediately after valve opening was plotted against mouth pressure (alveolar pressure) immediately before valve opening. This procedure was repeated a number of times at the same lung volume and then at different lung volumes. Thus, each curve presented in Figure 13–15 was constructed from multiple data points. Note that flow increased as effort increased until a critical ΔP was reached; thereafter, flow remained relatively constant (trace C in Fig. 13–13 had been reached). At the critical ΔP, where flow remained constant, the airways collapsed.

In Chapter 4 we discussed the pressure-flow relationships of collapsible tubes and presented a plot of flow against the difference between inflow and outflow pressures for a hypothetic example (see Fig. 4–10A). A comparison of Figure 13–15 with Figure 4–10A reveals marked simi-

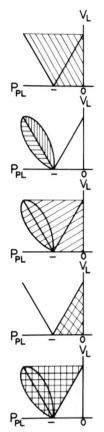

AREA A ($\backslash\backslash\backslash$) = WORK OF INSPIRATION FROM FRC TO OVERCOME RECOIL OF LUNG.

AREA B ($\equiv$) = WORK TO OVERCOME R_{AW} DURING INSPIRATION FROM FRC.

AREA C ($|||$) = ENERGY STORED IN ELASTIC TISSUES TO OVERCOME R_{AW} DURING EXPIRATION TO FRC.

AREA D ($\diagup\diagup$) = TOTAL WORK OF INSPIRATION FROM FRC TO OVERCOME RECOIL OF LUNG PLUS R_{AW}.

AREA E ($\times\!\times\!\times$) = ENERGY STORED IN CHEST WALL DURING EXPIRATION.

AREA F ($\#\#\#$) = NET INSPIRATORY WORK OF SYSTEM FROM FRC (LESS THAN JUST LUNGS–AREA D– BECAUSE OF HELP FROM CHEST WALL).

Fig. 13–16. Work of breathing. (From Green, J.F.: Mechanical Concepts in Cardiovascular and Pulmonary Physiology. Philadelpha, Lea & Febiger, 1977.)

larities. The figures are similar because they represent the same phenomenon.

WORK OF BREATHING

Work, defined as the product of pressure times volume, must be done for breathing to occur. This *work of breathing* results from energy expended by the respiratory muscles not only to expand the lung, but also to overcome airway resistance. Figure 13–16 defines the different types of work that are done during the process of breathing.

14

PULMONARY GAS EXCHANGE

GAS EXCHANGE THROUGH THE INDIVIDUAL PULMONARY CAPILLARY

The amount of gas exchanged by the lung is determined by the metabolic requirements of the body as a whole; however, gas exchange is accomplished by simple diffusion at the level of the pulmonary capillary. For gases, the driving force for diffusion is the difference in partial pressure of the gas (Stacy, 1955 and Brown, 1974). We can, thus, describe the diffusion of dissolved gases across the alveolar capillary membrane as follows:

$$J_{gas} = \frac{DA}{d} (P_1 - P_2),\qquad(14–1)$$

where J_{gas} is the flux of gas; D is the diffusion coefficient; d is the thickness of the alveolar membrane; A is the area of the membrane; and $P_1 - P_2$ is the difference in partial pressure of the gas. This equation is an expression of Fick's law of diffusion. The amount of gas transferred across the alveolar membrane as well as the partial pressure difference on both sides of the pulmonary capillary can usually be measured (or at least accurately estimated); however, the length of the diffusion path and the surface area of the diffusion membrane cannot be measured in the lung. Thus, the diffusion coefficient cannot be determined. Nevertheless, the overall diffusion characteristic of the lung can be assessed by lumping the quantities DA/d from Equation 14–1 into a single term called the *diffusion capacity* of the lung, D_L. Using oxygen as an important

example, one can obtain the following expression relating the determinants of oxygen transfer at each point along the pulmonary capillary:

$$\dot{V}_{O_2} = D_L \, (P_{AO_2} - P_{CO_2}), \tag{14-2}$$

where $\dot{V}_{O_2}$ is the amount of oxygen transferred per unit time; P_{AO_2} is
the partial pressure in the alveoli; and P_{CO_2} is the partial pressure of
oxygen in the capillary blood. Figure 14-1 presents a schematic representation of the expected moment-to-moment changes in the P_{O_2} of the
pulmonary blood along the course of the pulmonary capillary (heavy
line marked P_C). The oxygen transferred at *each point* along the capillary
can be described by Equation 14-2. In this example, the partial pressure
of oxygen in the alveoli (P_A) is 100 mm Hg. The pulmonary venous
blood entering the capillary has a P_{O_2} of 40 mm Hg. Thus, the P_{O_2}
difference across the alveolar wall at the beginning of the capillary is 60
mm Hg (100 − 40). This relatively large gradient initiates an immediate
and rapid transfer of oxygen, which decreases as the gradient decreases.
By the time the blood reaches the end of the capillary, the P_{O_2} is raised
almost to equilibrium with the alveolar gas. Because determining the
moment-to-moment change in P_{O_2} along the pulmonary capillary is impossible, thinking about the average transfer of oxygen along the pulmonary capillary is more useful. To accomplish this, we must only make
one small change in Equation 14-2 as follows:

$$\dot{V}_{O_2} = D_L \, (P_{AO_2} - P_{\overline{C}O_2}). \tag{14-3}$$

$P_{\overline{C}O_2}$ is the mean partial pressure oxygen in the pulmonary capillary,
and ($P_{AO_2} - P_{\overline{C}O_2}$) is the mean P_{O_2} difference across the alveolar-capillary wall. $P_{\overline{C}O_2}$ is the theoretic value of P_{O_2} that is needed to permit
the diffusion of the same amount of oxygen as actually occurs along the
capillary. The changing capillary oxygen tension (P_C) is shown by the
curve in Figure 14-1. The line marked $P_{\overline{C}}$ gives the mean value of capillary P_{O_2} for the example in Figure 14-1. The cross-hatched area below
this line shows the actual amount by which the rate of oxygen transfer
exceeds the mean rate at the beginning of the capillary. The cross-hatched
area above this line shows the amount by which the actual rate of oxygen
transfer falls below the mean rate at the end of the pulmonary capillary.
Note that the oxygen tension in the blood at the end of the pulmonary
capillary under normal conditions has almost, but not totally, achieved
equilibration with the oxygen in the alveolus. Thus, an alveolar-to-end-
capillary oxygen difference exists which represents a *diffusion limitation*.
Fortunately, when breathing room air (21 percent oxygen), this difference is physiologically insignificant (less than 1 mm Hg).

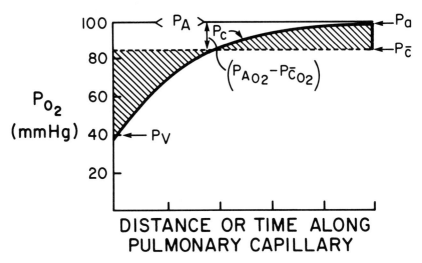

Fig. 14–1. Expected moment-to-moment changes in the partial pressure of oxygen along the course of a single pulmonary capillary in a person breathing room air. The various oxygen partial pressures are as follows: P_A = alveolar; P_C = capillary; P_V = mixed venous; P_a = arterial; $P_{\bar{C}}$ = mean capillary. Note the small alveolar-end capillary partial pressure gradient.

GAS EXCHANGE THROUGH THE LUNG AS A WHOLE

If all the blood that leaves the lungs were to pass through ideal gas exchange units, such as the ideal theoretic capillary depicted in Figure 14–1, the partial pressure of oxygen in the arterial blood (e.g., measured from the aorta) would, for all practical purposes, be equal to that in the alveoli (i.e., a gradient less than 1 mm Hg). Because the P_{O_2} of the arterial blood is, on the average, 9 mm Hg less than that in the end-capillary blood of an ideal unit, all blood that leaves the lungs does not come from ideal gas exchanging units. Two principal reasons account for this *alveolar-to-arterial (A-a) gradient*. First, some small amount of blood totally bypasses the gas exchange areas of the lung through *anatomic shunts*, which are direct communications from the right to the left side of the pulmonary circulation. A second and far more complicated reason for A-a gradients is related to the fact that all alveoli do not receive blood flow in proportion to their ventilation. In fact, ventilation-perfusion ratios are distributed throughout the lung (Fig. 14–2). When ventilation is less than perfusion, the equilibrium pressure of oxygen in the alveoli (P_{AO_2}) is less than (and the P_{ACO_2} higher than) that depicted in Figure 14–1, which assumes equal ventilation and blood flow. When ventilation is greater than perfusion, the end-capillary P_{O_2} is greater than (and the P_{CO_2} is less than) that of the ideal gas exchanging units. Because of the shape of the CO_2-dissociation curve (see the following), deviations of the ventilation to perfusion ratio away from unity have little effect on arterial P_{CO_2}. There is also little effect on arterial P_{O_2} when the venti-

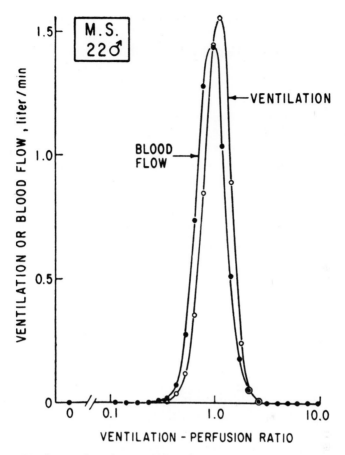

Fig. 14–2. Distribution of ventilation and blood flow in a normal 22-year-old man. Note that the curves are symmetric on a log scale with no areas of high or low ventilation-perfusion ratios. There is no shunt ($\dot{V}/\dot{Q} = 0$). (From Wagner, et al.: Continuous distribution of ventilation-perfusion ratios in normal subjects breathing air and 100% oxygen. J. Clin. Invest., *54*:54, 1974. Reproduced with permission of the publisher.)

lation-perfusion ratio exceeds unity as a result of the shape of the oxygen dissociation curve (see the following). Thus, the primary effect of ventilation-perfusion imbalance comes from the gas exchange units that have ventilation-perfusion ratios less than unity. Thus, when blood that is less than fully oxygenated is mixed with oxygenated blood, arterial P_{O_2} falls. In other words, the end result of a ventilation-perfusion imbalance is the same as an anatomic shunt; however, to distinguish it from anatomic shunt it is often called *alveolar shunt*. The depression of arterial P_{O_2} from both sources is usually lumped together and called *physiologic shunt* or *venous admixture*.

QUANTIFYING THE EFFECTS OF THE
VENTILATION-PERFUSION RELATIONSHIP

Because changes in ventilation and perfusion, or more precisely in the ratio of ventilation to perfusion, have immediate effects at the level of the local alveolar unit, we will first discuss how changes in ventilation and perfusion can affect gas exchange on the local level and will then show how these effects, when accumulated, can affect the gas exchange of the lung as a whole.

To get a feel for the effects of ventilation and perfusion, think of the individual alveolar unit as a mixing chamber. At constant alveolar ventilation ($\dot{V}_A$) and capillary blood flow ($\dot{Q}_C$),* gas tensions equilibrate by the time the blood reaches the end of the capillary. If we could somehow keep $\dot{Q}_C$ constant but increase $\dot{V}_A$, the partial pressure of CO_2 would fall whereas that of O_2 would rise. This would happen because the elevated ventilation would remove CO_2 from the alveolus faster than it could be delivered by the blood. Also, O_2 would be delivered to the alveolus faster than it could be removed by the blood (i.e., create a new equilibrium between blood and gas). If $\dot{V}_A$ remained constant while $\dot{Q}_C$ increased, P_{CO_2} would rise and P_{O_2} would fall.

The quantitative relationship of alveolar ventilation ($\dot{V}_A$) to capillary perfusion ($\dot{Q}_C$) can be demonstrated by simply applying a few mass balances. The amount of oxygen that crosses the alveolar-capillary membrane ($\dot{V}_{O_2}$) is equal to both the amount of oxygen lost by the alveolus and gained by the blood. On the alveolar side of the membrane, the amount of O_2 lost $\dot{V}_{O_2}$ is equal to the difference in the amount of oxygen inspired and the amount of oxygen expired from the given alveolus. Thus,

$$\dot{V}_A \, F_{I_{O_2}} - \dot{V}_A \, F_{A_{O_2}} = \dot{V}_{O_2}, \qquad (14\text{–}4)$$

where $F_{I_{O_2}}$ and $F_{A_{O_2}}$ are the fractions of oxygen in the inspired and alveolar air, respectively. On the blood side of the membrane, the amount of O_2 gained, $\dot{V}_{O_2}$ is equal to the difference between the amount of oxygen delivered to the alveolar unit in the mixed venous blood and the amount leaving in the end-capillary blood. Thus,

$$\dot{Q}_C \, C_{ca_{O_2}} - \dot{Q}_C \, C_{cv_{O_2}} = \dot{V}_{O_2}, \qquad (14\text{–}5)$$

where $C_{ca_{O_2}}$ and $C_{cv_{O_2}}$ are the contents of oxygen in the blood leaving (arterial) and entering (venous) the capillary, respectively. Because these

---

*To minimize words and to allow for the development of equations relating the many gas exchange variables, the use of symbols cannot be avoided. Wherever possible, the standard symbols listed in Appendix 1 are used. In the above derivation, the alveolus and blood regions of the individual alveolar units are distinguished by using the subscript "A" for the air side and "c" for the blood or capillary side. To further distinguish the various compartments of the lung, superscripts will be used. When in doubt, refer to Appendix 1 for clarification.

two relationships, representing the amount of oxygen that crosses the alveolar-capillary membrane, must be equal,

$$\dot{V}_A \, (F_{I_{O_2}} - F_{A_{O_2}}) = \dot{Q}_C \, (Cca_{O_2} - C_{CV_{O_2}}).$$

Solving for $\dot{V}_A/\dot{Q}_C$, yields

$$\frac{\dot{V}_A}{\dot{Q}_C} = \frac{Cca_{O_2} - C_{CV_{O_2}}}{F_{I_{O_2}} - F_{A_{O_2}}}. \tag{14-6}$$

A similar expression can be obtained for CO_2 (recalling that $F_{I_{CO_2}}$ equals zero):

$$\frac{\dot{V}_A}{\dot{Q}_C} = \frac{C_{CV_{CO_2}} - Cca_{CO_2}}{F_{A_{CO_2}}}. \tag{14-7}$$

From these relationships, we can see that for any given value of $F_{I_{O_2}}$, $C_{CV_{O_2}}$, and $C_{CV_{CO_2}}$, the values of $F_{A_{O_2}}$ and $F_{A_{CO_2}}$ and Cca_{O_2} and Cca_{CO_2} are a function of the ratio of ventilation to perfusion.

This relationship can be seen graphically with the aid of the *oxygen-carbon dioxide diagram* (Fig. 14–3). This diagram (derived in App. 3) shows all possible combinations of O_2 and CO_2 at different $\dot{V}_A/\dot{Q}_C$ ratios. The O_2-CO_2 diagram also illustrates another interesting fact; when $C_{CV_{O_2}}$, $C_{CV_{CO_2}}$, and $F_{I_{O_2}}$ remain constant, changes in $\dot{V}_A/\dot{Q}_C$ change the respi-

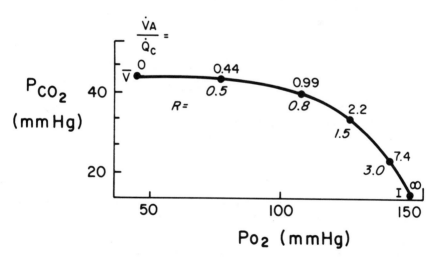

Fig. 14–3. Oxygen-carbon dioxide diagram representing all possible values of P_{CO_2} and P_{O_2} that are compatible with different ventilation-perfusion ratios ($\dot{V}_A/\dot{Q}_C$) and respiratory exchange ratios (R) in an alveolar unit receiving mixed venous blood with CO_2 and O_2 partial pressures equal to $\bar{v}$ and inspiratory gas CO_2 and O_2 partial pressures equal to I. (Redrawn from Cherniack, R.M., Cherniack, L., and Naimark, A.: Respiration in Health and Disease. 2nd Edition. Philadelphia, W. B. Saunders, 1972.)

ratory exchange ratio (R) of the individual alveolar unit. The reason for this change is simple—changing $\dot{V}_A/\dot{Q}_C$ changes $\dot{V}_{CO_2}$, $\dot{V}_{O_2}$ and, thus, the ratio of $\dot{V}_{CO_2}/\dot{V}_{O_2}$.

From the O_2-CO_2 diagram (see Fig. 14–3), one can see that lower-than-normal ventilation-perfusion ratios (less than approximately 1) depress arterial P_{O_2} in much the same way as does shunt flow. In fact, a ventilation-perfusion ratio of zero is, by definition, alveolar shunt. Similarly, one can see from the O_2-CO_2 diagram that greater-than-normal ventilation-perfusion ratios create alveolar gas tensions in the air leaving the lung that are similar to those that would occur if dead space was augmented above normal. In fact, a ventilation-perfusion ratio of infinity is, by definition, alveolar dead space.

THE "EFFECTIVE" COMPARTMENT

Because the blood that leaves the lung consists of blood from millions of individual alveolar units, each with separate ventilation-perfusion relationships, it is difficult to consider the effect of ventilation and perfusion without resorting to an intellectual trick that helps to conceptualize the process. Imagine that the arterial blood comes from only two compartments, one that consists of physiologic shunt and another in which all gas exchange occurs. This last compartment is called the *effective compartment*. Whereas the gas tensions in the blood leaving any individual alveolar unit are determined by the $\dot{V}_A/\dot{Q}_C$ ratio of the unit, the amount of oxygen and carbon dioxide that *must* be exchanged by the lung as a whole is determined by the metabolic needs of the body as a whole; that is, the R ratio of the body. Only one value of P_{O_2} and P_{CO_2} is compatible with the value of R. The effective compartment is then the imaginary compartment, *which would produce this P_{O_2} and P_{CO_2} if there were no ventilation-perfusion inhomogeneities and if no diffusion gradient existed.* (See App. 3 for a more detailed description of the effective P_{O_2} and P_{CO_2}.) Thus, when we think about the effective compartment of the lung, we recognize that, in many individual alveolar units, the $\dot{V}_A/\dot{Q}_C$ is greater than zero but less than normal and that the blood from these many units slightly depresses the arterial P_{O_2}.* The same effect would be produced if most of the alveoli were functioning with normal $\dot{V}_A/\dot{Q}_C$

Table 14–1.   Flows and Arterial Oxygen from a Hypothetic Six-Unit Lung

Alveolar Unit	1	2	3	4	5	6	Totals
Flow (L/min)	1.0	0.5	1.0	1.0	1.0	0.5	5
End-capillary O_2 content (vol %)	20	20	18	19	17	12	18

---

*In practice, alterations in $\dot{V}_A/\dot{Q}_C$ also affect CO_2 transport, but because of the shape of the CO_2 dissociation curve and the increase in ventilation that occurs, the P_{CO_2} in the arterial blood is virtually unchanged.

ratios, but a few with $\dot{V}_A/\dot{Q}_C$ ratios of zero. Thus, imagine that the entire depression of arterial P_{O_2} is caused by an alveolar shunt.* Consider the following hypothetic example. Suppose we had a lung with six different functioning alveolar units and with the flows and oxygen contents listed in Table 14–1. The total flow through this hypothetic lung is 5 L/min, and the oxygen content of the arterial blood is 18 vol %. A mass balance for this hypothetic lung can show how this arterial content is achieved: $1.0(20) + 0.5(20) + 1.0(18) + 1.0(19) + 1.0(17) + 0.5(12) = 5(18)$. Of course, in practice we would have no idea of the flow or oxygen content of each unit. We could, however, create an *as if* condition by assuming only two categories of alveoli: a perfect, effective category with no $\dot{V}_A/\dot{Q}_C$ mismatch and an alveolar shunt unit. If we assumed that the content of oxygen leaving the effective compartment was 20 vol %, we could then calculate that, if 4.5 L/min of flow from the effective compartment had mixed with 0.5 L/min of shunt flow, the same arterial content would have occurred. That is, $4.5(20) + 0.5(0)$ would equal $5(18)$. In other words, all our original six alveolar units that contributed to the depression in arterial P_{O_2} acted *as if* there were a true alveolar shunt of 0.5 L/min. In actual practice, we calculate values of the effective P_{O_2} and P_{CO_2} (by methods described later) and then, with the aid of the oxygen dissociation curve, find the arterial oxygen content to use in the calculation of shunt flow. The idea is, however, much the same as the mass balance from our hypothetic example.

In summary, A-a partial pressure differences of respiratory gases come from two sources: true anatomic shunts and blood leaving alveolar compartments with ventilation-perfusion imbalances. Blood from this latter compartment can be treated as an *as if* shunt, thereby allowing us to characterize the A-a difference as "physiologic" shunt.

CALCULATING PHYSIOLOGIC SHUNT

Because A-a partial pressure differences can be characterized as caused by physiologic shunts, it is useful to know how such shunts can be measured. This knowledge also allows us to illustrate how the shape of the O_2 and CO_2 dissociation curves affect gas exchange.

The total amount of oxygen that enters the systemic arterial system per unit time is the algebraic sum of that coming from the effective

---

*We can apply the same reasoning to demonstrate how $\dot{V}_A/\dot{Q}_C$ mismatches contribute to alveolar dead space.

compartment plus physiologic shunt. This can be shown by the following mass balance:

$$\dot{Q}_a\, C_{aO_2} = \dot{Q}_a^e\, C_{aO_2}^e + \dot{Q}_a^s\, C_{VO_2}, \qquad (14\text{–}8)$$

where C represents the content of oxygen (C_{aO_2} is arterial blood; $C_{aO_2}^e$ is effective compartment; and C_{VO_2} is mixed venous blood). A similar relationship can be written for CO_2:

$$\dot{Q}_a\, C_{aCO_2} = \dot{Q}_a^e\, C_{aCO_2}^e + \dot{Q}_a^s\, C_{VCO_2}. \qquad (14\text{–}9)$$

From these equations, one can easily see how adding shunt blood to the blood from the effective compartment lowers the content of oxygen in the arterial blood (because C_{VO_2} is less than $C_{aO_2}^e$) and raises the content of carbon dioxide (because C_{VCO_2} is greater than $C_{aCO_2}^e$). These relationships, in and of themselves, do not explain why the P_{O_2} of arterial blood is significantly lower than that of the blood from the effective compartment or why the P_{CO_2} remains virtually the same (as is the case). To understand this, one must appreciate the differences in the shapes of the oxygen and carbon dioxide dissociation curves (see Chap. 11).

Figure 14–4 presents an oxygen dissociation curve. To discover why shunt blood depresses the P_{aO_2}, consider a hypothetic example where a

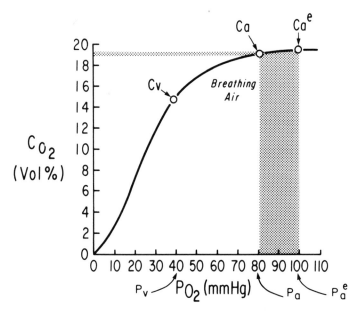

Fig. 14–4. Oxygen dissociation curve illustrating how a small amount of venous admixture (shunt blood) can depress the arterial P_{O_2} when the pulmonary system is "opening" on the flat upper portion of the dissociation curve. (Redrawn from Riley, R.L.: Gas exchange and transportation. *In* Physiology and Biophysics. 19th Edition. Edited by T. C. Ruch, and H. D. Patton. Philadelphia, W. B. Saunders, 1965.)

patient is breathing room air and 9 parts of blood from the effective compartment ($C_{aO_2}^e$ is 19.5) are mixed with 1 part of shunt blood (C_{VO_2} is 15). By mass balance, one sees that 9 (19.5) + 1 (15) = 10 (19). Thus, the content of the arterial blood is depressed by only 0.5 vol %. To find out what the changes are in the P_{O_2}, one must go to the oxygen dissociation curve (see Fig. 14–4). The $P_{aO_2}^e$ is equal to 100 mm Hg, and the P_{VO_2} is 40 mm Hg. Because we are "operating" on the flat upper portion of the dissociation curve, mixing these bloods results in a P_{aO_2} of 82 mm Hg. In other words, the nonlinear shape of the oxygen dissociation curve results in the depression of arterial P_{O_2}. A shunt of 10 percent, which depresses content by only 0.5 vol %, depresses P_{aO_2} nearly 20 mm Hg. It is important to emphasize that, when mixing bloods in a test tube or in our minds, we must *mix amounts* (contents), *not* partial pressures. Only contents are directly related to the number of oxygen molecules. Obviously, because the shape of the oxygen dissociation curves is so important, if we had started with a lower content in the blood from the effective compartment (i.e., because the patient was breathing air with a low percentage of oxygen) and had mixed shunt blood with this blood (with a still lower content), the depression in P_{O_2} would not have been as severe. This fact has important practical consequences when the diffusion capacity of the lung is measured by the oxygen method.

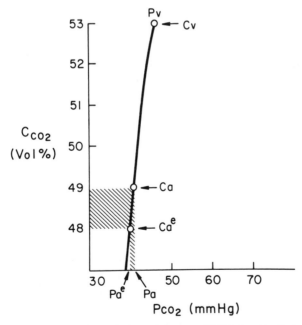

Fig. 14–5. Physiologic carbon dioxide dissociation curve illustrating the effect a small amount of venous admixture has on arterial P_{CO_2}. (Redrawn from Riley, R.L.: Gas exchange and transportation. *In* Physiology and Biophysics. 19th Edition. Edited by T. C. Ruch, and H. D. Patton. Philadelphia, W. B. Saunders, 1965.)

Because the *carbon dioxide* dissociation curve is steep over its operating range, the mixing of shunt blood with blood from the effective compartment does not significantly raise the P_{aCO_2}. Consider the hypothetic example illustrated in Figure 14–5. Mixing 4 parts of blood from the effective compartment ($C^e_{aCO_2}$ is 48) with 1 part of mixed venous blood (C_{VCO_2} is 53) results in the following mass balance: 4 (48) + 1 (53) equals 5 (49). This shunt is rather large (20 percent) and raises the CO_2 content in the arterial blood from the effective value of 48 to 49 vol %. Because of the linear carbon dioxide dissociation curve, the rise in P_{aCO_2} is somewhat less than 1 mm Hg (see Fig. 14–5).

To calculate the percentage of the total pulmonary blood flow (cardiac output) that can be attributed to shunt flow (alveolar plus anatomic), one must only remember that

$$\dot{Q}_a = \dot{Q}^e_a + \dot{Q}^s_a. \tag{14–10}$$

Solving Equation 14–10 for $\dot{Q}^e_a$ and substituting the result into Equation 14–8 yields, on rearrangement,

$$\frac{\dot{Q}^s_a}{\dot{Q}_a} = \frac{C^e_{aO_2} - C_{aO_2}}{C^e_{aO_2} - C_{VO_2}}. \tag{14–11}$$

Thus, if we measure three separate oxygen contents we can directly calculate the percentage shunt. We can sample arterial blood and thus measure C_{aO_2}, and we can sample mixed venous blood from the pulmonary artery* (with the aid of a Swan-Ganz catheter) and thus measure C_{VO_2}. However, sampling blood directly from the effective compartment is impossible. Fortunately, we can accurately calculate what $C^e_{aO_2}$ should be.

Determining Effective P_{CO_2} and P_{O_2} Values

As we just discussed large shunts have virtually no effect on the P_{CO_2} because of the shape of the carbon dioxide dissociation curve. Thus, we can consider the P_{CO_2} measured from the arterial blood (P_{aCO_2}) equal to that of the blood leaving the effective compartment ($P^e_{aCO_2}$). Given $P^e_{aCO_2}$, we could calculate $P^e_{aO_2}$ if we could find some easily measured relationship that relates the effective CO_2 and O_2 tensions. Fortunately, such a relationship can be found in the respiratory exchange ratio, R, which relates the amount of carbon dioxide produced by the body as a whole ($\dot{V}_{CO_2}$) to the oxygen consumption of the body as a whole ($\dot{V}_{O_2}$). Because the lungs subserve the needs of the body, the amount of gas exchanged by the lung is dictated by the metabolic requirements of the body. Effective gas exchange in the lungs can occur only where blood

---

*Venous blood does not become fully mixed until it passes through the right atrium.

and gas come together; that is, in the effective compartment. Because only one alveolar gas composition (P_{O_2} and P_{CO_2}) is compatible with the metabolic requirements of the body as a whole, this alveolar gas composition must be the effective value. Therefore, by relating the alveolar P_{O_2} and P_{CO_2} to the respiratory exchange ratio, we can determine the effective P_{O_2}. The relationship that makes this determination possible is the *alveolar gas equation*. This equation is nothing more than a rearrangement of the CO_2/O_2 exchange ratio in which the ratio is expressed in terms of the alveolar gases in the effective compartment. The full derivation of the alveolar gas equation (found in Appendix 3), although straightforward, requires algebra because various substitutions and corrections must be performed, such as for the differences in volume between inspiratory and expiratory gases. When all the algebra is complete, the following precise form of the alveolar gas equation results:

$$P^e_{E_{O_2}} = P_{I_{O_2}} - \left[F_{I_{O_2}} + \frac{1 - F_{I_{O_2}}}{R} \right] P^e_{E_{CO_2}}. \qquad (14\text{--}12)$$

$P^e_{E_{O_2}}$ and $P^e_{E_{CO_2}}$ are the partial pressures of oxygen and carbon dioxide in the effective compartment of the expired air,* $F_{I_{O_2}}$ is the inspired oxygen concentration, expressed as a fraction of the total; and R is the respiratory exchange ratio ($\dot{Q}_{CO_2}/\dot{V}_{O_2}$). R can be easily calculated by collecting a patient's expired air over a period of time and determining his oxygen uptake and carbon dioxide production. Because, for practical purposes, P_{aCO_2} equals $P^e_{aCO_2}$, which equals $P^e_{E_{CO_2}}$, we can directly substitute P_{aCO_2} for $P^e_{E_{CO_2}}$ in Equation 14–12 and, thus, calculate $P^e_{E_{O_2}}$. We can then determine the oxygen content in the blood leaving the effective compartment ($C^e_{aO_2}$) from the oxygen dissociation curve, assuming that $P^e_{E_{O_2}}$ equals $P^e_{aO_2}$.

Calculating Physiologic Dead Space

Physiologic dead space can be determined in a manner completely analogous to the calculation of shunt flow. We must first recognize that the total amount of carbon dioxide that enters the expired air is the algebraic sum of that coming from the effective compartment plus dead space (anatomic and alveolar). This amount can be shown by the following mass balance:

$$V_E F_{E_{CO_2}} = V^e_E F^e_{E_{CO_2}} + V^D_E F_{I_{CO_2}}, \qquad (14\text{--}13)$$

---

*Note: To distinguish between the alveolar and blood regions of the lung, we will use the subscripts "E" for the air side and "a" for the blood side. The "E" represents *expired air* because, in practice, all alveolar gas samples are measured from the expired air.

where F represents the fractional concentration of carbon dioxide ($F_{E_{CO_2}}$ = expired air; $F^e_{E_{CO_2}}$ = effective compartment; $F_{I_{CO_2}}$ = inspired air). Next, we must remember that

$$V_E = V^e_E + V^D_E. \qquad (14\text{–}14)$$

Solving Equation 14–14 for V^e_E and substituting the result into Equation 14–13 yields on rearrangement (after recognizing that $F_{I_{CO_2}} = 0$):

$$\frac{V^D_E}{V_E} = \frac{F^e_{E_{CO_2}} - F_{E_{CO_2}}}{F^e_{E_{CO_2}}}. \qquad (14\text{–}15)$$

Equation 14–15 can also be expressed in terms of partial pressures because F_{CO_2} equals $P_{CO_2}/(P_B - P_{H_2O})$.* Substituting this partial pressure statement into Equation 14–15, yields,

$$\frac{V^D_E}{V_E} = \frac{P^e_{E_{CO_2}} - P_{E_{CO_2}}}{P^e_{E_{CO_2}}}. \qquad (14\text{–}16)$$

Because $P^e_{E_{CO_2}}$ equals $P_{a_{CO_2}}$, we need only measure the P_{CO_2} in arterial blood and the expired air to calculate the dead space ratio.

Alveolar Ventilation Equation

As a direct consequence of our discussions about ventilation-perfusion relationships, we can derive an important relationship that allows one to assess the appropriateness of an individual's ventilation. Remembering that gas exchange occurs exclusively in the effective compartment and that, normally, CO_2 is not in the inspired air, we see that CO_2 output is the product of ventilation from the effective compartment ($\dot{V}^e_E$) and the fractional concentration of CO_2 in the gas. Thus,

$$\dot{V}_{CO_2} = \dot{V}^e_E \, F^e_{E_{CO_2}}. \qquad (14\text{–}17)$$

To express this relationship in terms of partial pressures, we simply substitute $F^e_{E_{CO_2}} = P^e_{E_{CO_2}}/(P_B - P_{H_2O})$ into Equation 14–17. We can further substitute $P_{a_{CO_2}}$ for $P^e_{E_{CO_2}}$, introduce the appropriate numeric values for P_B and P_{H_2O}, and add a factor to account for the dissimilar units in which $\dot{V}_{CO_2}$ and $\dot{V}^e_E$ are usually expressed.† The *alveolar ventilation equation* results:

$$P_{a_{CO_2}} = \frac{\dot{V}_{CO_2}}{\dot{V}^e_E} (.864). \qquad (14\text{–}18)$$

A normal value for $P_{a_{CO_2}}$ is approximately 40 mm Hg and means that

---

*P_B = barometric pressure and P_{H_2O} = water vapor pressure.
†$\dot{V}_{CO_2}$ is conventionally expressed in units of STPD (standard temperature, pressure and dry) whereas $\dot{V}^e_E$ is expressed in units of BTPS (body temperature, pressure and saturated with water vapors).

ventilation of the effective compartment is appropriate to the metabolic production of CO_2. This relationship is used commonly in clinical practice to appropriately adjust the frequency and tidal volume of a ventilator that is breathing for a patient. If the patient's P_{aCO_2} is above 40 mm Hg, $\dot{V}_E^e$ is generally inadequate; if P_{aCO_2} is lower than 40 mm Hg, $\dot{V}_E^e$ is usually not proportional to CO_2 production. Of course, clinical judgment dictates the appropriate limits for these values.

Measuring the Diffusion Capacity of the Lung

We began our discussion of pulmonary gas exchange by pointing out that the amount of gas exchange across the alveolar-capillary membrane is proportional to the average partial pressures on both sides of the membrane and that the constant of proportionality is called the diffusion capacity of the lung, D_L. In effect, D_L measures a kind of resistance of the path through which the gas passes. This pathway includes the diffusion across the alveolar membrane itself, across the interstitial fluid between the alveolus and the capillary, through the capillary membrane, through the plasma, and finally into the red blood cell. The units of D_L are ml of gas transferred per min per mm Hg pressure difference between the alveolar gas and the pulmonary capillary blood. D_L is useful because it can change from normal during various disease states when (1) the alveolar and/or capillary membrane is thickened or separated by excess fluid or (2) the surface area for exchange changes. The diffusion capacity also can be affected by the rate of chemical reaction of the gas with hemoglobin. In theory, a value of D_L can be calculated for any gas passing the alveolar-capillary membrane; however, for practical purposes related to ease of measurement, D_L is usually measured for carbon monoxide (CO) even though it is not a physiologic gas. Carbon monoxide is used to measure D_L because, until it reacts with hemoglobin, its behavior (i.e., mixing and diffusing properties) is much like that of oxygen. Two additional important properties make CO ideal for measuring D_L—its affinity for hemoglobin is about 210 times as great as that of O_2 and it is usually not present in venous blood (in nonsmokers). Thus, as soon as it enters the blood (in low concentrations), it becomes bound to hemoglobin and its partial pressure in the blood remains virtually zero. Consequently, the mean capillary P_{CO} can be considered zero, thereby greatly simplifying the calculation of D_L because the mean alveolar-capillary partial pressure differences ($P_{ACO_2} - P_{\bar{C}O_2}$) become simply P_{ACO}. The carbon monoxide diffusion capacity of the lung can then be measured as:

$$D_L = \frac{\dot{V}_{CO}}{P_{ACO}},\qquad (14\text{--}19)$$

where both $\dot{V}_{CO}$ and P_{ACO} are easily measured.

Causes for the Normally Occurring Ventilation-Perfusion Ratio

As was discussed in Chapter 9, gravity causes both pulmonary artery and pulmonary venous pressure to increase 1 cm H_2O pressure for each cm distance down the lung. This distribution of pressures results in the distribution of blood flow within the lungs to three major zones, depending on the magnitudes of these pressures (see Fig. 9–2). In the upper third of the lung (zone I), the alveolar pressure is greater than or equal to pulmonary artery pressure and there is no flow ($\dot{V}_A/\dot{Q}_C = \infty$). In the middle zone (zone II), pulmonary arterial pressure is greater than alveolar pressure, which is greater than pulmonary venous pressure. In zone II, flow through the pulmonary capillaries is proportional to the difference between pulmonary arterial and alveolar pressure and increases down the lung as this pressure difference increases (i.e., pulmonary artery pressure increases). In the dependent region of the lung (zone III), pulmonary artery pressure is greater than pulmonary venous pressure, which is also greater than alveolar pressure. In this region, flow is proportional to the difference between pulmonary artery and pulmonary venous pressure. Because both of these pressures increase equally for each cm distance down the lung, the driving pressure for flow does not change in successively lower portions of zone III. Nevertheless, blood continues to increase down zone III because the increasing transmural pressure causes a decrease in pulmonary vascular resistance. Thus, in general, blood flow per unit volume of lung (or in each successive horizontal layer of lung) continues to increase from apex to dependent regions.

Ventilation also increases from the apex to the base of the lung. However, this increase is not as marked as the increase with blood flow. The reason for this increase in ventilation is related to the magnitude of pleural pressure, which increases about 0.25 cm H_2O per cm of distance down the lung. The increasing pleural pressure (presumably caused by gravity) *decreases* the transpulmonary pressure from the apex to the base of the lung. If the lung is 30 cm high, the transpulmonary pressure at the top of lung is about 7.5 cm H_2O greater than that at the base. This means that the upper and lower parts of the lung operate on different portions of the pressure-volume curve (i.e., alveoli at the base are less expanded relative to those at the top). Furthermore, because the pressure-volume curve of the lung is alinear (see Fig. 13–10), the alveoli at the base of the lung expand more than those at the top for any given change in transpulmonary pressure. These effects result in a larger ventilation per unit alveolar volume at the base of the lung compared to that at the top.

Because both blood flow and ventilation increase down the lung, but blood flow increases more than ventilation, the ratio of ventilation to perfusion decreases from apex to base. Thus, there is an overall distribution of ventilation-perfusion ratios even in the normal individual (i.e., ventilation is not perfectly matched in *each* alveolar unit). Fortunately, in the normal individual, this distribution of ventilation-perfusion ratios does not cause a significant depression in arterial P_{O_2}. Of the 9 mm Hg A-a oxygen gradient that is normally present, about 8 mm Hg can be attributed to venous admixture. These quantitative relationships, however, can change markedly with disease.

DETERMINING VENTILATION-PERFUSION DISTRIBUTIONS

Ever since lungs were recognized to contain a distribution of ventilation-perfusion ratios there has been a need to measure this distribution in both normal humans and patients. In the absence of a suitable method, the conceptual treatment of the lungs as either a two- or three-compartment model gave the physiologist and physician a method of rationally treating the effects of ventilation-perfusion imbalances. For most individuals, these methods are still the primary means of understanding gas exchange problems. However, in recent years, the distribution of ventilation and perfusion has been measured through the application of computer methods (Farhi, 1967; Farhi and Yakoyama, 1967; Hlastala and Robertson, 1978; Wagner, et al., 1974a, 1974b; West, 1977). The technique involves the continuous injection of a solution of six inert gases dissolved in saline (sulfur hexafluoride, ethane, cyclopropane, halothane, diethyl ether, and acetone) into a peripheral arm vein. After 10 to 20 minutes, samples of arterial blood, mixed venous blood, and expired gas are collected. The concentration of inert gases is then measured by gas chromatography. Cardiac output and total ventilation are also measured. From these data, two graphs are made. The first is a plot

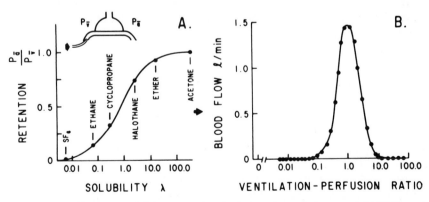

Fig. 14–6. *A*: Retention-solubility curve showing inert gas retentions measured with the multiple inert gas technique. *B*: A distribution of ventilation-perfusion ratios derived from the retention solubility curve. P_a = inert gas partial pressure in arterial blood; $P_{\bar{v}}$ = inert gas partial pressure in mixed venous blood. (From West, J.B.: Ventilation-perfusion relationships. Am. Rev. Resp. Dis., *116*:919–943, 1977.)

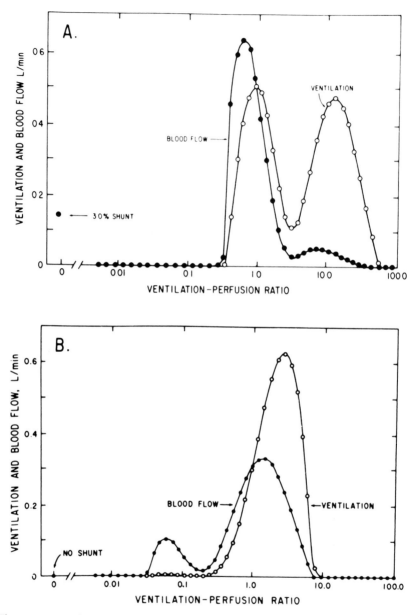

Fig. 14–7. Distribution of ventilation-perfusion ratios measured in patients with chronic obstructive lung disease. *A:* A patient with predominantly emphysema. *B:* A patient with predominantly chronic bronchitis. (From Wagner, et al.: Ventilation perfusion inequality in chronic
obstructive pulmonary disease. J. Clin. Invest., *59:*203, 1977.)

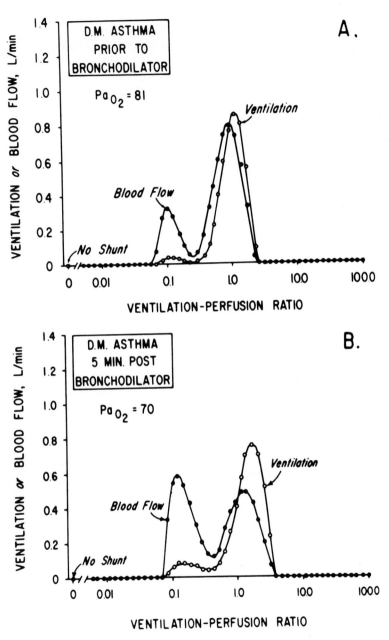

Fig. 14–8. Distribution of ventilation and perfusion in patients with asthma before, *A*, and after, *B*, bronchodilator therapy. (From West, J.B.: Ventilation-perfusion relationships. Am. Rev. Resp. Dis., *116*:919–943, 1977.)

of inert *gas retention* (arterial divided by mixed venous partial pressures) against the solubility of each of the six gases. The second is a plot of inert *gas excretion* (mixed expired divided by mixed venous partial pressure) against solubility. The key feature of this method is that important information about the distribution of ventilation-perfusion ratios can be derived from the shape of the retention-solubility curves. If a distribution contains shunt ($\dot{V}/\dot{Q}$ equals 0), the retention of the least soluble gas (sulfur hexafluoride) increases. Likewise, if the distribution has a significant amount of lung units with high ventilation-perfusion ratios, the retention of the high solubility gas decreases. The method uses the measured inert gas retention and determines, by computer analysis, the distribution of ventilation and perfusion that is most consistent with that given pattern. An example of a retention-solubility curve is shown in Figure 14–6; also shown is a derived distribution curve. For details of this method, the reader is referred to Hlastala and Robertson, 1978 and Wagner, Saltzman and West, 1974.

This method has been applied to the study of ventilation-perfusion relationships in both normal humans and in patients with various types of pulmonary diseases. An example of a normal distribution is presented in Figure 14–2. Figure 14–7 illustrates the type of distribution obtained from patients with chronic obstructive diseases. The results in Figure 14–7A are from a patient believed to have emphysema. The distribution pattern is bimodal, and a large amount of ventilation goes to units with high ventilation-perfusion ratios and a small amount of blood flow to units with low ratios. There was also a 3 percent shunt. This pattern suggests large dead space with low shunt presumably caused by areas of parenchymal destruction. The results in Figure 14–7B are from a patient with chronic bronchitis. Blood flow is considerable to areas with low ventilation-perfusion ratios but without shunt. This pattern is consistent with the hypoxemia seen in this group of patients. The type of distribution pattern found in patients with asthma is seen in Figure 14–8. Figure 14–8A, obtained before bronchodilator therapy, shows a bimodal distribution of blood flow with about 25 percent of the blood flow going to lung units with low ventilation-perfusion ratios. Following bronchodilation with isoproterenol (Fig. 14–8B), the amount of blood flow to areas of low ventilation-perfusion ratios markedly increased. This change in the distribution pattern helps to explain the decrease in arterial P_{O_2} that is often seen in asthmatic patients following bronchodilator therapy.

15

LUNG WATER

Fluid balance in the lung is governed by the general principles discussed in Chapter 8, yet the magnitude of the Starling forces involved is considerably different. Furthermore, fluid balance in the lung must be considered separately because of the lung's functionally different anatomy. Figure 15–1 presents an electron micrograph of the alveolar-capillary membrane. When fluid leaves the capillary it can enter not only the interstitial spaces but also the alveolar space. The capillary endothelium is highly permeable to water and many solutes (i.e., small molecules and ions). It is also *relatively* leaky to protein molecules. Consequently, the amount of protein in the interstitial spaces (e.g., the concentration of protein in the lymph leaving the lungs) is about twice that in the interstitial spaces of the peripheral tissues (4 g/L versus 2 g/L). By contrast, the alveolar epithelium is much less permeable to proteins and even to small ions; however, the alveolar wall is still highly permeable to water.

STARLING FORCES

The fluid flow across the wall of the pulmonary capillary, $\dot{Q}_C$, is described by the Starling hypothesis; thus,

$$\dot{Q}_c = CFC\left[(P_c - P_i) - (\pi_p - \pi_i)\right], \qquad (8\text{–}3)$$

where P_c and P_i are the pulmonary capillary and interstitial hydrostatic pressures; π_p and π_i are the plasma and interstitial colloid osmotic pressures in the lung; and CFC, the pulmonary capillary filtration coefficient. Under normal conditions, the pulmonary capillary pressure is believed to be approximately 7 mm Hg (recall that the mean pulmonary artery pressure is only about 13 mm Hg). The plasma colloid osmotic pressure is 28 mm Hg. The pressures in the interstitial spaces are open to considerable speculation. However, recent attempts to measure both P_i and

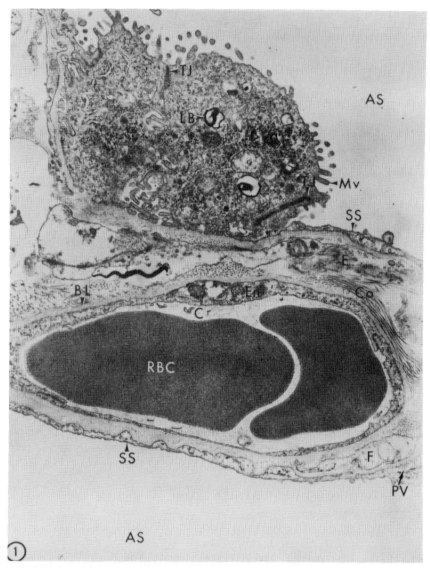

Fig. 15–1. Electron micrograph of the alveolar-capillary membrane. Note the close proximity of the simple squamous (SS) epithelium lining the alveolar space (AS) and that of the endothelial (En) wall of the capillary (C). Pinocytotic vesicles (PV) can be found in both membranes. Two erythrocytes (RBC) are seen in the capillary. A thin basal lamina (BL) surrounds the capillary. Both collagenous (Co) and elastic (E) fibers can be found in the interstitial spaces; fibroblasts (F) are also present. Secretory cells separated by tight junctions (TJ) are seen in the upper alveolar space; microvilli (Mv) project from the cells. Lamellar bodies (LB) believed to be phospholipid surfactant can also be seen in the secretory cells. (Human; ×7000.) (From Matthews, J.L., and Martin, J.H.: Atlas of Human Histology and Ultrastructure. Philadelphia, Lea & Febiger, 1971.)

π_i have given us considerable insight into the magnitude of these forces. Measurement of interstitial pressure with the capsule technique of Guyton (Meyer, et al., 1968) has yielded values of P_i that are approximately 6 mm Hg subatmospheric. Measurement of the protein concentration in lymph leaving the lungs suggests that π_i is probably about 16 mm Hg, somewhat higher than the interstitial oncotic pressure believed to exist in the peripheral tissues. This difference is understandable however considering the relatively high concentration of protein in the lung lymph. The cause of the negative interstitial pressure in the lung, as elsewhere in the body, is unknown. Nevertheless, a negative P_i is easier to accept in the lungs because of the well-recognized, elastic recoil forces that yield the negative pleural pressure.

When these Starling forces are balanced, a net force of about 1 mm Hg apparently drives fluid out of the pulmonary capillaries. This net filtration force is believed to cause a continual flow of fluid into the interstitial spaces which, under normal conditions, is rapidly returned to the circulation by the pulmonary lymphatic system.

PULMONARY EDEMA

The excess accumulation of lung water (interstitial or alveolar), known as *pulmonary edema*, is caused by factors that upset the normal Starling balance (e.g., increase P_c, decrease π_c, lymphatic blockage). One of the most common causes of pulmonary edema is a rise in pulmonary capillary pressure, secondary to heart disease (e.g., acute myocardial infarction, left ventricular failure caused by hypertension). Pulmonary capillary pressure can also be increased by noncardiogenic causes, such as overinfusions of blood or saline. An excessive amount of saline can create complications by causing a fall in the plasma oncotic pressure and a rise in capillary pressure. It is interesting to note that, in situations where pulmonary capillary pressure rises slowly over a period of years (e.g., mitral stenosis), much higher values of capillary pressure can occur before clinical signs of edema appear. Presumably, this higher capillary pressure is the result of an increase in the lymphatic drainage; thus, fluid movement is not prevented by a slowly rising capillary pressure and the lung "learns" to tolerate a higher-than-normal fluid flux because it can maintain its low interstitial hydrostatic pressure.

Pulmonary edema can be produced by an increase in capillary permeability. This type of edema is usually caused when toxins are either inhaled (e.g., sulfur dioxide, chlorine) or circulated (e.g., endotoxins from bacterial infections). Pulmonary edema may also appear when the normal lymphatic drainage system is distorted or obstructed such as occurs in diseases like silicosis or lung cancer.

When sufficient lung water accumulates so that edema is recognizable, two types of edema can occur, depending on severity. In the early stages of pulmonary edema, lung water collects almost exclusively in the interstitial space; this type of edema is known as *interstitial edema*. As edema progresses in severity, portions of the edema fluid break through the alveolar wall and collect in the alveolar spaces, thereby forming *alveolar edema*.

With interstitial edema most fluid collects in the loose connective tissues surrounding the blood vessels and bronchioles in the so-called *perivascular* and *peribronchial* spaces. The tight interstitial spaces of the *interalveolar septa* rarely accumulate significant amounts of edema fluid. When the interstitial edema becomes severe, the edema fluid begins to appear in the alveolar spaces. Because the permeability of the alveolar wall is low, alveolar edema is believed to result from rupture of the alveolar wall rather than from filtration. The frequent appearance of erythrocytes in alveolar edema fluid supports this idea.

The effects of pulmonary edema depend on the type and severity of the edema. Gas exchange is only slightly affected by interstitial edema, but alveolar edema can cause hypoxemia because of ventilation-perfusion abnormalities (i.e., alveolar edema stops ventilation in the flooded alveolus, producing alveolar shunt flow). Pulmonary edema (both interstitial and alveolar) decreases the lung compliance by increasing surface tension forces and possibly by directly altering the elastic properties of the lung. Airway resistance can also be increased, particularly with alveolar edema.

These problems show themselves clinically with *dyspnea* (difficulty or distress in breathing). In the early stages of edema, coughing is frequent but dry; later, coughing often produces a pink foaming type of sputum *(fulminant edema)*. In severe pulmonary edema, cyanosis is present.

16

CONTROL OF RESPIRATION

In Chapter 7 we discussed the mechanisms controlling vascular tone. We saw that they could be categorized as either local or neurogenic in origin. Regarding the regulation of respiration, the body's demand for oxygen and the elimination of carbon dioxide involves such a diverse integration of responses that most of what we will be discussing centers around the neural control that achieves this complex integration. We will begin our discussion of respiratory control by reviewing how the central nervous system establishes our normal breathing pattern, i.e., the rate and depth of each breath.

Unfortunately, we know far less about the control of respiration than we would like. New experiments are constantly changing basic concepts. Furthermore there is no single theory that explains all aspects of respiratory control (Wyman, 1977; Sant'Ambrogio, 1982; Coleridge, 1984). What is presented here is based on what the author believes is the most widely held views concerning the control of respiration. These views may be superseded at any time by more current information and better understood mechanisms.

CENTRAL CONTROL CENTERS

The natural rhythm of respiration is controlled by neurons located in the medulla and pons, known collectively as the *respiratory centers* (Euler, 1986). Within the medullary there are two groups of neurons that appear to be important in the control of breathing: (1) the *dorsal respiratory group* and (2) the *ventral respiratory group*. The dorsal region appears to receive and integrate sensory information and to then initiate a motor response. The primary function of the ventral region appears to augment inspiration and to facilitate an active expiration. Axons originating in the dorsal respiratory group project to the contralateral spinal cord where they pass to the phrenic nerve (and hence to the diaphragm). They also

229

pass to the ventral respiratory group and interact with other neurons there. Because of these interactions the respiratory centers should not be thought of as a discrete center but rather a collection of widely divergent neurons.

Rhythm Generation

The intrinsic respiratory rhythm appears to originate in the dorsal respiratory group within cells of the ventrolateral nucleus of the solitary tract. These cells act as a *central inspiratory excitation* (CIE). When left alone, the CIE produces an increasing number of action potentials which continues to increase as a ramp function until a critical level, called the *off-switch* is reached. When the off-switch is reached the CIE abruptly ceases its discharge. The CIE sends its "output" to the phrenic nerve where the increasing number of action potentials which occur before the off-switch is reached produce what is known as the *phrenic volley or burst* which directly drives the diaphragm. The greater the amplitude (voltage) of the phrenic burst the greater will be the tidal volume, for any given period of discharge, called the *inspiratory time.* The actual mechanism for the off-switch is believed to reside in the lower pons in an area called the "nucleus parabrachialis".

An important aspect of this control mechanism is that sensory input from the vagus nerves can terminate the phrenic burst prematurely. The mechanism behind this phenomenon is far from understood, but it appears that the vagal input in some way sums with the output from the CIE, without altering the level of the off-switch. Thus the off-switch receives at least two inputs (and probably more of unknown origin), one from the CIE and one from the vagi; when the combined inputs from these sources sum to reach the off-switch, the phrenic burst and therefore inspiration is terminated. When acting alone the CIE rises as a ramp function; therefore, the amount of activity necessary to reach the off-switch steadily decreases with time during inspiration. This means that to terminate an inspiration prematurely vagal input, which somehow gets added to the CIE output to reach the off-switch must be greater duiring the earlier parts of inspiration than during the later parts. The sensory input from the vagus nerves is believed to originate from the slowly adapting pulmonary stretch receptors (see below) which senses the size of each tidal volume. Thus, when we tend to take large breaths, such as during exercise, the pulmonary stretch receptors discharge at a greater frequency, afferent vagal input is greater and this input sums with the CIE to reach the off-switch earlier, terminating inspiration earlier. The stretch receptor feedback, which is such an integral part of the mechanism which we just discussed is called the *Hering-Breuer reflex.*

Ways of Altering Tidal Volume and Frequency

From the preceding discussion we can see that the factors that are important in determining the rate and depth of breathing are (1) the rate of rise of the CIE, (2) the level of the off-switch, and (3) the amount of vagal feedback. For example, when the off-switch rises (becomes less sensitive) the sum of the CIE plus vagal feedback must rise to a higher level before inspiration is terminated, therefore tidal volume becomes greater. If, on the other hand, the off-switch does not change but the rate of rise of the CIE increases, the tidal volume increases as the inspiratory time decreases. Thus, changes in the level of the off-switch primarily affects the tidal volume, while changing either the rate of rise of the CIE or the amount of vagal feedback can change both the tidal volume and the respiratory frequency. It is important to note that the length of a respiratory cycle (and therefore the breathing frequency) is a sum of the inspiratory and expiratory times. The inspiratory time is determined by when the off-switch is triggered. The determinants of expiratory time are less well understood but appear to be proportional to the inspiratory time. Because the determinants of tidal volume and frequency are so closely associated with the central mechanisms which are currently so incompletely understood, most investigators have chosen to investigate the control of breathing by simply measuring the factors which affect the total minute ventilation. Thus much of our remaining discussion of the control of breathing will center around minute ventilation. Just remember that minute ventilation is merely tidal volume times frequency.

We will now turn our attention to the many respiratory receptors which continually monitor the body's respiratory variables (i.e., P_{CO_2}, P_{O_2}, and pH). This information is fed to the neural control centers in the brain, where it is synthesized in such a way as to ultimately affect the mechanisms discussed above; namely, that which determines the rate and depth of breathing.

CHEMORECEPTORS

Peripheral Chemoreceptors

The peripheral chemoreceptors are of two types: the *carotid bodies* and the *aortic bodies* (Comroe, 1964; Fitzgerald and Lahiri, 1986). The former are located near the bifurcation of the common carotid artery, and the latter can be found (1) above the aortic arch and between the right subclavian and right common carotid arteries, (2) between the left subclavian and left common carotid arteries, and (3) between the aortic arch and the pulmonary artery. Figure 7–9 presents a schematic of the location and innervation of baroreceptors and chemoreceptors in the carotid and aortic regions of the dog and cat.

The carotid bodies are composed of two principal types of cells. The *glomus cells* (type 1), which have numerous nerve endings, and the *supporting cells* (type 2), which have cytoplasmic extensions that ensheathe

the glomus cells. The axons that contact the glomus cells are believed to be primarily afferent branches of the *carotid sinus nerve*, a branch of the *glossopharyngeal nerve* (nerve 9). There are also a few efferent sympathetic fibers from the *superior cervical ganglion*. The carotid bodies receive their arterial blood supply from branches of the common carotid artery.

Relatively little is known about the aortic chemoreceptors in humans. They can be found either as discrete organs resembling small carotid bodies (i.e., in cats) or as loose aggregates of glomus cells distributed in diffuse and irregular patterns along branches of the vagus nerve (i.e., in dogs). Afferent innervation of the aortic bodies occurs by way of the *vagus nerve* (cranial nerve 10). The aortic bodies receive their arterial blood supply primarily from small branches of the aorta and from brachiocephalic arteries.

The blood flow to the chemoreceptors on a weight basis is the highest of any organ in the body. For instance, in a cat with a normal blood pressure, an average of 40 c.mm. of blood per minute passes through the carotid body (Daly, 1954). Because the weight of the carotid body of the cat is only about 2 mg, this represents a blood flow equivalent to approximately 2000 ml/min per 100 gm of tissue. For comparison, the blood flow through the brain is only about 50 ml/min per 100 gm of tissue.

Teleologically speaking, the chemoreceptors "sample" the chemical composition of the body fluids. The peripheral chemoreceptor samples several quantities, although the carotid and aortic bodies respond somewhat differently. The *chief* stimulant to both the carotid and the aortic bodies is *hypoxia* (low arterial P_{O_2}). They also respond to elevated P_{CO_2} and to reduced pH (increase in $[H^+]$), but it is difficult to separate the effects of these stimuli. Nevertheless, during experiments where actual pH was held constant as arterial P_{CO_2} was varied, changes in P_{CO_2} apparently acted mainly through its effect on pH, e.g., $CO_2 + H_2O \rightleftharpoons H_2CO_3 \rightleftharpoons H^+ + HCO_3^-$ (Hornbein, 1963). When both hypoxia and hypercapnea affect the peripheral chemoreceptors their combined effect is synergistic; that is, the increase in ventilation is greater than would occur if either stimulus acted alone.

I should emphasize here that the primary stimulus for the peripheral chemoreceptors is low arterial oxygen tension; hypoxia does not affect the central chemoreceptors (see the following). However, carbon dioxide has a profound effect on the central chemoreceptors. Consequently, it has been difficult to separate the effects of the various stimulants on respiration.

As previously noted, the response of the carotid and aortic chemoreceptors to stimulation appears different (and sometimes even antagonistic).* For example, specific carotid body stimulation causes hyperpnea (increased ventilation), bradycardia, and hypotension; however, specific aortic body stimulation causes hyperpnea, tachycardia, and hypertension. Under normal conditions, both sets of peripheral chemoreceptors are stimulated together, and the ventilatory and circulatory responses result from the net effect of all the different afferent impulses.

Figure 16–1 illustrates an hypoxic response curve obtained by requesting an individual to breathe different concentrations of oxygen. As the inspired oxygen concentration is progressively decreased, the individual's ventilatory drive increases at any given level of $P_{A_{CO_2}}$. If the alveolar P_{CO_2} is allowed to fall (as it normally does under such condi-

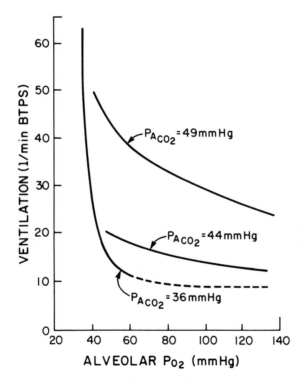

Fig. 16–1. Pulmonary ventilation as a function of alveolar P_{O_2} at different levels of alveolar P_{CO_2} (Redrawn from data of Loeschcke, H.H., and Gertz, K.H., 1958.)

---

*Differences apparently occur between species also. For example, patients who have had their carotid chemoreceptors surgically removed (but whose aortic chemoreceptors have remained intact) in an attempt to relieve bronchial asthma do not respond to mild or moderate hypoxia with the expected increase in ventilation (Lugliani, et al., 1971). Thus, in humans, the carotid bodies apparently are more important than the aortic bodies in initiating a physiologic response to hypoxia.

tions), less hyperventilation occurs. The flattening of the hypoxic response curve as P_{CO_2} is lowered is believed to occur because the lowered P_{CO_2} depresses ventilation through its action on the central chemoreceptors (see the following). The hypocapnia that normally occurs with hyperventilation consequently offsets much of the direct stimulating effect of hypoxia on the peripheral chemoreceptors except at low levels of $P_{A_{O_2}}$.

The synergistic effects of hypoxia and hypercapnia can also be seen with the CO_2-*response curve* (Fig. 16–2). This curve is obtained by asking an individual to breathe increasing concentrations of P_{CO_2} (at constant $P_{A_{O_2}}$) while recording his ventilation. Figure 16–2 shows several response curves obtained at different levels of $P_{A_{O_2}}$. Two observations can be made. First, at any given level of alveolar oxygen tension, the greater the $P_{A_{CO_2}}$, the greater the ventilation. Second, at any level of $P_{A_{CO_2}}$, the ventilation is greater as the alveolar oxygen tension is lowered. The additive effects of hypoxia can be eliminated by total denervation of the

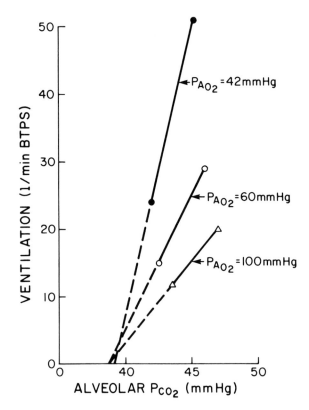

Fig. 16–2. CO_2 response curves. Pulmonary ventilation as a function of alveolar P_{CO_2} at different levels of $P_{A_{O_2}}$ (Drawn from data taken from experiment No. 26 of Lloyd, et al., 1958.)

peripheral chemoreceptors,* but the ventilatory response to CO_2 remains because hypoxia is the chief stimulant for the peripheral chemoreceptors, whereas P_{CO_2} acts predominantly on the central chemoreceptors.†

Central Chemoreceptors

Chemosensitive areas (collectively termed chemoreceptors) have been identified in the ventrolateral region of the medulla, between 200 to 600 μ below the surface, either by the direct application of various chemicals or by changing the composition of the cerebrospinal fluid that bathes the surface of the medulla. There is, however, no anatomic evidence of any specialized receptor cells in this or any other location on the brain. The current view is that the various respiratory stimulants are directly sensed by the neurons that influence respiration. The most important stimulus for the central chemoreceptors is hydrogen ions; increasing $[H^+]$ stimulates ventilation whereas decreasing $[H^+]$ depresses ventilation.

The central chemoreceptors are bathed in *cerebrospinal fluid* (CSF), which is formed in the choroid plexus of the lateral cerebral ventricles. The CSF is separated from the blood by a *blood-brain barrier*, which is relatively impermeable to the large ions, such as H^+ and HCO_3^-, but is easily crossed by molecular CO_2. CSF is not an ultrafiltrate of plasma. The composition of CSF is compared in Table 16–1 with that of plasma. Because of the extremely low concentration of protein in CSF, bicarbonate is the principal buffer in cerebrospinal fluid. Therefore, the changes

Table 16–1. Comparison of the Normal Composition of Cerebrospinal Fluid and Plasma*

Substance	CSF†	Plasma†
Na	141.2	140.6
K	2.96	4.46
Ca	2.43	5.23
Mg	2.40	1.94
Cl	127	103
HCO_3^-	21.5	24.8
Protein	15–45 mg/100 ml	6.6–8.6 gm/100 ml
Glucose	45–70 mg/100 ml	70–105 mg/100 ml
P_{CO_2}	50.2 mm Hg	39.5 mm Hg
pH	7.336	7.409

*Data from Murray, J.F.: The Normal Lung. Philadelphia, W. B. Saunders, 1976.
†Expressed as mEq/L unless otherwise stated.

---

*Hypoxia, which occurs following total peripheral chemoreceptor denervation, can actually depress ventilation because of its direct effect on the central nervous system.
†It has been estimated that about 20 percent of the ventilatory drive induced by hypercapnia can be attributed to carbon dioxide's effect on the peripheral chemoreceptors.

in CSF pH are governed almost solely by the Henderson-Hasselbalch equation, which relates CSF pH, [HCO_3^-], and P_{CO_2} as follows:

$$pH = pK + \log \frac{[HCO_3^-]}{[\alpha \cdot P_{CO_2}]}, \qquad (16\text{–}1)$$

where the pK is the dissociation constant and α is the solubility of CO_2 in CSF. Because the bicarbonate concentration ([HCO_3^-]) is about the same in both CSF and plasma, the lower CSF pH is mainly owing to the higher P_{CO_2} (about 9 mm Hg higher).

The Henderson-Hasselbalch equation (see Eq. 16–1) allows us to understand both the acute and the chronic effects of P_{CO_2} on CSF [H^+] and, therefore, the centrally stimulated ventilatory drive. We saw from the CO_2 response curve that, when P_{ACO_2} (and therefore P_{ACO_2} is increased acutely, ventilation increases even when the peripheral chemoreceptors are totally denervated. This increase occurs because CO_2 freely diffuses across the blood-brain barrier and, through the hydration of CO_2 and water ($CO_2 + H_2O \rightleftharpoons H_2CO_3 \rightleftharpoons H^+ + HCO_3^-$, forms hydrogen ions which stimulate the central chemoreceptors.

In some chronic situations, such as in patients with long-standing CO_2 retention, CSF pH is normal. This normalcy is believed to occur because active transport of HCO_3^- across the blood-brain barrier restores the ratio of Equation 16–1, [HCO_3^-]/[$\alpha \cdot P_{CO_2}$], to normal. In such cases, the patient would have an abnormally low ventilation for his arterial P_{CO_2}.

PULMONARY RECEPTORS

There are three basic types of pulmonary receptors whose afferent fibers traverse the vagus nerve and which play important roles in the normal control of breathing and in the pulmonary defense response (see below). Two of these receptors are myelinated A-fibers and are distributed throughout the tracheobronchial tree: the *slowly adapting and rapidly adapting pulmonary stretch receptors* (Sant'Ambrogio, 1982). The other type of pulmonary receptor is the nonmyelinated *pulmonary C-fiber* which is distributed throughout the tracheobronchial tree and located within the lung interstitium (Coleridge, 1984; Coleridge and Coleridge, 1986).

Slowly Adapting Pulmonary Stretch Receptors

The primary stimulus for these fibers is a change in lung volume. They discharge at high frequency with the rhythmic inflation of the lung. They are believed to provide the negative feedback which sums with the central inspiratory excitation in the medulla to terminate inspiration (see above), i.e., the Hering-Breuer Reflex.

Rapidly Adapting Pulmonary Stretch Receptor (Irritant Receptor)

These receptors which are inactive during quiet breathing discharge at high frequency, but only in response to rapid changes in transpulmonary pressure, thus they discharge more in exercise and when the lung compliance decreases (becomes stiff). They provide a positive feedback to the central centers to excite inspiratory neurons. When the lungs begin to collapse they cause an occasional sigh or "augmentd breath" which serves to re-expand collapsed alveoli. In certain species, notably the rabbit, these fibers have been shown to be sensitive to noxious gases and other irritants such as cigarette smoke. Some physiologists therefore refer to them as irritant receptors. This is perhaps a misnomer in other mammals such as the dog and possibly man, because pulmonary C-fibers appear to sense various irritants (see below).

Pulmonary C-fibers

These fibers provide low frequency, irregular input to the central nervous system during quiet breathing. They are believed to be stimulated by pulmonary congestion, pulmonary edema and various products of inflammation such as histamine, bradykinin and the prostaglandins. C-fibers located in the airway mucosa are highly sensitive to chemical irritants. When stimulated, pulmonary C-fibers cause rapid shallow breathing. They are thought to be responsible for the sensations of dyspnea in exercise and play an important role in the pulmonary defense reflexes (see below).

Pulmonary Defense Reflexes

The pulmonary defense reflexes are part of the "pulmonary defense response", which has both non-reflex and reflex components. The non-reflex components consist largely of release, in airway walls, of physiologically active chemicals (e.g., prostaglandins, kinins, histamine, etc.) and mobilize cellular defense mechanisms. A "defense reflex" is one that operates in emergencies when life itself is threatened. It must be contrasted with normal reflexes that operate in normal circumstances termed "regulatory reflexes", such as the Hering-Breuer Inflation Reflex. The pulmonary defense reflexes include: (1) rapid, shallow breathing (with an initial apnea if the stimulus is intense), (2) bronchoconstriction, (3) increased mucosal secretion, (4) cough, and (5) bradycardia, if the stimulus is intense. The pulmonary defense reflexes are evoked by irritant chemicals such as air pollutants (e.g., SO_2) and by chemicals released locally in the airway walls (e.g., prostaglandins, bradykinin and histamine), all of which stimulate afferent pulmonary C-fibers.

The pulmonary defense reflexes are protective. The combination of responses protects the respiratory tract from possible harmful effects of inhaled irritants. The rapid shallow breathing pattern promotes turbulence of airflow so irritants tend to settle out at proximal bronchial bi-furcations, are diluted by secretions and expelled by coughing. The coughing is believed to be caused by rapidly adapting receptors; the rest of the reflexes are probably initiated by pulmonary C-fibers.

EFFECTOR ORGAN

The effector organ of respiration is, of course, the muscles of respiration: the diaphragm and the intercostal muscles. During quiet breathing, the diaphragm is responsible for 70 to 90 percent of the tidal volume; expiration is passive (see Chap. 13). With moderately increased ventilation (50 L/min), the diaphragm is assisted by the lower intercostal muscles; expiration is still largely passive but is helped near the end of expiration by the antero-lateral abdominal and internal intercostal muscles. When ventilation exceeds 50 L/min, the diaphragm and all the accessory muscles (i.e., scaleni, sternocleidomastoids, etc.) are active; expiration is active and all the abdominal muscles are participating.

The diaphragm and intercostal muscles are connected to the higher-level respiratory centers by motor neurons in the phrenic and intercostal nerves, which descend down the spinal cord in tracts that run in the ventral parts of the lateral columns of the spinal cord.

The final common path to the muscles of respiration from the spinal cord is the *alpha motor neuron*. The impulses along this nerve represent the total integrated results of all neural influences from supraspinal levels plus the final modulating influences that originate as spinal reflexes (e.g., from muscle spindles). In this latter regard, the respiratory muscle contains two types of fibers: (1) the main *extrafusal fibers*, which do most of the real work of shortening, and (2) the *muscle spindles*, which are specialized organs of proprioception. The extrafusal fibers are innervated by the *alpha motor neurons* whereas the muscle spindles are innervated by the *gamma motor neurons*. When muscle shortening is opposed (i.e., by a decrease in lung or chest wall compliance), the muscle spindles reflexly stimulate the alpha motor neurons and the extrafusal fibers shorten further. This system represents a final compensation mechanism that helps to stabilize ventilation when mechanical conditions can change.

LANGUAGE

The symbols used by physiologists have always been confusing. The reason is simple: different physiologists used different symbols to represent the same parameter. Fortunately, in 1950, a group of physiologists agreed to a standard set of symbols and abbreviations. This reduced the confusion tremendously but did not eliminate it. For example, some physiologists use the symbol V to mean blood volume; others use Q. In preparing this text, an attempt was made to use the symbols most commonly used today. Those for gases and blood were adapted by the 1950 convention (Fed. Proc., 9:602–605, 1950) and are listed below. A dash (—) above a symbol indicates a mean value; a dot ($\cdot$) above a symbol means a time derivative.

SYMBOLS

General Variables

V   volume, gas
$\dot{V}$ a gas volume per unit time
Q   volume, blood
$\dot{Q}$ volume flow of blood per unit time
P   a gas pressure, or partial pressure
F   fractional concentration in dry gas phase
C   concentration of gas in blood
S O_2 saturation of blood
R   exchange ratio (CO_2 output divided by O_2 uptake)
D   diffusing capacity
f   frequency of breathing (lower case to avoid confusion with fractional concentration)

Symbols Used to Modify the Above

I	inspired gas	a	arterial blood
E	expired gas	c	capillary blood
A	alveolar gas	v	venous blood
D	dead space gas	p	plasma
S	shunt blood	ac	alveolar component
B	barometric	e	effective
L	lung		

HEMODYNAMICS

Hydraulics is the study of fluids in motion. Because Newton's second law of motion ($F = m \times a$) must be obeyed by each and every particle of fluid, hydraulics can become one of the most complex branches of mechanics if the proper conditions are not fulfilled. If the conditions are fulfilled, the flow of fluid is of a relatively simple type called streamline or steady flow, and equations of motion may be relatively simply derived. In streamline flow, every particle of fluid passing a particular point follows exactly the same path as the preceding particles that had passed that same point. These paths are called lines of flow or streamlines. The fundamental relationships of hydraulics are defined by the *Bernoulli equation*, which relates pressure, velocity, and elevation at points along the streamline. The Bernoulli equation is essentially an application of the principle of conservation of energy to fluid flow (i.e., the work done on a particle of fluid must equal the sum of its initial and final energies).

For the moment, let us consider the flow through a rigid conduit of a nonviscous, incompressible fluid. Figure A2–1 represents a portion of such a conduit. Let us follow a small bolus of fluid, indicated by shading, as it passes from one point to another along the conduit.

Let h_1 be the elevation of the first point above some reference level, v_1 the velocity at that point, A_1 the cross-sectional area of the conduit, and P_1 the pressure. All of these quantities may vary from point to point, and H_2, v_2, A_2, and P_2 are their values at a second point.

Because the fluid is under pressure at all points, inward forces shown by the heavy arrows are exerted against both faces of the bolus. As the element moves from point one to point two, work is done on it by the force acting on its left face, and work is done *by* it against the force acting on its right face. The net work done on the bolus (i.e., difference between these quantities) equals the gain in its kinetic and potential energy.

If A represents the cross-sectional area of the conduit at any point and P represents the corresponding pressure, the force against a face of the bolus at any point is $P \times A$. The work done on the element in the motion in the diagram is

$$\int_a^c Fds = \int_a^c P\,Ads,$$

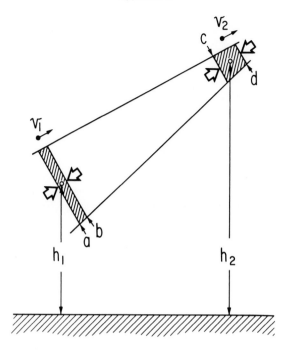

Fig. A2–1. Portion of a rigid conduit through which flows a nonviscous incompressible fluid. See text for details. (From Green, J.F.: Mechanical Concepts in Cardiovascular and Pulmonary Physiology. Philadelphia, Lea & Febiger, 1977.)

where ds is any short distance measured along the tube, and the limits are from A to C because these are the initial and final positions of the left face. This integral may be written

$$\int_a^c P\,A\,ds = \int_a^b P\,A\,ds + \int_b^c P\,A\,ds.$$

Similarily, the work done *by* the element in its motion is

$$\int_b^d P\,A\,ds = \int_b^c P\,A\,ds + \int_c^d P\,A\,ds.$$

The net work done on the element is

$$\int_a^b P\,A\,ds + \int_b^c P\,A\,ds - \int_b^c P\,A\,ds - \int_c^d P\,A\,ds = \int_a^b P\,A\,ds - \int_c^d P\,A\,ds.$$

The distances from A to B and from C to D are sufficiently small so that the pressures and areas may be considered constant along these limits. Therefore,

$$\int_a^b P \, Ads = P_1 \, A_1 \, \Delta S_1, \text{ and}$$

$$\int_c^d P \, Ads = P_2 \, A_2 \, \Delta S_2.$$

However, $A_1 \Delta S_1 = A_2 \Delta S_2 = V$, where V is the volume of the bolus. Hence,

$$\text{net work} = (P_1 - P_2) \, V. \tag{A2–1}$$

Let ρ be the density of the liquid and m be the mass of the bolus. Then V equals $\dfrac{m}{\rho}$, and Equation A2–1 becomes

$$\text{net work} = (P_1 - P_2) \, \frac{M}{\rho}.$$

We now equate the net work on the element to the sum of the increases in its kinetic and potential energy:

$$(P_1 - P_2) \, \frac{m}{\rho} = (\tfrac{1}{2} \, mv_2^2 - \tfrac{1}{2} \, mv_1^2) + (mgh_2 - mgh_1).$$

Rearranging yields

$$(P_1 - P_2) \, \frac{m}{\rho} + (\tfrac{1}{2} \, mv_1^2 + mgh_1) = (\tfrac{1}{2} \, mv_2^2 + mgh_2). \tag{A2–2}$$

Equation A2–2 states that the work done on the bolus plus the initial energy of the bolus must equal the final energy of the bolus. Thus, energy has been conserved. After cancelling m and rearranging terms, we obtain

$$P_1 + \frac{1}{2} \, \rho v_1^2 + \rho g h_1 = P_2 + \frac{1}{2} \, \rho v_2^2 + \rho g h_2. \tag{A2–3}$$

Equation A2–3 states that, as a nonviscous bolus flows from point one to point two, the total energy at point one equals the total energy at point two. Because the subscripts 1 and 2 refer to any two points along the conduit we may write

$$P + \frac{1}{2}\rho v^2 + \rho gh = \text{constant total fluid energy.} \quad \text{(A2–4)}$$

Either Equation A2–3 or Equation A2–4 is known as the Bernoulli equation. Note that P is the absolute (not measured) pressure and must be expressed in dynes per square centimeter (not mm Hg), and the density must be expressed in grams per cubic centimeter. Thus, assuming the fluid perfusing our conduit is nonviscous, the total fluid energy at any two points is the same. This, however, is unrealistic because most fluids, especially those found in biologic systems, such as blood, possess at least some degree of viscosity. Viscosity may be thought of as the internal friction of a fluid. Because of viscosity, a force must be exerted to cause one layer of fluid to slide past another or to slide past the surface of a conduit. Because a force must be exerted to overcome the internal friction of the fluid (the viscosity), the total fluid energy at two points along the conduit in reality cannot be the same, for the fluid energy at the upstream end must be greater than the fluid energy at the downstream end by an amount necessary to overcome the internal friction. That is, the total fluid energy at point two, E_{T2} must equal the total fluid energy at point one, E_{T1}, minus some amounts of energy due to frictional losses, E_f. This is symbolized by

$$E_{T2} = E_{T1} - E_f. \quad \text{(A2–5)}$$

This does not mean that energy has been destroyed, because heat is developed whenever friction forces are present. By measuring this heat, one can show that it is exactly equivalent to the decrease in total fluid energy; hence, the work done against friction, E_f, is the same as energy converted to heat. (Note: the total energy of any single point for a viscous fluid can still be described by Equation A2–4; however, the total energy at point two will be less than that at point one by an amount equal to the energy lost to friction.) The force, F_f, that is necessary to overcome the internal friction of a fluid has been found experimentally to be proportional to the wall area of a conduit, A, and the gradient of velocity which occurs at right angles to the direction of flow, $\frac{dv}{dr}$, where dv is a small difference in velocity between two points and dr is a small difference in radius between these two points. This relationship is expressed as

$$F_f = \eta A \frac{dv}{dr}. \quad \text{(A2–6)}$$

The proportionality constant is called the *coefficient of viscosity*, or simply the *viscosity.* The unit of viscosity is that of force times distance divided by area times velocity, or, in the cgs system, 1 dyne · sec/cm^2. A viscosity of 1 dyne · sec/cm^2 is called a *poise.* Small viscosities are usually expressed in *centipoises* (1 cp $=$ 10^{-2} poise). With this quantitative expression for viscosity, we can now modify the Bernoulli equation to derive an expression that adequately and realistically relates the driving energy for flow to the resulting flow. Consider a rigid, horizontal conduit of internal radius, r, and length, L. Liquid is flowing from point one to point two. Applying Equation A2–5, we obtain the following relationship for the difference in total fluid energy between point one and point two:

$$P_2 + \frac{1}{2}\rho v_2^2 + \rho g h_2 = P_1 + \frac{1}{2}\rho v_1^2 + \rho g h_1 - E_f. \qquad (A2–7)$$

Because the conduit is horizontal and of constant radius ($r_1 = r_2$ and $h_1 = h_2$), the kinetic energy and hydrostatic potential energy terms cancel from Equation A2–7. Therefore, the equation reduces to the following expression, which states that the difference in pressure energy between point one and point two is equal to the energy lost due to friction, thus

$$(P_1 - P_2) = E_f.$$

If these energy terms are now expressed as forces, the driving force is

$$(P_1 - P_2)\pi r^2.$$

(Pressure equals force per unit area; therefore, force equals pressure times area.) The viscous force from Equation A2–6 is

$$F_f = -\eta A \frac{dv}{dr} = -\eta 2\pi r L \frac{dv}{dr},$$

where the minus sign is introduced because v decreases as r increases. That is, the velocity in the center of the tube is the greatest and the velocity at the liquid-surface junction is the least. Equating these forces, we find that

$$-\frac{dv}{dr} = (P_1 - P_2)\frac{r}{2\eta L}, \text{ and}$$

$$-dv = \frac{P_1 - P_2}{2\eta L} r dr.$$

Integration of this equation gives

$$- v = \frac{P_1 - P_2}{4\eta L} r^2 + C.$$

Let R equal complete radius of the tube. Because v equals O when r equals R

$$- C = \frac{P_1 - P_2}{4\eta L} R^2$$

and, therefore,

$$v = \frac{P_1 - P_2}{4\eta L} (R^2 - r^2),$$

where is the equation for a parabola. Because the discharge rate, $\dot{Q}$, is

$$d\dot{Q} = vdA = \frac{P_1 - P_2}{4\eta L} (R^2 - r^2) \times 2\pi rdr$$

and,

$$\dot{Q} = \int_0^R d\dot{Q} = 2\pi \frac{P_1 - P_2}{4\eta L} \int_0^R (R^2 - r^2) \, rdr, \qquad (A2\text{–}8)$$

then

$$\dot{Q} = \frac{\pi R^4}{8\eta L} (P_1 - P_2).$$

Equation A2–8 is known as *Poiseuille's law.* Because "R" is generally used to denote the quantity known as resistance to flow (see below), "R" from Equation A2–8 is generally replaced with "r," used to denote the radius. Rearranging the equation, we have

$$\frac{P_1 - P_2}{\dot{Q}} = \frac{8\eta L}{\pi r^4}.$$

Thus, the ratio of the total pressure drop of flow is proportional to the viscosity and the length and inversely proportional to the fourth power of the radius. The quantity, $\frac{8\eta L}{\pi r^4}$, is generally referred to as the *resistance to flow,* R, because it represents those factors that tend to retard flow. In the cgs system, the unit for resistance is dynes · sec/cm⁵, pressure being expressed as dynes/sq cm and flow in cm³/sec.

This simple relationship has been the foundation on which modern hemodynamics is based. Because the length remains constant in most vascular systems and, at normal rates of flow, the viscosity also remains constant, a change in the resistance is generally interpreted as a change in the vessel's diameter (2r). An increasing diameter results in the fall of vascular resistance, and a decreasing diameter results in an increase in the vascular resistance. It should be emphasized at this point that these relationships hold only for streamline (steady) flow.

APPENDIX 3

VENTILATION-PERFUSION RELATIONSHIPS

The principles set forth in this Appendix are based on the three-compartment model of pulmonary gas exchange (Riley 1946, 1949, 1965). Therefore, before proceeding with the derivation of the alveolar gas equation and the O_2–CO_2 distribution curve, we will briefly discuss this model.

The Three-Compartment Model of Pulmonary Gas Exchange

In an attempt to understand the sometimes complicated mechanisms that can produce significant A-a oxygen partial pressures differences, it is helpful to use yet another conceptual model (Fig. A3–1). The lung can be thought of as consisting of three functional parts or compartments. In one compartment, the alveoli are ventilated, but there is no blood perfusing through the capillaries. The second compartment is both ventilated and perfused, and the third compartment is perfused but not ventilated. Because blood and gas have contact in only the second compartment, the *effective* gas exchange occurs here. This *effective compartment* functions like the ideal capillary functioned in Figure 14–1. The volume of gas per minute that ventilates the effective compartment is symbolized by $\dot{V}_E^e$. The volume of blood per minute contributed to the cardiac output by this compartment is symbolized as $\dot{Q}_a^e$. The volume of gas per minute that ventilates the nonperfused compartment is represented by $\dot{V}_E^{D\,alv}$ Because there is no blood to be oxygenated in this compartment, this ventilation is actually wasted and is called *alveolar dead space*, thus the superscript D alv. The composition of gas in this compartment is close to that of the inspired air. The last of the three primary compartments of the lung is perfused but not ventilated. The blood per minute contributed from this compartment to the cardiac output is represented by $\dot{Q}_a^{S\,alv}$. Because the blood actually passes by alveoli (even though these alveoli are not ventilated), this blood is called the *alveolar shunt contribution*. Its composition is the same as that of mixed venous blood. It should be emphasized that the *alveolar* shunt blood ($\dot{Q}_a^{S\,alv}$) comes from different channels within the lung (i.e., nonventilated alveoli) rather than from the true *anatomic* shunts ($\dot{Q}_A^{S\,anat}$) even though the end result is the same (i.e., a depression of the arterial P_{O_2}).

The previous discussion defined the gas and blood components of the three primary lung compartments. Yet the mixed expired air and the

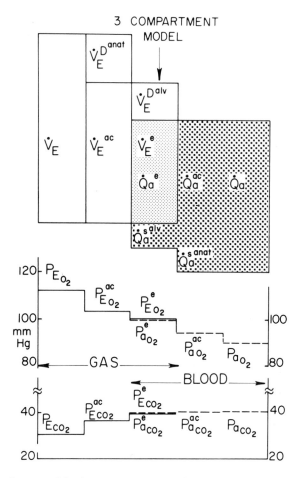

Fig. A3–1. Schematic of the three-compartment model of pulmonary gas exchange.

blood leaving the lungs consist of not only a mixture of the components of the primary compartments but also of components from the anatomic dead space and anatomic shunt. Let us refer again to Figure A3–1 to illustrate this concept. The air side contains an alveolar component of the expired air ($\dot{V}_E^{ac}$), which is made up of air from the effective compartment ($\dot{V}_E^e$) and the alveolar dead space ($\dot{V}_E^{D\ alv}$). The expired air from the alveolar compartment thus mixes with the air from the anatomic dead space ($\dot{V}_E^{D\ anat}$). This air never reaches the alveoli; e.g., air in the nose, trachea, and bronchi (see Chap. 12). Its composition is the same as that of the inspired gas. There is a similar mixing of compartments on the blood side. Like in the air side, there is an alveolar compartment for the blood ($\dot{Q}_a^{ac}$) made up of blood from the effective compartment ($\dot{Q}_a^e$) and the alveolar shunt compartment ($\dot{Q}_a^{S\ alv}$). The blood from the alveolar compartment then mixes with the true anatomic shunt blood ($\dot{Q}_a^{S\,anat}$) to form the arterial blood leaving the lung. The composition of both $\dot{Q}_a^{S\,alv}$ and $\dot{Q}_a^{S\,anat}$ is equal to mixed venous blood. Note that $\dot{V}_E^{D\,alv}$ is analogous to $\dot{Q}_a^{S\,alv}$ and that $\dot{V}_E^{D\,anat}$ is analogous to $\dot{Q}_a^{D\,anat}$. In other words, $\dot{V}_E^{D\,alv}$ and $\dot{V}_E^{D\,anat}$ have the same effect on the expired air as do $\dot{Q}_a^{S\,alv}$ and $\dot{Q}_a^{S\,anat}$ on the arterial blood. Let us now examine this effect.

The lower portion of Figure A3–1 shows the normal values for the partial pressures of oxygen and carbon dioxide in the various compartments of the lung for both expired air and arterial blood. The symbolism is much the same as that used for the air and blood flow. For example, the partial pressures of oxygen and carbon dioxide of the gas from the effective compartment are represented by $P_{EO_2}^e$ and $P_{ECO_2}^e$, respectively. Again the "E" means expired air because the partial pressures are measured from samples taken from expired air. For similar reasons, the partial pressures in the blood are $P_{aO_2}^e$ and $P_{aCO_2}^e$, respectively. Starting at the effective compartment, we see that the partial pressure for oxygen in the blood leaving the effective compartment ($P_{aO_2}^e$) is essentially equilibrated with that in the alveoli ($P_{EO_2}^e$); that is, there is an A–a gradient owing only to diffusion limitation. Thus, the effective compartment functions like the ideal capillary previously discussed (see Chap. 14). When the blood leaves the effective compartment, its oxygen tension progressively falls because progressively more mixed venous blood (with a P_{O2} near 40 mm Hg) is added, first from alveolar shunts and then from anatomic shunts. The story regarding carbon dioxide is different. The blood P_{CO2} values remain virtually unchanged as the blood becomes arterialized despite significant additions of shunt blood. The reason for this is related to the shape of the CO_2 dissociation curve, which was discussed in Chapter 14.

On the air side of our lungs, the partial pressure of oxygen progressively increases as the gas moves from the effective compartment to become expired air. This increase occurs because progressively more dead space air with a P_{O2} near 150 mm Hg is added. The P_{CO2} in the expired air is, however, less than that in the air coming from the effective compartment because the partial pressure of carbon dioxide in the inspired air (and, therefore, in the dead space compartments) is essentially zero. Thus, as a rule of thumb, we can state that, under normal conditions, $P_{EO_2}^e$ equals $P_{aO_2}^e$ which is greater than P_{aO_2}, whereas $P_{EO_2}^e$, $P_{aO_2}^e$, $P_{aCO_2}^{ac}$ and P_{aCO_2} are all equal.

The near identity of P_{aCO_2} and $P_{ECO_2}^e$ makes P_{aCO_2} of tremendous practical significance in studies of pulmonary function because arterial blood can be readily sampled and analyzed whereas the effective value cannot be determined directly.

Alveolar Gas Equation

This relationship results from a rearrangement of the CO_2/O_2 exchange ratio (R) when this ratio is expressed in terms of the alveolar gases in

GAS R LINES

THE ALVEOLAR EQUATION:

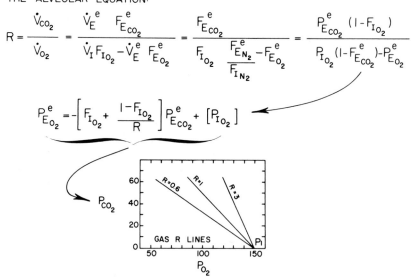

$$R = \frac{\dot{V}_{CO_2}}{\dot{V}_{O_2}} = \frac{\dot{V}_E^e \, F_{E_{CO_2}}^e}{\dot{V}_I F_{I_{O_2}} - \dot{V}_E^e \, F_{E_{O_2}}^e} = \frac{F_{E_{CO_2}}^e}{F_{I_{O_2}} \dfrac{F_{E_{N_2}}^e - F_{E_{O_2}}^e}{F_{I_{N_2}}}} = \frac{P_{E_{CO_2}}^e (1 - F_{I_{O_2}})}{P_{I_{O_2}} (1 - F_{E_{CO_2}}^e) - P_{E_{O_2}}^e}$$

$$P_{E_{O_2}}^e = -\left[F_{I_{O_2}} + \frac{1 - F_{I_{O_2}}}{R} \right] P_{E_{CO_2}}^e + [P_{I_{O_2}}]$$

Fig. A3–2. Derivation of the gas R Lines. (Redrawn from Riley, R.L.: Gas exchange and transportation. *In* Physiology and Biophysics. 19th Edition. Edited by T. C. Ruch, and H. D. Patton. Philadelphia, W. B. Saunders, 1965.)

the effective compartment (see Fig. A3–2). This rearrangement is done as follows:

$$R = \frac{\dot{V}_{CO_2}}{\dot{V}_{O_2}} = \frac{\dot{V}_E^e \, (F_{E_{CO_2}}^e - F_{I_{CO_2}})}{\dot{V}_E^e \, (F_{I_{O_2}} - (F_{E_{O_2}}^e)}. \tag{A3–1}$$

Recalling that $F_{I_{CO_2}}$ equals zero and making the appropriate substitutions for the F terms (i.e., $P/P_B - P_{H_2O}$) yields the following simple form of the alveolar gas equation after rearrangement of Equation A3–1:

$$P_{E_{O_2}}^e = P_{I_{O_2}} - \frac{P_{E_{CO_2}}^e}{R}. \tag{A3–2}$$

When one takes into account the differences in inspired and expired volumes (see Riley, 1965), the following precise form of the alveolar gas equation results:

$$P_{E_{O_2}}^e = \left[F_{I_{O_2}} + \frac{1 - F_{I_{O_2}}}{R} \right] P_{E_{CO_2}}^e + [P_{I_{O_2}}]. \tag{A3–3}$$

The terms within the left brackets equal zero when R equals 1 and seldom exceed 2 or 3 mm Hg. For any constant values of R, $F_{I_{O_2}}$, and $P_{I_{O_2}}$, a linear relationship exists between $P^e_{E_{CO_2}}$ and $P^e_{E_{O_2}}$ (see Fig. A3–2). Thus, a graphic representation of the gas equation is a family of straight lines (gas R lines) originating at the inspired air point. Each line passes through all possible values of $P^e_{E_{O_2}}$ and $P^e_{E_{CO_2}}$ for the specified value of R and $P_{I_{O_2}}$.

Note that the coordinates in Figure A3–2 have been labeled simply as P_{CO_2} and P_{O_2} because the exact same relationship can be used to describe the alveolar P_{O_2} and P_{CO_2} in any given single alveolar unit (single alveolus perfused by a single capillary) with its own separate R value (see the following). The partial pressures that form the *gas R lines* in Figure A3–2 become the effective values when the R used to compute the curves represents the CO_2/O_2 exchange ratio for the entire lung.

Blood R Lines

The difference between the amount of gas in the mixed venous blood entering the effective compartment and in the capillary blood leaving the effective compartment is the amount of gas exchanged. This is a statement of the Fick principle, which we can use to determine blood $\dot{V}_{CO_2}$ and $\dot{V}_{O_2}$. We may then use these values to compute a blood R line (Fig. A3–3). If the resulting R relationship is plotted using C_{CO_2} and C_{O_2} as coordinates, when C_v and R are held constant, the equation describes a straight line whose slope is determined by R. Thus, a family of R lines can be generated using different values of R, all originating at the mixed venous point. Each line passes through all possible values of $C^e_{a_{O_2}}$ and $C^e_{a_{CO_2}}$ for a given value of R and C_v.

The equations from which the blood R lines are generated cannot be easily expressed in terms of partial pressures because of the alinear dissociation curves. In Figure A3–3, blood R lines have been plotted in terms of partial pressures by taking successive points along each blood R line and converting the contents to partial pressures using the appropriate dissociation curves.

Note again that the coordinates in Figure A3–3 have been labeled simply as C_{CO_2}, C_{O_2}, P_{CO_2} and P_{O_2} because, like the gas R lines, these same relationships can be used to describe capillary blood C_{CO_2}, C_{O_2}, P_{CO_2}, and P_{O_2} in any given alveolar unit possessing its own separate R value (see the following). The contents and partial pressures used to form the blood R lines in Figure A3–3 become the effective values when the R used to compute these curves represents the CO_2/O_2 exchange ratio for the entire lung.

BLOOD R LINES

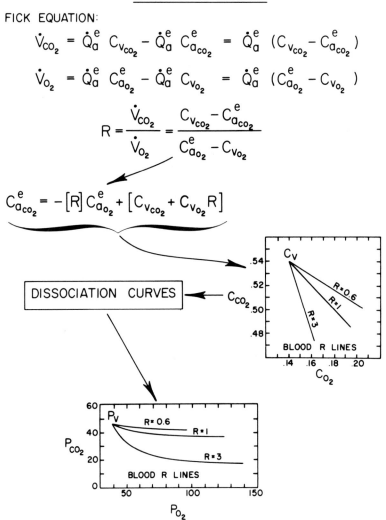

FICK EQUATION:

$$\dot{V}_{CO_2} = \dot{Q}_a^e \, C_{V_{CO_2}} - \dot{Q}_a^e \, C_{a_{CO_2}}^e = \dot{Q}_a^e \, (C_{V_{CO_2}} - C_{a_{CO_2}}^e)$$

$$\dot{V}_{O_2} = \dot{Q}_a^e \, C_{a_{O_2}}^e - \dot{Q}_a^e \, C_{V_{O_2}} = \dot{Q}_a^e \, (C_{a_{O_2}}^e - C_{V_{O_2}})$$

$$R = \frac{\dot{V}_{CO_2}}{\dot{V}_{O_2}} = \frac{C_{V_{CO_2}} - C_{a_{CO_2}}^e}{C_{a_{O_2}}^e - C_{V_{O_2}}}$$

$$C_{a_{CO_2}}^e = -[R]\, C_{a_{O_2}}^e + [C_{V_{CO_2}} + C_{V_{O_2}} R]$$

DISSOCIATION CURVES

C_{CO_2}

C_V

.54

.52

.50

.48

R=0.6

R=1

R=3

BLOOD R LINES

.14 .16 .18 .20

C_{O_2}

P_{CO_2}

60

P_V

40

R=0.6

R=1

20

R=3

0

BLOOD R LINES

50   100   150

P_{O_2}

Fig. A3–3. Derivation of the blood R Lines. (Redrawn from Riley, R.L.: Gas exchange and transportation. *In* Physiology and Biophysics. 19th Edition. Edited by T. C. Ruch, and H. D. Patton. Philadelphia, W. B. Saunders, 1965.)

DISTRIBUTION CURVE

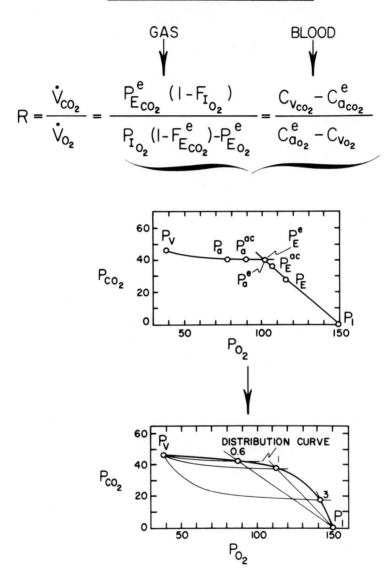

$$R = \frac{\dot{V}_{CO_2}}{\dot{V}_{O_2}} = \frac{\overset{\text{GAS}}{\overbrace{P^e_{E_{CO_2}}(1-F_{I_{O_2}})}}}{P_{I_{O_2}}(1-F^e_{E_{CO_2}})-P^e_{E_{O_2}}} = \frac{\overset{\text{BLOOD}}{\overbrace{C_{V_{CO_2}}-C^e_{a_{CO_2}}}}}{C^e_{a_{O_2}}-C_{V_{O_2}}}$$

Fig. A3–4.   Derivation of the distribution curve (CO_2–O_2 diagram). (Redrawn from Riley, R.L.: Gas exchange and transportation. *In* Physiology and Biophysics. 19th Edition. Edited by T. C. Ruch, and H. D. Patton. Philadelphia, W. B. Saunders, 1965.)

The Distribution Curve

Each R line in Figure A3–2 and A3–3 defines all possible values of
P_{O_2} and P_{CO_2} in the blood and gas leaving an individual alveolar unit
(or the effective compartment) that are compatible with any given value
of R at the specified values of P_{IO_2}, C_{vO_2}, and C_{vCO_2}. Yet, one and only
one R line represents the respiratory exchange ratio of the body as a
whole. When the gas and blood R lines, which represent the whole body
R values, are plotted on the same coordinates (that is, the simultaneous
solution of gas and blood equations for the whole body R), the point of
intersection identifies the only values of P_{O_2} and P_{CO_2} that are compatible
with the R value of the body as a whole (Fig. A3–4). These values are,
by definition, the effective values. In other words, given a certain CO_2
production and a certain O_2 consumption and given a specified C_{vO_2}
and C_{vCO_2}, the effective P_{O_2} and P_{CO_2} values are fixed.*

If every alveolus-capillary gas exchanging unit in the lung received
the exact same ventilation and the exact same perfusion, each and every
unit would have the effective P_{O_2} and P_{CO_2} values and there would be
no need to conceptualize a three-compartment model. This is not the
case, and innumerable different alveolar values exist in different specific
localities of the lung as a result of differences in the local alveolar ventilation and capillary perfusion. Each local ventilation-perfusion ratio is
associated with a different local R value. In each separate alveolus with
its own R, the composition of the gas and blood is determined by the
intersection of the appropriate gas and blood R line for that alveolus.
In Figure A3–4, three different gas and blood R lines are plotted and
their points of intersection are connected, forming the *distribution curve*.
This curve passes through all possible values for alveolar gas and end
capillary blood in the absence of an end-capillary diffusion gradient in
a lung in which the inspired and mixed venous points are fixed and are
as indicated in this figure. Alveolar dead space and alveolar shunt are
represented at the extremes of the distribution curve where the ventilation and perfusion ratios are infinite and zero, respectively. The effective value is one point on this curve.

Because individual alveolar ventilation-perfusion ratios are widely distributed, the individual alveolar units are scattered widely over the distribution curve. Furthermore, because the alveolar components of the
blood and gas are diluted by alveolar shunt and dead space, respectively,
they do not lie at the intersection of the blood and gas R lines for the
lung as a whole (as do the effective values). Nevertheless, the alveolar
component of the expired air and the alveolar component of the arterial
blood must be consistent with the gas exchange requirements of the

---

*Changing C_{vO_2}, C_{vCO_2}, or P_{IO_2} repositions these curves with respect to each other. They
would thus intersect at different points and yield different effective P_{O_2} and P_{CO_2} values.

lung as a whole. Therefore, they lie on the gas and blood R lines which represent the CO_2/O_2 exchange ratio of the lung as a whole, even though they represent a mixture of many small contributions for individual alveolar units that do lie on the distribution curve. The alveolar component of the expired gas (P_E^{ac}) lies to the right of the effective value along the R line for the lung as a whole whereas the alveolar component of the arterial blood (P_a^{ac}) lies to the left (see Figure A3–4).

REFERENCES

Ahlquist, R.P.: A study of the adrenotropic receptors. Am. J. Physiol., *153*:586, 1948.

Alexander, J.K., Dennis, E.W., Smith, W.G., et al.: Blood volume, cardiac output and distribution of systemic blood flow in extreme obesity. Cardiovasc. Res. Cent. Bull., *1*:39, 1962.

Bartlestone, H.J.: Role of the veins in venous return. Circ. Res., *8*:1059, 1960.

Bernard, C.: Leçons sur les Phénomènes de la Vie Communes aux Animaux et aux Vegetaux. Paris, B. Bailliere et Fils, 1879.

Berne, R.M.: Myocardial blood flow: metabolic determinants. *In* The Peripheral Circulations. Edited by R. Zelis. New York, Grune & Stratton, 1975.

Bevan, J.A., Bevan, R.D., and Duckles, S.P.: Adrenergic regulation of vascular smooth muscle. *In* Handbook of Physiology. Sect. 2, The Cardiovascular System. Vol. II, Vascular Smooth Muscle. Edited by D.F. Bohr, A.P. Somlyo, and H.V. Sparks, Jr. Bethesda, MD, American Physiological Society, 1980, pp. 515–566.

Brady, A.J.: Mechanical properties of cardiac fibers. *In* Handbook of Physiology. Sect. 2, The Cardiovascular System. Vol. I, The Heart. Edited by S.R. Berne, N. Sperelakis, and S.R. Geiger. Bethesda, MD, American Physiological Society, 1979, pp. 461–474.

Brooks, C., Hoffman, B.F., and Suckling, E.E.: Excitability of the Heart. New York, Grune & Stratton, 1955.

Brown, A.C.: Passive and active transport. *In* Physiology and Biophysics. Edited by T.C. Ruch and H.D. Patton. Philadelphia, W.B. Saunders, 1974.

Bülbring, E., Broding, A.F., Jones, A.W., and Tomita, T. (editors): Smooth Muscles. Baltimore, Williams & Wilkins, 1970.

Burnstock, G.: Cholinergic and purinergic regulation of blood vessels. *In* Handbook of Physiology. Sect. 2, The Cardiovascular System. Vol. II, Vascular Smooth Muscle. Edited by D.F. Bohr, A.P. Somlyo, and H.V. Sparks, Jr. Bethesda, MD, American Physiological Society, 1980, pp. 567–612.

Burton, A.C.: On the physical equilibrium of small blood vessels. Am. J. Physiol. *164*:319, 1951.

Burton, A.C.: Relation of structure to function of the tissue of the wall of blood vessels. Physiol. Rev., *34*(4):619, 1954.

Caldini, P., Permutt, S., Waddell, J.A., and Riley, R.L.: Effect of epinephrine on pressure, flow and volume relationships in the systemic circulation of the dog. Circ. Res., *34*:606, 1974.

Celander, O.: The range of control exercised by the sympathico-adrenal system. Acta Physiol. Scand. [Suppl. 116], *34*:1, 1954.

Channon, W.B.: Organization for physiological homeostasis. Physiol. Rev., *9*:399, 1929.

Christensen, E.H., and Mitteilung, V.: Minutenvolumen und Schlagvolumen des Herzens wahrend schwerer korperlicher arbeit. Arbeitphysiologie, *4*:470, 1931.

Coleridge, H.M., and Coleridge, J.C.G.: Reflexes evoked from tracheobronchial tree and lungs. *In* Handbook of Physiology. Sect. 3, The Respiratory System. Vol. II, Control of Breathing. Edited by A.F. Fishman, N.S. Cherniack, J.G. Widdicombe, and S.R. Geiger. Bethesda, MD, American Physiological Society, 1986, pp. 395–429.

Coleridge, J.C.G., and Coleridge, H.M.: Afferent vagal C fibre innervation of the lungs and airways and its functional significance. Rev. Physiol. Biochem. Pharmacol., *99*:1, 1984.

Coleridge, J.C.G., and Coleridge, H.M.: Chemoreflex regulation of the heart. *In* Handbook of Physiology. Sect. 2, The Cardiovascular System. Vol. 1, The Heart. Edited by R.M. Berne, N. Sperelakis, and S.R. Geiger. Bethesda, MD, American Physiological Society, 1979, pp. 653–689.

Coleridge, J.C.G., and Kidd, C.: Electrophysiological evidence of baroreceptors in the pulmonary artery of the dog. J. Physiol., 150:319, 1960.

Comroe, J.H., Jr.: Peripheral chemoreceptors. In Handbook of Physiology. Sect. 3, Respiration. Vol. I. Edited by W.O. Fenn, and H. Rahn. Bethesda, MD, American Physiological Society, 1964, pp. 557–583.

Comroe, J.H., Jr., Farster, R.E., Dubois, A.B., et al.: The Lung: Clinical Physiology and Pulmonary Function Tests. 2nd ed. Chicago, Year Book Medical Publishers, Inc., 1965.

Crone, C., Kruhoffer, P., Lassen, N.A., and Ussings, H.H.: Alfred Benzon Symposium II on Capillary Permeability. Copenhagen, Munksgaard International Publishers, 1970.

Daly, I. de B., and Hebb, C.O.: Pulmonary and Bronchial Vascular Systems. Baltimore, Williams & Wilkins, 1967.

Daly, M. de B., Lambertsen, C.J., and Schweitzer, A.: Observation of the volume of blood flow and oxygen utilization of the carotid body in the cat. J. Physiol., 125:67, 1954.

Dexter, L., Whittenberger, J.L., Haynes, F.W., et al.: Effect of exercise on circulatory dynamics of normal individuals. J. Appl. Physiol., 3:439, 1951.

Donald, K.W., Bishop, J.M., Cumming, G., and Wade, O.L.: The effect of exercise on the cardiac output and circulatory dynamics of normal subjects. Clin. Sci., 14:37, 1955.

Douglas, C.G., and Haldane, J.S.: The regulation of the general circulation role in man. J. Physiol., 56:69, 1922.

Downing, S.E.: Baroreceptor regulation of the heart. In Handbook of Physiology. Sect. 2, The Cardiovascular System. Vol. I, The Heart. Edited by R.M. Berne, N. Sperelakis, and S.R. Geiger. Bethesda, MD, American Physiological Society, 1979, pp. 621–652.

Drees, J.A., and Rothe, C.F.: Reflex venoconstriction and capacity vessel pressure-volume relationships in dogs. Circ. Res., 34:360, 1974.

Duomarco, J.L., and Rimini, R.: Energy and hydraulic gradients along systemic veins. Am. J. Physiol., 178:215, 1954.

Ehrlich, W., Schrijen, F.V., Solomon, T.A., et al.: Arterial pressure-flow relationships in the awake standing dog. Am. J. Physiol., 229:1261, 1975.

Einthoven, W., Fahr, G., and de Waart, A.: Uber die Richtung und die manifeste Grosse der Potentialschwankungen im menschlichen Herzen und uber den Einfluss der Herzlage auf die Form des Elektrokardiogramms. Arch. Ges. Physiol., 150:275, 1913. (English translation by H.H. Hoff, and P. Sekelj, Am. Heart J., 40:163, 1950.)

Engelberg, J., and Du Bois, A.B.: Mechanics of pulmonary circulation in isolated rabbit lungs. Am. J. Physiol., 186:401, 1959.

Euler, C.V.: Brain stem mechanisms for generation and control of breathing pattern. In Handbook of Physiology. Sect. 3, The Respiratory System. Vol. II, Control of Breathing. Edited by A.P. Fishman, N.S. Cherniack, J.G. Widdicombe, and S.R. Geiger. Bethesda, MD, American Physiological Society, 1986, pp. 1–67.

Farhi, L.E.: Elimination of inert gas by the lung. Respir. Physiol., 3:1, 1967.

Farhi, L.E., and Yakoyama, T.: Effects of ventilation-perfusion inequality on elimination of inert gases. Respir. Physiol., 3:12, 1967.

Feigl, E.O.: Carotid sinus reflex control of coronary blood flow. Circ. Res., 23:223, 1968.

Feigl, E.O.: Parasympathetic control of coronary blood flow in dogs. Circ. Res., 25:509, 1969.

Fishman, A.P.: Pulmonary circulation. In Handbook of Physiology. Sect. 3, The Respiratory System. Vol. I, Circulation and Nonrespiratory Functions. Edited by A.P. Fishman, A.B. Fisher, and S.R. Geiger. Bethesda, MD, American Physiological Society, 1986, pp. 93–165.

Fishman, N.H., Phillipson, E.A., and Nadel, J.A.: Effect of differential vagal cold blockade on breathing pattern in conscious dogs. J. Appl. Physiol., 34:754, 1973.

Fitzgerald, R.S., and Lahiri, S.: Reflex responses to chemoreceptor stimulation. In Handbook of Physiology. Sect. 3, The Respiratory System. Vol. II, Control of Breathing. Edited by A.P. Fishman, N.S. Cherniack, J.G. Widdicombe, and S.R. Geiger. Bethesda, MD, American Physiological Society, 1986, pp. 313–362.

Glazier, J.B., Hughes, J.M.B., Maloney, J.E., and West, J.B.: Measurements of capillary dimensions and blood volume in rapidly frozen lungs. J. Appl. Physiol., 26:65, 1969.

Gow, B.S.: Circulatory correlates: vascular impedance, resistance, and capacity. In Handbook of Physiology. Sect. 2, The Cardiovascular System. Vol. II, Vascular Smooth Muscle. Edited by D.F. Bohr, A.P. Somlyo, and H.V. Sparks, Jr. Bethesda, MD, American Physiological Society, 1980, pp. 353–408.

Green, J.F.: Determinants of systemic blood flow. *In* International Review of Physiology, Cardiovascular Physiology III. Vol. 18. Edited by A.C. Guyton and D.B. Young. Baltimore, University Park Press, 1979, pp. 33–65.

Green, J.F.: Mechanical Concepts in Cardiovascular and Pulmonary Physiology. Philadelphia, Lea & Febiger, 1977.

Green, J.F.: Mechanism of action of isoproterenol on venous return. Am. J. Physiol., 232:H152, 1977.

Green, J.F.: The pulmonary circulation. *In* The Peripheral Circulation. Edited by R. Zelis. New York, Grune & Stratton, 1975.

Green, J.F., and Attix, E.: Volume-pressure hysteresis in the peripheral venous system of the dog. Fed. Proc., 33(3):333, 1974.

Grodins, F.S.: Some simple principles and complex realities of cardiopulmonary control in exercise. Circ. Res., 20(Suppl. 1):171, 1967.

Gupta, P.D., Henry, J.P., Sinclair, R., and von Baumgarten, R.: Responses of atrial and aortic baroreceptors to nonhypotensive hemorrhage and transfusion. Am. J. Physiol., 211:1429, 1966.

Guyton, A.C.: Interstitial fluid pressure. II. Pressure-volume curves of interstitial space. Circ. Res., 16:452, 1965.

Guyton, A.C., Jones, C.E., and Coleman, T.C.: Circulatory Physiology: Cardiac Output and its Regulation. Philadelphia, W.B. Saunders, 1973.

Guyton, A.C., Taylor, A.E., and Granger, H.J.: Circulatory Physiology II: Dynamics and Control of the Body Fluids. Philadelphia, W.B. Saunders, 1975.

Hackett, J.G., Abboud, F.M., Mark, A.L., et al.: Coronary vascular responses to stimulation of chemoreceptors and baroreceptors. Evidence for reflex activation of vagal cholinergic innervation. Circ. Res., 31:8, 1972.

Heymans, C., and Neil, E.: Reflexogenic Areas of the Cardiovascular System. Boston, Little, Brown, 1958.

Hlastala, M.P., and Robertson, H.T.: Inert gas elimination characteristics of the normal and abnormal lung. J. Appl. Physiol., 44(2):258, 1978.

Hodgkin, A.L., and Hurley, A.F.: A quantitative description of membrane current and its application to conduction and excitation in nerve. J. Physiol., 117:500, 1952.

Holt, J.P.: The collapse factor in the measurement of venous pressure: the flow through collapsible tubes. Am. J. Physiol., 134:292, 1941.

Hornbein, T.F., and Roos, A.: Specificity of H ion concentration as a carotid chemoreceptor stimulus. J. Appl. Physiol., 18:580, 1963.

Howell, J.B., Permutt, S., Proctor, P.F., and Riley, R.L.: Effect of inflation of the lung on different parts of pulmonary vascular bed. J. Appl. Physiol., 16:71, 1961.

Hsieh, A.C.L.: The cutaneous circulation. *In* The Peripheral Circulations. Edited by R. Zelis. New York, Grune & Stratton, 1975.

Hughes, J.M.B., Glazier, J.B., Maloney, J.E., and West, J.B.: Effect of lung volume on the distribution of pulmonary blood flow in man. Respir. Physiol., 4:58, 1968.

Intaglietta, M., Pawula, R.F., and Tompkins, W.R.: Pressure measurements in the mammalian microvasculature. Microvasc. Res., 2:212, 1970.

Jackman, A.P., and Green, J.F.: Arterial pressure-flow relationships in the anesthetized dog. Ann. Biomed. Eng., 5:384, 1977.

Johnson, P.C.: The myogenic response. *In* Handbook of Physiology, Sect. 2, The Cardiovascular System. Vol. II, Vascular Smooth Muscle. Edited by D.F. Bohr, A.P. Somlyo, and H.V. Sparks, Jr. Bethesda, MD, American Physiological Society, 1980, pp. 409–442.

Johnson, P.C.: Review of previous studies and current theories of autoregulation. Circ. Res., Suppl. to Vols. 14 and 15, I–2 to I–9, 1964.

Katchalsky, A., and Curran, P.F.: Non-equilibrium Thermodynamics in Biophysics. Cambridge, Harvard University Press, 1965.

Kedem, O., and Katchalsky, A.: A physical interpretation of the phenomenological coefficients of membrane permeability. J. Gen Physiol., 45:143, 1961.

Kedem, O., and Katchalsky, A.: Thermodynamic analysis of the permeability of biological membranes to non electrolytes. Biochim. Biophys. Acta, 27:229, 1958.

Knowlton, F.P., and Starling, E.H.: The influence of variations in temperature and blood pressure on the performance of the isolated mammalian heart. J. Physiol. (Lond.), 64:206, 1912.

Korner, P.I.: Central nervous control of autonomic cardiovascular function. *In* Handbook of Physiology. Sect. 2, The Cardiovascular System. Vol. I, The Heart. Edited by R.M. Berne, N. Sperelakis, and S.R. Geiger, Bethesda, MD, American Physiological Society, 1979, pp. 691–739.

Krogh, A.: Regulation of the supply of blood to the right heart (with a description of a new circulation model). Scand. Arch. Physiol., 27:227, 1912.

Landis, E.M., and Pappenheimer, J.R.: Exchange of substances through the capillary walls. *In* Handbook of Physiology. Sect. II. Vol. 2. Circulation. Bethesda, MD, American Physiological Society, 1963, pp. 961–1034.

Levy, M.N., and Martin, P.J.: Neural control of the heart. *In* Handbook of Physiology. Sect. 2, The Cardiovascular System. Vol. I, The Heart. Edited by R.M. Berne, N. Sperelakis, and S.R. Geiger. Bethesda, MD, American Physiological Society, 1979, pp. 581–620.

Lewis, T.: The Mechanism and Graphic Registration of the Heart Beat. London, Shaw & Sons, 1925.

Lewis, T.: Observations upon the reactions of the vessels of the human skin to cold. Heart, 15:177, 1930.

Marey, E.J.: Excitations électriques du coeur physiologie experimentale. Travaux du Laboratoire de M. Marey, Paris, Masson & Cie, Vol, 2, p. 63, 1876.

Mark, A.L., and Abboud, F.M.: Myocardial blood flow: neuro-humoral determinants. *In* The Peripheral Circulation. Edited by R Zelis. New York, Grune & Stratton, 1975.

Maseri, A., Caldini, P., Howard, P., et al.: Determinants of pulmonary vascular volume-recruitment versus distensibility. Circ. Res., 31:218, 1972.

Master, A.M., Garfield, C.I., and Walters, M.B.: Normal Blood Pressure and Hypertension. Philadelphia, Lea & Febiger, 1952.

Mellander, S.: Comparative studies on the adrenergic neuro-hormonal control of resistance and capacitance blood vessels in the cat. Acta Physiol. Scand., 50 (Suppl. 176):1, 1960.

Mellander, S., and Johansson, B.: Control of resistance, exchange and capacitance functions in the peripheral circulation. Pharmacol. Rev., 20:117, 1968.

Meyer, B.J., Meyer, A., and Guyton, A.C.: Interstitial fluid pressure V. Negative pressure in the lungs. Circ. Res., 22:263, 1968.

Milnor, W.R.: Pulmonary hemodynamics. *In* Cardiovascular Fluid Dynamics. Vol. 2. Edited by D.H. Bergel. New York, Academic Press, 1972.

Murray, J.F.: The Normal Lung, 2nd ed. Philadelphia, W.B. Saunders, 1986.

Nichol, J.T., Girling, F., Jerrard, W., et al.: Fundamental instability of small blood vessels and critical closing pressures in vascular beds. Am. J. Physiol., 164:330, 1951.

Permutt, S., Bromberger-Barnea, B., and Bane, H.N.: Alveolar pressure, pulmonary venous pressure, and the vascular waterfall. Med. Thorac., 19:239, 1962.

Permutt, S., and Riley, R.L.: Hemodynamics of collapsible vessels with tone: the vascular waterfall. J. Appl. Physiol., 18:924, 1963.

Perry, R.H., and Chilton, C.H.: Chemical Engineers Handbook. New York, McGraw-Hill, 1973.

Remington, J.W.: Hysteresis loop behavior of the aorta and other extensible tissues. Am. J. Physiol., 180:83, 1955.

Rhodin, J.A.G.: Architecture of the vessel wall. *In* Handbook of Physiology. Sect. 2, The Cardiovascular System. Vol. II. Vascular Smooth Muscle. Edited by D.F. Bohr, A.P. Somlyo, and H.V. Sparks, Jr. Bethesda, MD, American Physiological Society, 1980, pp. 1–31.

Richardson, T.Q., Stallings, J.O., and Guyton, A.C.: Pressure-volume curves in live intact dogs. Am. J. Physiol., 201:471, 1961.

Riley, R.L.: Gas exchange and transportation. *In* Physiology and Biophysics. 19th Ed. Edited by T.C. Ruch, and H.D. Patton. Philadelphia, W.B. Saunders, 1965.

Riley, R.L., and Cournand, H.: Ideal alveolar air and the analysis of ventilation-perfusion relationships in the lung. J. Appl. Physiol., 1:825, 1949.

Riley, R.L., Lilienthal, J.L., Proemmel, D.D., and Franke, R.E.: On the determination of the physiologically effective pressures of O_2 and CO_2 in the alveolar air. Am. J. Physiol., 147:191, 1946.

Rodbard, S.: Flow through collapsible tubes: augmented flow produced by resistance at the outlet. Circulation, 11:280, 1955.

Rothe, C.F.: Reflex control of veins and vascular capacitance. Physiol. Rev., 63:1281, 1983.

Rowell, L.B.: The splanchnic circulation. *In* The Peripheral Circulation. New York, Grune & Stratton, 1975.

Roy, C.S., and Brown, J.G.: The blood pressure and its variations in the arterioles, capillary and smaller veins. J. Physiol. (Lond.), 2:223, 1879.

Sant'Ambrogio, G.: Information arising from the tracheobronchial tree of mammals. Physiol. Rev., 62:531, 1982.

Scheinberg, P.: The cerebral circulation. *In* The Peripheral Circulations. Edited by R. Zelis. New York, Grune & Stratton, 1975.

Shepherd, J.T., and Vanhoutte, P.M.: Skeletal muscle blood flow: neurogenic determinants. *In* The Peripheral Circulations. Edited by R. Zelis. New York, Grune & Stratton, 1975.

Shoukas, A.A., and Sagawa, K.: Control of total systemic vascular capacity by the carotid sinus baroreceptor reflex. Circ. Res., 33:23, 1973.

Shoukas, A.A., and Sagawa, K.: Total systemic vascular compliance measured as incremental volume-pressure ratio. Circ. Res., 28:277, 1971.

Skinner, N.S.: Skeletal muscle blood flow: metabolic determinants. *In* The Peripheral Circulations. Edited by R. Zelis. New York, Grune & Stratton, 1975.

Sparks, H.V., Jr.: Effect of local metabolic factors on vascular smooth muscle. *In* Handbook of Physiology. Sect. 2, The Cardiovascular System. Vol. II, Vascular Smooth Muscle. Edited by D.F. Bohr, A.P. Somlyo, and H.V. Sparks, Jr. Bethesda, MD, American Physiological Society, 1980, pp. 475–513.

Starling, E.H.: On the absorption of fluids from the connective tissue spaces. J. Physiol. (Lond.), 19:312, 1896.

Starling, E.H.: Some points in the pathology of heart disease. Effects of heart failure on the circulation. Lancet, 1:652, 1897.

Stephens, N.L.: Smooth Muscle Contraction. New York, Marcel Dekker, Inc., 1984.

von Neergaard, K.: Neue Auffassungen uber einen Grundbegriff der Atemmechanik. Die Retraktionkraft der Lunge, abhangig von der Oberflachenspannung in den Alveolen. Z. Ges. Exp. Med., 66:373, 1929.

Wade, O.L., and Bishop, J.M.: Cardiac output and regional blood flow. Oxford, Blackwell Scientific Publications, 1962.

Wagner, P.D., Laravuso, R.B., Uhl, R.R., and West, J.B.: Continuous distributions of ventilation-perfusion ratios in normal subjects breathing air and 100% O_2. J. Clin. Invest., 54:54, 1974.

Wagner, P.D., Saltzman, H.A., and West, J.B. Measurement of continuous distributions of ventilation-perfusion ratios: theory. J. Appl. Physiol., 36(5):588, 1974.

West, J.B.: Ventilation/Blood Flow and Gas Exchange. Oxford, Blackwell Scientific Publications, 1965.

West, J.B.: Ventilation-perfusion relationships. Am. Rev. Respir. Dis., 116:919, 1977.

West, J.B., and Dollery, C.T.: Distribution of blood flow and the pressure-flow relations of the whole lung. J. Appl. Physiol., 20:175, 1965.

West, J.B., and Dollery, C.T.: Distribution of blood flow and ventilation-perfusion ratio in the lung, measured with radioactive CO_2. J. Appl. Physiol., 15:405, 1960.

West, J.B., Dollery, C.T., and Naimark, A.: Distribution of blood flow in isolated lung; relative to vascular and alveolar pressures. J. Appl. Physiol., 19:713, 1964.

Wiederhielm, C.A., Woodbury, J.W., Kirk, S., and Rushmer, R.F.: Pulsatile pressure in the microcirculation of frog's mesentery. Am. J. Physiol., 207:173, 1964.

Wyman, R.J.: Neural generation of the breathing rhythm. *In* Ann. Rev. Physiol. Edited by E. Knobil, R.R. Sonnenschein, and I.S. Edelman. Palo Alto, CA. Annual Reviews, Inc., 1977, pp. 417–418.

INDEX

Page numbers in italics indicate figures; numbers followed by t indicate tabular material.

A band, 41
A wave, of venous pulse, 57
A-a gradient. *See* Alveolar-to-arterial gradient
Absolute refractory period. *See* Effective
   refractory period
Absorption. *See* Filtration-absorption
Acetylcholine, pharmacomechanical coupling
   and, 107
   vagal stimulation mimicked by, 115
   vascular smooth muscle and, 107
Acidosis, effects on pulmonary and systemic
   circulations, 149
Actin, 40
Actin filaments, 41, 43
   of vascular smooth muscle, 105-106
Action potential, 17-24, 26. *See also* Potential,
   action
   characterization of, 19-24
   ionic basis of, 17-19
Activation gates, 22-23
Actomyosin, 41
Adam's apple, 177
Adenosine, coronary blood flow and, 153
   pharmacomechanical coupling and, 107
Adenosine triphosphate (ATP), splitting of, 41,
   43
ADH. *See* Antidiuretic hormone
Admixture, venous, 209
Adrenergic receptors, 112-113. *See also* Alpha-
   adrenergic receptors; Beta-adrenergic
   receptors
Adventitia. *See* Tunica media
Afferent inputs, cardiovascular centers and, 121
A-fibers, rapidly adapting, 236, 237
   slowly adapting, 236
Afterload, 45
   cardiac function curve and, 51, *54*
   ventricular, 47
      effect on pressure-volume curve, 47-48, *49*
Agonists, alpha-adrenergic, 107
Airway(s). *See* Pulmonary airways
Albumin, 160
Aldosterone, blood volume and, 166-167
Alpha motor neuron, muscles of respiration
   and, 238
Alpha-adrenergic agonists, 107
Alpha-adrenergic receptors, differentiation from
   beta-adrenergic receptors, 112-113, 113t
   in coronary vasculature, 151-152
   in pulmonary vasculature, 148
   in skeletal muscle vasculature, 153, 154
   in splanchnic vasculature, 157
   in vascular smooth muscle, 107

Alveolar compliance. *See* Compliance,
   pulmonary
Alveolar dead space, 247
Alveolar edema, 228. *See also* Pulmonary edema
Alveolar gas equation, 217, 249-251
Alveolar phagocytes, 179, *180*
Alveolar pressure, 198-200, *199*
   during forced expiration, 200
Alveolar shunt, 209, 247
Alveolar ventilation equation, 218-219
Alveolar-capillary membrane, 225, *226*
Alveolar-to-arterial (A-a) gradient, 208
   physiologic shunt and, 213-214
Alveolus(i), 175, 178-179, *179*, *180*
   compliance of, 185, 187-190
   epithelial permeability of, 225
   recruitment and derecruitment of, 183
   structure of, 179, *180*
   surface forces of, 184-185
   ventilation-perfusion relationship and, 210-212
Anastomoses, arteriovenous, cutaneous
   circulation and, 158
Anatomic shunts, 208, 247
Angina, pain of, 126
Angiocardiogram, venous, *6*
Angiotensin, blood volume and, 167
   pharmacomechanical coupling and, 107
Anomalous rectification, 24
Anterior cardiac veins, 150, 151
Anterior longitudinal sulcus, 5
Antidiuresis, plasma volume and, 166
Antidiuretic hormone (ADH), atria receptors
   and, 126
   plasma volume and, 166
Aorta, 5
   function of, 77
Aortic bodies, 124, *125*, 125, 231, 232-235
   innervation of, 232
   stimulation of, 233-235
Aortic depressor nerve, 124
Aortic pressure, cardiac cycle and, 56
   coronary blood flow and, 151
Aortic valve, 5
Arterial pressure, 96-104
   baroreceptors and, 124
   effective back pressure and, 98-100
   mean, 75, 97-98, 100-101
   normal values of, *103*, 104, 104t
   pressure-flow relationships and, 96-98
   prolonged reductions in, 134
   pulse, 101-103
   systemic, 75, 97-98
      control of, 123
   urinary output and, 166
Arterial resistance, chemoreceptor stimulation
   and, 125
   splanchnic, 156

Arteriole(s), 10, 77
Arterioluminal vessels, 150
Arteriovenous anastomoses, cutaneous
    circulation and, 158
Artery(ies), 10
    carotid, 124, 232
    compliance of, 66
    coronary, 5, 150
    elastic, 11
    muscular, 11
    pulmonary, 5
    walls of, 11
Asthma, ventilation-perfusion relationships in,
    223, 224
Atelectasis, 179
ATP. *See* Adenosine triphosphate
Atria receptors, 126
Atrial pressure, as coupler, 86-89
    cardiac cycle and, 53
    elevations in, 135
Atrioventricular (AV) node, 25
Atrioventricular bundle, 25
Atrioventricular septum, 25
Atrioventricular valves, 5
    cardiac cycle and, 53-54, 56
Atrium(a), 5, *7*
    left, 5
    right, 5
Atropine, coronary blood flow and, 152
    skeletal muscle circulation and, 154
Autonomic nervous system, contraction and,
    115
Autoregulation, 108
Autoregulatory escape, splanchnic vasculature
    and, 157
AV node. *See* Atrioventricular node
AV ring, 5
Axon reflex, 158

Back pressure, 98-100
Baroreceptors, 122-124, *125*
    arterial pressure and, 124
    blood volume and, 165
    coronary blood flow and, 152
    low pressure, 126
    splanchnic circulation and, 156
Basal tone, 108
    maintenance of, metabolic hypothesis of, 109-
        110, *110*
    myogenic hypothesis of, 108-109, *109*
    of pulmonary vessels, 148
    of skeletal muscle vasculature, 154, 155
    of splanchnic vasculature, 157
Basement membrane, 11
Basophils, 163
Bernoulli equation, 240, 242-243
Beta-adrenergic agonists, 107
Beta-adrenergic receptors, differentiation from
        alpha-adrenergic receptors, 112-113, 113t
    in coronary vasculature, 152
    in skeletal muscle vasculature, 153-154
    in splanchnic vasculature, 157
    in vascular smooth muscle, 107
Bicarbonate ion, 170
Blood, 10, 160-171
    alveolar shunt and, 247

composition of, 160-164
    physical chemistry of, 167-171
    volume of, normal values of, 164, 164t
        regulation of, 164-167
Blood flow. *See also* Pressure-flow relationships
    at rest and under maximal vasodilation, 108,
        109
    cerebral, 155-156
    coronary, 150-153
        distribution of, 150-151
        mechanical determinants of, 151
        metabolic determinants of, 152-153
        neurohumoral determinants of, 151-152
    cutaneous, 157-159
    in carotid artery, 124
    normal, 57-58, 58t
    pulmonary, 140-149
        distention hypothesis and, 144-145
        local determinants of, 148-149
        lung inflation and, 146-147
        mechanical determinants of, 140-148
        neurogenic determinants of, 148
        recruitment hypothesis and, 145
        Starling resistor concept and, 140-145
        vascular resistance and, 145
        venous return and, 147-148
    respiratory chemoreceptors and, 232
    skeletal muscles and, 153-155
        local determinants of, 154-155
        neurohumoral determinants of, 153-154
    splanchnic, 156-157
        local determinants of, 157
        neurohumoral determinants of, 156-157
    systemic, 81-95
        cardiac output and, 85-95
        venous return and, 81-84
    vascular smooth muscle and, 106
Blood platelets, *161*, 164
Blood pressure. *See* Pressure
Blood R lines, 251, *252*
    distribution curve and, *253*, 254-255
Blood-brain barrier, 235
Body mass, blood volume and, 164, *165*
Bradycardia, arterial pressure and, 124
    as defense reflex, 237
    cardioinhibitory center and, 120
    chemoreceptor stimulation and, 125
    respiratory chemoreceptor stimulation and,
        233
Bradykinin, capillary permeability and, 135
    C-fibers and, 237
    defense reflexes and, 237
    vagal receptors and, 126
Brain, blood flow to, 155-156
Breathing. *See also* Respiration
    work of, 205
Bronchial smooth muscle, 178
Bronchial tree, 177-178, *178*
Bronchioles, 177-178
    respiratory, 178, *179*
    terminal, 178
Bronchitis, ventilation-perfusion relationships
    in, *222*, 224
Bronchoconstriction, as defense reflex, 237
Bronchus(i), 176, 177
Bundle of His, 25

C wave, of venous pulse, 57
Calcium, in excitation-contraction mechanism, 43
Capacitance vessels, 78
Capacity, diffusion, 206, 219
  functional residual, 181, 193-194, *194*
  inspiratory, 181
  total lung, 181
  vital, 181
Capillary(ies), 10, 11, *12*
  as Starling resistors, 73
  continuous, 11, *13*
  cytopempsis and, 139
  diffusion and, 138-139
  discontinuous, 12, *13*, *14*
  edema formation and, 135-136
  fenestrated, 11-12, *13*, *14*
  filtration-absorption process and, 134-135
  lymphatic, 13, *15*, 137-138
  pulmonary, 225
    epithelial permeability of, 225
    gas exchange through, 206-207
    permeability of, 227
    pressure of, 227
    ventilation-perfusion relationship and, 210-212
  Starling principle of fluid balance and, 130, 131-133
Capillary bed, 11, *12*
Capillary filtration coefficient, 130, 134
  changing, 135
Capillary oxygen tension, 207, *208*
Capillary pressure, blood volume and, 165-166
  determinants of, 128-130
  pulmonary, pulmonary edema and, 227
Carbon dioxide, cardiovascular centers and, 121
  cerebral circulation and, 155-156
  chemoreceptor stimulation and, 125
  coronary blood flow and, 153
  determining pressure of, 216-217
  diffusion of, 138
  given off during respiration, 175
  respiratory chemoreceptors and, 232
  stimulation by, 118
Carbon dioxide dissociation curve, *215*, 216
Carbon dioxide-response curve, *234*, 234-235
Carbon dioxide transport, *170*, 170-171
Carbonic acid, 170
Carbonic anhydrase, 171
Cardiac contraction, changes in dimensions of heart during, *9*
  depolarization and onset of, *19*, 19-20
  determinants of performance and, 45-46
  excitation-contraction coupling and, 43
  isovolumic phase of, 54
  length-tension relationship and, 43-45, *44*
  sliding filament model of, 40-43
Cardiac cycle, 29, 52-56
  action of valves during, *8*
  excitability of heart during, 29, *30*, 31, *31*
  hemodynamic events of, 52-54, *55*
  normal pressure and flow during, 57-58, 58t
Cardiac function, control of, 115-127
Cardiac function curve. *See also* Cardiac output function curve; Ventricular function curve
  for hypereffective heart, *89*, 89-90
  for hypoeffective heart, *89*, 89-90

with output as function of right atrial pressure, 87, *88*, 89
Cardiac index, 58
Cardiac muscle. *See* Myocardium
Cardiac output, 85-95
  controlling mechanisms of, 91-93
  distribution of, 93-95
  duality of control of, 85-86
  factors influencing venous return and, 89-90
  fluid balance and, 135
  right atrial pressure as coupler and, 86-89
  systemic factors influencing, 90-91
  venous return and, 85
Cardiac output function curve, 50, *52*, *53*
Cardiac performance, indexes of, 49-50
Cardiac tetanization, 29
Cardiac valves. *See* Valves
Cardiac veins, anterior, 150, 151
Cardioaccelerating center, 120
Cardioinhibitory center, 120
Cardiovascular centers, 118, 120-121
Cardiovascular function, neural control of, 118, 120-127
  levels of, 118, 120-121
  peripheral receptors and, 121-127
Cardiovascular reflexes, 118
Cardiovascular system, control of, 105-127
  subdivisions of, 76
Carotid artery, baroreceptors and, 124
  blood flow in, 124
  common, 232
Carotid bodies, 124, *125*, 231-235
  innervation of, 232
  stimulation of, 233-235
Carotid sinus, 124
Carotid sinus hypotension, 152
Carotid sinus nerve, 124-125, 232
  coronary blood flow and, 152
Carotid sinus pressure, skeletal muscle circulation and, 154
Catecholamines, adrenergic receptors and, 114
  hypereffective heart and, 52
  stimulation by, 117
Cell membrane, permeability of, 18, 23, 24
Centipoises, 244
Central inspiratory excitation (CIE), 230
  tidal volume and, 231
Central nervous system, control of cardiovascular function and, 121, *123*
  control of respiration and, 229-231
    rhythm generation and, 230
    tidal volume and frequency and, 230-231
Cerebral cortex, cardiovascular centers and, 121
Cerebral vasculature, 155-156
Cerebrospinal fluid (CSF), composition compared with plasma, 235, 235t
  respiratory chemoreceptors and, 235-236
C-fibers, 236, 237
Chemical control mechanisms, 113-115, 119t
Chemoreceptors, 122-123, 124-125, *125*
  coronary blood flow and, 152
  respiratory, 231-236
    central, 235-236
    peripheral, 231-235
  splanchnic circulation and, 156
Chest wall, compliance of, 190, *191*, *192*, 192-193

Chest wall *(Continued)*
  compliance of lung plus, 194-195, *196,* 197
  position of heart in relation to, *4*
  pressure-volume curve of, 193-194, *195*
Chest wall recoil, 190, *191*
Cholinergic sympathetic nerves, 112
Chordae tendineae, 5
Chronic obstructive diseases, ventilation-
      perfusion relationships in, *222,* 224
Chronotropic effect, 46
CIE. *See* Central inspiratory excitation
Circulation. *See also* Blood flow; Microcirculation
  central, 76
  function of, 3-4
  greater, 11
  interdependence with heart, 4
  lesser, 11
  mechanics of, 59-80
  pulmonary, 11
  systemic, 11, 76
    properties of serial sections of, 77t, 77-78
Circulatory parameters, for systemic and
      pulmonary venous systems compared,
      147-148, 148t
Circulatory system, basic anatomy of, *10,* 10-16
  conceptual model of, 75-80
  hydraulic model of, 79-80, *80*
  lumped parameter model of, *79,* 79-80
Coefficient of viscosity, 243-244
Cold-induced vasodilation, 158
Collapsible tubes, flow through, 69-73, *71*
Collateral ventilation, 179
Colloid osmotic pressures, 131
  fluid balance and, 130
  lymphatic system and, 138
  measurement of, 133
Common carotid artery, 232
Compensatory pause, 29
Compliance, 61-63
  defined, 63
  of chest wall, 190, *191, 192,* 192-193
    lung plus, 194-195, *196,* 197
  of circulatory system, 77
  of lungs, plus chest wall, 194-195, *196,* 197
    pulmonary edema and, 228
  of pulmonary and systemic systems
      compared, 66-68, *67,* 147, 148t
  pulmonary, 185, 187-190
  vascular. *See* Vascular compliance
Conduction, velocity of, 28
Conductivity, as property of heart muscle, 9, 9t
Conduit. *See* Tube(s)
Congestive heart failure, 227
Continuous capillaries, 11, *13*
Contractility, myocardial. *See* Myocardium,
      contractility of
Contraction. *See* Cardiac contraction
Control, of cardiac output, 85-86
Control mechanisms, extrinsic, 115
  intrinsic, 115
Coronary arteries, 5, 150
Coronary sinus, 5, 150, 151
Coronary sulcus, 5
Coronary veins, 5, 150, 151
Cough, as defense reflex, 237
Countercurrent heat exchange, 157, 158
Cranial nerves, ninth, 124, 232
  tenth. *See* Vagus nerve

Critical closing pressure, 98
  defined, 99
Cross-bridges, 41, 43
  length-tension relationship and, 43-45
Crystalloid therapy, filtration-absorption process
      and, 135
CSF. *See* Cerebrospinal fluid
Cyanide, coronary blood flow and, 152
Cyanosis, pulmonary edema and, 228
Cytopempsis, 139

Dalton's law, 167
DCI. *See* Dichloroisoproterenol
Dead space, alveolar, 247
  physiologic, 217-218
Defense reflexes, pulmonary, 237-238
Deflections, electrocardiographic, 33-36, *35, 36*
Depolarization, 19-20, 22
  in pacemaker cell, 26-27
  of atrial muscle, 33
  of sarcolemma, 43
  of ventricular muscle, 35
  onset of contraction and, *19,* 19-20
Depressants, hypoeffective heart and, 52
Depressor area, in medial reticular formation,
      118, 120, *120*
Diaphragm, 230, 238
Diastasis, 56
Diastole, 29, 52
  cardiac cycle and, 53-54
  coronary blood flow and, 151
Diastolic potential, maximum, 22
Diastolic pressure, 101
Diastolic run-off, 101
Dibenzyline (phenoxybenzamine
      hydrochloride), adrenergic receptors and,
      113
  skeletal muscle circulation and, 153
Dichloroisoproterenol (DCI), adrenergic
      receptors and, 113
Dicrotic notch, pulse pressure and, 101, *102*
Diffusion, across capillary walls, 138-139
  Fick's law of, 138, 206
  measuring lung capacity for, 219
Diffusion capacity, 206, 219
Diffusion limitation, 207
Digitalis, myocardial contractility and, 46
Dipole, 32
  electrical field generated by, 32, *33*
  equivalent, 36
Discontinuous capillaries, 12, *13, 14*
Disk, intercalated, 39
Distention hypothesis, 144-145
Distribution curve, *253,* 254-255
Dorsal respiratory group, 229
  rhythm generation and, 230
Drug(s). *See also specific drugs*
  adrenergic receptors and, 114
  hypoeffective heart and, 52
  myocardial contractility increased by, 46
  sympathetic stimulation mimicked by, 117-118
  vascular smooth muscle and, 107
"Dub" heart sound, 57
Ducts, lymphatic, right, 15
  thoracic, 15
Dyad, 43

Dyspnea, C-fibers and, 237
  pulmonary edema and, 228

Ectopic foci, 25-26
Edema, alveolar, 228
  fluid balance and, 135-136
  fulminant, 228
  interstitial, 228
  pulmonary. *See* Pulmonary edema
  safety factor against, 136
Effective compartment, 247
  alveolar gases in, *250*, 250-251
  of lung, 212-213
Effective refractory period, 29
  ionic basis for, 31
Effector organ, pulmonary, 238
Efferent autonomic innervation, of heart, 115,
  116
Einthoven's triangle, 33, *34*
Elastance, 62
Elastic arteries, 11
Elastic behavior, 59-63
  compliance and, 61-63
Elastic membranes, internal and external, 11
Elasticity, definition of, 59-60
  measuring, *61*, 61-62
Electrocardiogram, 32-38
  deflections and, 33-36, *35*, *36*
  dipole and, 32, *33*
  electrical axis of heart and, 36
  precordial leads and, 37, 37t, *38*
  standard lead system for, 32-33, *34*
Electrodes, unipolar, 37
Emphysema, ventilation-perfusion relationships
  in, *222*, 224
End-systolic pressure-volume curve, 47
Eosinophils, 163
Epiglottis, 177
Epinephrine, adrenergic receptors and, 112, 113,
  114-115
  contractile enhancement by, 23
  myocardial contractility and, 46
  splanchnic blood flow and, 157
  stimulation by, 117-118
  vascular smooth muscle and, 107
Equilibrium potential, 18
Equivalent dipole, 36
Erythrocyte(s), 160, *161*, *162*, 163
  carbon dioxide transport and, 171
  oxygen transport and, 168-170
Erythrocyte volume, regulation of, 167
Erythropoiesis, 167
Erythropoietin, 167
Excitability, 29-32
  as property of heart muscle, 8
  normal, period of, 29
Excitation-contraction coupling mechanism, 43
Exercise, cardiac output and, 91, *92*, 93-95, *94*,
  95t
Expiration, determinants of, 231
  muscles of respiration and, 238
  pressure-flow relationships during, 197, 198-
  200, *199*
  rhythm of, 230
Expiratory reserve volume, 181
Expiratory volume-flow curve, 201, *201*, 204

External elastic membrane, 11
Extrafusal fibers, of respiratory muscle, 238
Extrasystole, 29
Extrinsic control mechanisms, 115

Feedback, negative, 122-123
  respiratory rhythm generation and, 230
Fick's law of diffusion, 138, 206
  blood R lines and, 251
Filling, rapid and slow phases of, 56
Filtration-absorption, 130-139
  blood volume regulation and, 164-166
  capillary filtration coefficient and, 134
  colloid osmotic pressures and, 131
  cytopempsis and, 139
  diffusion and, 138-139
  edema formation and, 135-136
  process of, 134-135
  role of lymphatic system in, 137-138
  Starling balance and, 130, 131-133, *133*
Flow. *See* Blood flow; Pressure-flow
  relationships
Fluid, Bernoulli equation and, 240, 242-243
  cerebrospinal, 235t, 235-236
  exchange of. *See* Filtration-absorption
  flow through collapsible tubes, 69-73, *71*
  flow through rigid tubes, 68-69, *69*, 240-243,
  241
  hemodynamics and, 240-246
  interstitial. *See* Interstitial fluid
  renal regulation of, 166-167
Fluid balance, in lung, 225-228
  Starling principle of. *See* Starling principle of
  fluid balance
Formed elements, in blood, 160, *161*, *162*, 163-
  164
FRC. *See* Functional residual capacity
Fulminant edema, 228
Functional residual capacity (FRC), 181, 193-194,
  194

Gamma motor neuron, muscles of respiration
  and, 238
Ganglion, stellate, 148
  superior cervical, 232
Gas chromatography, determination of
  ventilation-perfusion ratios by, 221
Gas exchange, 175, 206-224
  effective, 247
  individual pulmonary capillary and, 206-207
  lung as a whole and, 208-213
  physiologic shunt and, 213-221
  pulmonary edema and, 228
  three-compartment model of, 247-249, *248*
  ventilation-perfusion distributions and, 221,
  221, *222*, *223*, 224
Gas excretion, *221*, 224
Gas R lines, *250*, 250-251
  distribution curve and, *253*, 254-255
Gas retention, *221*, 224
Gates, sodium and potassium channels and, 22-
  23
Gating potentials, 22
Globin, 163
Glomus cells, 231

Glossopharyngeal nerve, 124, 232
Glottis, 177
Goldman constant-field equation, 19
Granular leukocytes, 163
Gravity, effect on pulmonary pressures, 142-144
Greater circulation, 11

H band, 41
H gates, 22-23
Haldane effect, 171
Heart, 10
  action potential of, 17-24
    ionic basis of, 17-19
  as pump, 39-58
  basic anatomy of, 4, 5-7, 6
  changes in dimensions during contraction, 9
  conductive system of, 25, 26
  electrocardiogram and, 32-38
  electrophysiology of, 17-38
  excitability of, 29-32
  function of, 3-4
  hypereffective, 50, 51-52
    cardiac function curve for, 89, 89-90
    cardiac output function and, 53
    factors leading to, 51-52
  hypoeffective, 50, 51, 52
    cardiac function curve for, 89, 89-90
    cardiac output function and, 53
    factors leading to, 52
  innervation of, 115
  interdependence with circulation, 4
  left and right, 76-77
  origin of heartbeat and, 25-28
  position in relation to chest wall, 4
  pressure-volume curve of, 47-48
  Starling's law of, 48-49, 51
  velocity of conduction and, 28
  ventricular function curve of, 48-52
Heart failure, congestive, pulmonary edema
    and, 227
  right, filtration-absorption process and, 134-
    135
Heart muscle. See Myocardium
Heart rate, 45
  control of, 117
  elevated, 53-54
  nervous control of, 115
Heart sounds, 56-57
  cardiac cycle and, 54, 56
Heart valves. See Valves
Heart wall, 5
Heartbeat, origin of, 25-28
Heme, 163
Hemodynamics, 240-246
Hemoglobin, 163
  carbon dioxide transport and, 171
  oxygen transport and, 168-170
Hemorrhage, blood volume and, 165
  filtration-absorption process and, 134
Henderson-Hasselbalch equation, 236
Henry's law, 167
Heparin, production of, 163
Hering-Breuer reflex, 126, 230, 236, 237
Histamine, capillary permeability and, 135
  C-fibers and, 237
  coronary blood flow and, 153

defense reflexes and, 237
  effects on pulmonary and systemic
    circulations, 149
  pharmacomechanical coupling and, 107
  production of, 163
  triple response of Lewis and, 159
Homeostatic process, 3
Hooke's law, 59-61
Hormones, antidiuretic, 126, 156
  vascular smooth muscle and, 107
Hyaline cartilage, 177
Hydraulic model, of circulatory system, 79-80,
    80
Hydraulics, 240
Hydrodynamics, 68
Hydrogen ions, coronary blood flow and, 153
  respiratory chemoreceptor stimulation and,
    235
Hydrostatic pressure, fluid balance and, 130
  interstitial, negative, 132
Hypercapnia, effects on pulmonary and
    systemic circulations, 149
  respiratory chemoreceptors and, 232, 234,
    234-235
Hypereffective heart. See Heart, hypereffective
Hyperemia, reactive, 108, 155
Hyperpnea, respiratory chemoreceptor
    stimulation and, 233
Hyperpolarization, 117
Hypertension, respiratory chemoreceptor
    stimulation and, 233
Hyperventilation, respiratory chemoreceptor
    stimulation and, 234
Hypocapnia, respiratory chemoreceptor
    stimulation and, 234
Hypoeffective heart. See Heart, hypoeffective
Hypotension, carotid sinus, 152
  respiratory chemoreceptor stimulation and,
    233
Hypothalamus, cardiovascular centers and, 121
Hypoxemia, pulmonary edema and, 228
Hypoxia, brain and, 155
  chemoreceptor stimulation and, 125
  coronary blood flow and, 153
  effects on pulmonary and systemic
    circulations, 149
  erythropoiesis and, 167
  respiratory chemoreceptors and, 232, 233,
    233-235, 234
  splanchnic circulation and, 156
Hysteresis, volume-pressure, 183-185, 184

I bands, 41
Ideal collapsible tube. See Starling resistor
Inactivation gates, 22-23
Innervation, of aortic bodies, 232
  of carotid bodies, 232
  of cerebral vessels, 155
  of coronary vasculature, 151-152
  of cutaneous vasculature, 158
  of heart, 115
  of kidney, 111
  of pulmonary vasculature, 148
  of skeletal muscle vasculature, 153-154
  of splanchnic circulation, 156
  of vascular smooth muscle, 107, 110-115

Inotropic agents, hypereffective heart and, 52
Inotropic effect, 46
Inspiration, determinants of, 231
    pressure-flow relationships during, 197, 198-200, *199*
Inspiratory capacity, 181
Inspiratory excitation, central, 230
Inspiratory reserve volume, 181
Inspiratory time, 230
Interalveolar septum, 179, 228
Interatrial septum, 5, *7*
Intercalated disk, 39
Intercostal muscles, 238
Intercostal nerve, muscles of respiration and, 238
Interdependence, cardiac and circulatory, 4
Internal elastic membrane, 11
Interstitial edema, 228
Interstitial fluid, colloid osmotic pressure and, 130, 131, 133, 138
    formation of edema and, 135-136, *136*
    lymphatic collection of, 15-16, *16*
    of lungs, 225, 227
    proteins in, 225, 227
Interstitial hydrostatic pressure, 132
    negative, 138
Interventricular septum, 5, *7*, 25
Intravascular pressure, 64-65
Intraventricular pressure, cardiac cycle and, 54
Intrinsic control mechanisms, 115
Ions, 17-19. *See also* Hydrogen ions; Potassium; Sodium
    refractory periods and, 31
    resting potential and, 17-19
Irritant receptor, pulmonary, 237
Isometric contraction, 44-45
Isoproterenol, adrenergic receptors and, 112, 113
    coronary blood flow and, 152
    skeletal muscle circulation and, 153-154
    splanchnic blood flow and, 157
    vascular smooth muscle and, 107
Isovolume pressure-flow relationship, *202, 203,* 204
Isovolumic phase of contraction, 54
Isovolumic relaxation phase, 56

Kallidin, 112
Kallikrein, action of, 112
Kidney, innervation of, 111
    regulation of plasma volume by, 166-167
Kinins, defense reflexes and, 237

Lactic acid, coronary blood flow and, 153
Language, 239
Laplace's law, 99
Laryngeal cavity, 177
Laryngeal prominence, 177
Larynx, 175, *176*, 177
Latent pacemakers, 25-26
Lead(s), for electrocardiogram, precordial, 37, 37t, *38*
    standard, 32-33, *34*
Length-tension relationship, in cardiac contraction, 43-45, *44*

Lesser circulation, 11
Leukocyte, *162*, 163
    granular, 163
    nongranular, 163
    polymorphonuclear, 163
Lewis, triple response of, 158-159
Lipid-insoluble molecules, cytopempsis and, 139
Lipid-soluble molecules, diffusion of, 138
Lobes, of lung, 177
Lobules, 177
Local currents, 28
Low pressure baroreceptors, 126. *See also* Baroreceptors
"Lubb" heart sound, 56-57
"Lubb-dub" heart sound, 56
Lumped parameter model, of circulatory system, *79*, 79-80
    of pulmonary airways, 197, *197*
Lung(s), 175, *176*, 177-179, *178*. *See also* Respiration
    blood flow of. *See* Blood flow, pulmonary
    compliance of, pulmonary edema and, 228
    compliance of chest wall plus, 194-195, *196*, 197
    diffusion capacity of, 206, 219
    effective compartment of, 212-213, 247, *250*, 250-251
    fluid balance in, 225-228
    gas exchange and. *See* Gas exchange
    inflation of, effect on pressure-flow relationships, 146-147
        reflex vasodilation caused by, 126
    lobes of, 177
    pressure-flow relationships of. *See* Pressure-flow relationships, pulmonary
    three compartments of, 247-249, *248*
    volume-pressure relationships of. *See* Volume-pressure relationships, of lung
    zones of, 142-144, *143*
        ventilation-perfusion ratio and, 220-221
Lung reflex, 126
Lung volumes, *181*, 181-182, 182t
    altering, 230-231
    functional residual capacity and, 181, 193-194, *194*
    unstressed, 63, 190
Lung water, 225-228
    pulmonary edema and, 227-228
    pressure-volume curve of. *See* Pressure-volume relationships, pulmonary
    Starling forces and, 225, 227
Lymph, 15. *See also* Interstitial fluid
Lymph nodes, 15
Lymph vessels, 15
Lymphatic capillaries, 13, 15, 137-138
Lymphatic duct, right, 15
Lymphatic system, anatomy of, 13, 15-16
    fluid balance and, 137-138
Lymphocytes, *161, 162*, 163

M gates, 22-23
M line, 41
Mass, body, blood volume and, 164, *165*
Maximum diastolic potential, 22
Mean systemic pressure, 64-65, 83-84, *90*, 90-91, 97

Mechanoreceptors, 124. *See also* Baroreceptors
Mediastinum, 5
Medulla, electrical stimulation of, 118, 120, *120*
  respiratory chemoreceptors of, 235
  respiratory control and, 229-230
Megakaryocytes, 164
Membrane(s), alveolar-capillary, 225, *226*
  basement, 11
  elastic, of arteries, 11
  permeability of, 18, 23, 24
  threshold of, 23
Membrane receptors, in vascular smooth
    muscle, 107
Metabolic activity, as determinant of coronary
    blood flow, 151-153
  control mechanisms and, 114
Metabolic hypothesis of basal tone, 109-110, *110*
Metabolic pump, 18
Metabolic requirements, distribution of cardiac
    output according to, 93-95
Metabolites, coronary blood flow and, 151-153
  skeletal muscle circulation and, 154-155
Metoprolol, adrenergic receptors and, 113
Microcirculation, 128-139
  determinants of capillary pressure and, 128-
    130
  filtration-absorption and, 130-139
Micropinocytosis, 139
Milieu interieur, 3, 128
Mitral valve, 5
Molecule size, diffusion and, 138-139
Monocytes, *162*, 163
Motor neurons, muscles of respiration and, 238
Multiunit smooth muscle, 106-107
Muscle(s). *See also* Myocardium
  of respiration, 238
  papillary, 5
  respiratory, chest wall compliance and, 193
  smooth, bronchial, 178
    multiunit, 106-107
    unitary, 106
  vascular. *See* Vascular smooth muscle
Muscle spindle, of respiratory muscle, 238
Muscular arteries, 11
Myocardium, 39-40, *40. See also* Cardiac
    contraction
  atrial, 33
  conductivity of, 9, 9t
  contractility of, 9, 9t, 45-46
    cardiac function curve and, 51, *54*
    nervous control of, 115
  excitability of, 8
  inherent rhythmicity of, 8-9, 9t
  loss of, hypoeffective heart and, 52
  preload of, 45
  ventricular, 35
    fiber arrangement of, 5, 7
    pressure-volume curve and, 47-48
Myofibrils, 39-40, *41*
Myofilaments, 39-40
  of vascular smooth muscle, 105
Myogenic hypothesis of basal tone, 108-109, *109*
Myosin, 40
  splitting of ATP by, 41, 43
Myosin filaments, 41

Naris, 177
Nasal septum, 177
Nasopharynx, 177
Negative feedback, peripheral receptors and,
    122-123
Nernst equation, 18
Nerve(s). *See also* Innervation; Vagus nerve;
    names of nervous systems
  aortic depressor, 124
  carotid sinus, 124-125, 232
  cholinergic sympathetic, 112
  glossopharyngeal, 124, 132
  intercostal, 238
  of Hering, 124-125, 232
  olfactory, 177
  phrenic, 229, 230, 238
  splanchnic, 156
Neurogenic control mechanisms, 113-115, 119t
Neurons, motor, 238
Neutrophils, 163
Nicotine, coronary blood flow and, 152
Nodes, atrioventricular, 25
  lymph, 15
  sinoatrial, 25-26
Nongranular leukocytes, 163
Nonnutrient channels, 154
Nonpacemaker potential, *21*, 21-24
Norepinephrine, adrenergic receptors and, 112,
    113
  effects on pulmonary and systemic
      circulations, 149
  skeletal muscle circulation and, 153
  splanchnic blood flow and, 157
  stimulation by, 117, 118
  vascular smooth muscle and, 107
Normal excitability, period of, 29
"Nucleus parabrachialis," 230

Off-switch, respiratory rhythm generation and,
    230
  tidal volume and, 231
Olfactory cells, 177
Olfactory nerve, 177
Olfactory region, 177
Oncotic pressures. *See* Colloid osmotic pressures
Osmolality regulatory system, plasma volume
    and, 166
Osmolarity, coronary blood flow and, 153
Osmoreceptors, plasma volume and, 166
Osmotic pressures. *See* Pressure(s), osmotic
Oxygen. *See also* Hypoxia
  cardiovascular centers and, 121
  chemoreceptor stimulation and, 125
  determining pressure of, 216-217
  diffusion of, 138
  stimulation by, 118
  transfer through pulmonary capillary, 207
  uptake of, 175
Oxygen consumption, coronary blood flow and,
    153
Oxygen dissociation curve, 168-170, *169*, *214*,
    214-215
Oxygen transport, blood chemistry and, 168-170
Oxygen-carbon dioxide diagram, *211*, 211-212
Oxyhemoglobin, 168

P wave, 33, *35*, 53
Pacemaker(s), latent, 25-26
Pacemaker cells, changes in frequency of
  discharge of, *27*, 27-28
  depolarization in, 26-27
Pacemaker potential, 21, *21*, 22, 24, 26-27
Papillary muscles, 5
Paranasal sinuses, 177
Parasympathetic nervous system, 112
  coronary vasculature innervation by, 151, 152
  heart rate and contractility and, 115, 117
  of pulmonary vasculature innervation by, 148
Partial pressures. *See also* Carbon dioxide;
    Oxygen
  in blood, 167-168
Perfusion. *See* Ventilation-perfusion ratios
Peribronchial spaces, fluid in, 228
Period of normal excitability, 29
Period of supernormality, 29
Perivascular spaces, fluid in, 228
Permeability, of cell membrane, 18, 23, 24
pH, respiratory chemoreceptors and, 232
Phagocytes, alveolar, 179, *180*
Pharmacomechanical coupling, 107
Pharynx, 176
Phase of rapid filling, 56
Phase of slow filling, 56
Phenoxybenzamine hydrochloride. *See*
    Dibenzyline
Phentolamine, coronary blood flow and, 152
  skeletal muscle circulation and, 153
Phrenic nerve, muscles of respiration and, 238
  role in control of respiration, 229, 230
Phrenic volley, 230
Physiologic carbon dioxide dissociation curve,
  171, *171*
Physiologic dead space, 217-218
Physiologic depressants, hypoeffective heart
  and, 52
Physiologic shunt, 209, 212, 213
  alveolar ventilation equation and, 218-219
  calculating, 213-221
  causes for normally-occurring ventilation-
    perfusion ratio and, 220-221
  diffusion capacity of lung and, 219
  effective carbon dioxide and oxygen pressures
    and, 216-217
  physiologic dead space and, 217-218
Plasma, 160
  composition compared with CSF, 235, 235t
  volume of. *See* Blood, volume of
Plasma proteins, 160
Plateau phase, of nonpacemaker potential, 23-24
Platelets, *161*, 164
Pleural pressure, 190
  during forced expiration, 200-201
Poiseuille's law, 70, 245
  applied to capillaries, 128
  distribution of cardiac output and, 93
  pulmonary vascular resistance and, 145
Polymorphonuclear leukocytes, 163
Pore(s), alveolar, 179
  capillary, diffusion and, 138-139
  in continuous capillaries, 11
Posterior longitudinal sulcus, 5
Potassium, coronary blood flow and, 153
  permeability of cell membrane to, 24

resting potential and, 17-19
Potassium channels, 22-23
Potential, action. *See* Action potential
  diastolic, maximum, 22
  equilibrium, 18
  gating, 22
  nonpacemaker, *21*, 21-24
  pacemaker, 21, *21*, 22, 24, 26-27
  resting, 17-19, 28
Potential difference, 32-33
P-QRS interval, 35
P-R interval, 35
Practolol, coronary blood flow and, 151-152
Precapillary sphincter, 11, 111
Precordial leads, 37, 37t, *38*
Preload, 45
  cardiac function curve and, 51, *54*
  indirect measurement of, 49
  ventricular, 47
Pressor area, in lateral reticular formation, 118,
    120, *120*
Pressure. *See also* Volume-pressure hysteresis;
    Volume-pressure relationships; *specific
    types of pressures*
  back, 98-100
  baroreceptors and. *See* Baroreceptors
  closing, critical, 98, 99
  diastolic, 101
  hydrostatic, interstitial, 132
  in carotid sinus, skeletal muscle circulation
    and, 154
  intravascular, 64-65
  intraventricular, 54
  normal, 57-58, 58t
  of oxygen and carbon dioxide, determining,
    216-217
  oncotic, 130, 131, 133, 138
  osmotic, colloid, 130, 131, 133, 138
  partial. *See also* Carbon dioxide; Oxygen
    in blood, 167-168
  systemic, mean, 64-65, 83-84, 97
    venous return curves and, *90*, 90-91
  systolic, 101
  ventricular, cardiac cycle and, 53
Pressure gradient, for venous return, 83-84
Pressure load, 71
Pressure-flow curve, 75
Pressure-flow relationships, pulmonary, *141*,
    141-148, 197-205
  effect of inflation on, 146-147
  forced expiration and, 200-201, *202*, *203*,
    204-205
  isovolume, *202*, *203*, 204
  spontaneous ventilation and, *197*, 197-200,
    199
  work of breathing and, 205
  vascular, 68-75
    arterial, 96-98
    basics of, 68-73
    effective back pressure and, 99, *100*
    resistance and, 73, 75
    venous, 83-84, *85*
Pressure-volume curves, of heart, end-systolic,
    47
  ventricular, 46, *46*, 47-48
  of interstitial spaces, 136, *137*

Pressure-volume relationships. *See* Volume-pressure relationships
Propranolol, coronary blood flow and, 152
  skeletal muscle circulation and, 154
Prostaglandins, C-fibers and, 237
  defense reflexes and, 237
  pharmacomechanical coupling and, 107
  vagal receptors and, 126
Protein(s), in interstitial fluid, 225, 227
  in plasma, 160
  loss from capillaries, 135
  return to circulation, 137-138
Pseudostratified columnar ciliated epithelium, 177
Pulmonary airways, anatomy of, *176,* 176-177
  as Starling resistor, 201
  lumped parameter model of, 197, *197*
  resistance of, pulmonary edema and, 228
Pulmonary artery, 5
Pulmonary blood flow. *See* Blood flow, pulmonary
Pulmonary capillary. *See* Capillary(ies), pulmonary
Pulmonary congestion, C-fibers and, 237
Pulmonary defense reflexes, 237-238
  C-fibers and, 237-238
Pulmonary edema, C-fibers and, 237
  fluid balance and, 227-228
  fulminant, 228
  types of, 227-228
Pulmonary gas exchange. *See* Gas exchange
Pulmonary mechanics, 183-205
  pressure-flow relationships of pulmonary airways and, 197-205
  volume-pressure relationships of lung and, 183-197
Pulmonary pressure. *See also* Pressure-flow relationships, pulmonary
  gravity and, 142-144
  pulmonary edema and, 227
  ventilation-perfusion ratio and, 220-221
Pulmonary receptors, 236-238
  C-fiber, 236, 237
  defense reflexes and, 237-238
  stretch, rapidly adapting, 236, 237
    slowly adapting, 236
Pulmonary surfactant, 179, 185, *186*
Pulmonary system, 175-182
  basic anatomy of, 176-179
  function of, 175-176
  lung volumes and, *181,* 181-182, 182t
Pulmonary veins, 5
Pulmonary ventilation. *See* Ventilation; Ventilation-perfusion ratios
Pulmonic valve, 5
Pulse, venous, 57
Pulse pressure, arterial, 101-103
  transmission of, *102,* 102-103
Purkinje's fibers, 25

Q wave, 35
QRS complex, 33, 35
  cardiac cycle and, 54
Q-T interval, 35-36

R lines, blood, 251, *252*
  distribution curve and, *253,* 254-255
  gas, *250,* 250-251
R wave, 35, 36
Rapid filling, phase of, 56
Rapidly adapting pulmonary stretch receptors, 236, 237
Reactive hyperemia, 108, 155
Receptor(s). *See also* Alpha-adrenergic receptors; Beta-adrenergic receptors; Stretch receptor(s)
  atria, 126
  peripheral, 121-127
  pulmonary, 236-238
  sympathetic, 126
  vagal, 125-126
  ventricular, 126
Recoil, of chest wall, 190, *191*
Recruitment hypothesis, 145
Rectification, anomalous, 24
Red blood cell. *See* Erythrocyte(s)
Red flare, 158
Red reaction, 158
Reflex(es), axon, 158
  cardiovascular, 118
  defense, 237-238
  Hering-Breuer, 126, 230, 236, 237
  lung, 126
  regulatory, 238
  spinal, 238
Reflex adjustment, vascular smooth muscle and, 107
Reflex vasodilation, lung inflation and, 126
Refractory periods, effective, 29, 31
  relative, 29, 31
  tetanization and, 29
Regulatory reflexes, pulmonary, 237
Relative refractory period, 29
  ionic basis for, 31
Renin, blood volume and, 167
Renin-angiotensin system, blood volume and, 167
Repolarization, 21. *See also* Depolarization
  of atria, 35
  partial, 22
Residual capacity, functional, 181, 193-194, *194*
Residual volume, 181
Resistance. *See also specific types*
  measure of, 73
  of airways, pulmonary edema and, 228
  of circulatory system, 77
  peripheral, total, 75, 97
  systemic, mean, 84
  to flow, 68, 245
Respiration, 175. *See also* Alveolus(i); Lung(s); Pulmonary system
  control of, 229-238
    central control centers and, 229-231
    chemoreceptors and, 231-236
    pulmonary receptors and, 236-238
  frequency of, altering, 230-231
Respiratory airways. *See* Pulmonary airways
Respiratory bronchioles, 178, *179*
Respiratory centers, 229-230
Respiratory muscles, 238
  chest wall compliance and, 193
Respiratory rhythm, control of, 230

Resting potential, 17-19
  velocity of conduction and, 28
Retention-solubility curve, *221*, 224
Reticular formation, pressor and depressor areas in, 118, 120, *120*
Rhythm, respiratory, control of, 230
Rhythmicity, as property of heart muscle, 8-9, 9t
Rigid tubes, flow through, 68-69, *69*, 240-243, *241*

S wave, 35
SA node. *See* Sinoatrial node
Safety factor against edema, 136
Saline, pulmonary edema and, 227
Sarcolemma, 39
  depolarization of, 43
Sarcomere, 39
  in sliding filament model, *40*, 40-43
  length-tension relationship and, 45
  shortening of, 41, *42*, 43
Sarcoplasmic reticulum, 43
Semilunar valves, 5
Septal cells, 179, *180*, 185
Septum(a), atrioventricular, 25
  interatrial, 5, *7*
  interventricular, 5, *7*, 25
Serotonin, effects on pulmonary and systemic circulations, 149
  pharmacomechanical coupling and, 107
Set point, 123
Shunts. *See also* Physiologic shunt
  alveolar, 209, 247
  anatomic, 208, 247
Sinoatrial (SA) node, 25
  cells of, 25
  heartbeat and, 25-26
Sinus, carotid, 124
  coronary, 5, 150, 151
  paranasal, 177
Skeletal muscles, blood flow in, 153-154
Skin, blood flow in, 157-159
Sliding filament model, 40-43
  excitation-contraction coupling and, 43
  length-tension relationship and, 43-45
Slow filling, phase of, 56
Slowly adapting pulmonary stretch receptors, 236
Smooth muscle, bronchial, 178
  multiunit, 106-107
  unitary, 106
  vascular. *See* Vascular smooth muscle
Sodium, blood volume and, 167
  pulmonary edema and, 227
  resting potential and, 17-19
Sodium channels, 22-23
  fast, 22-23, 24
  slow, 22, 23-24
Sphincter, precapillary, 11, 111
Spinal reflexes, 238
Splanchnic blood flow, 156-157
Splanchnic nerve, 156
Squamous pulmonary epithelial cells, 179
Standard limb leads, 33, *34*
Starling balance, pulmonary edema and, 227

Starling principle of fluid balance, 130, *131*, 131-133, *133*
  conventional, *131*, 131-132
  edema and, 136
  lung water and, 225, 227
  new, 132-133, *133*
Starling resistor, 70-73, *71*
  pressure-flow relationships through, 70-73, *74*
  pulmonary airway as, 201
  pulmonary circulation and, 140-145
Starling's law of the heart, 48-49, *51*
Stellate ganglion, 148
Stimulation, nervous, effects of, 115, 117
  of respiratory chemoreceptors, 232-235
  sympathetic, 117
    drugs mimicking, 117-118
Stretch receptor(s), 124
  pulmonary, 236, 237
  respiratory rhythm generation and, 230
Stroke volume (SV), 47
Stroke-volume principle, 81, *82*
Subsarcolemmal cisternae, *41*, 43
Sulcus(i), anterior longitudinal, 5
  coronary, 5
  posterior longitudinal, 5
Superior cervical ganglion, 232
Supernormality, period of, 29
Supporting cells, 231-232
Surface tension, alveolar, 184-185
Surfactant, pulmonary, 185, *186*
  secreted by septal cells, 179
SV. *See* Stroke volume
Symbols, physiologic, defined, 239
Sympathetic nervous system, cerebral vessel innervation and, 155
  coronary vasculature innervation by, 151-152
  cutaneous vasculature innervation by, 158
  heart rate and contractility and, 115
  hypoeffective heart and, 52
  pulmonary vasculature innervation by, 148
  skeletal muscle vasculature innervation by, 153-154
  splanchnic circulation innervation by, 156
  stimulation of, 117
    drugs mimicking, 117-118
  vascular smooth muscle innervation by, 110-112
  vasodilator pathways of, central and peripheral extensions of, 121, *122*
Sympathetic receptors, 126
Systemic circulation, 11
  properties of serial sections of, 77t, 77-78
Systemic veins, 5
Systole, 29, 53
  cardiac cycle and, 54, 56
  coronary blood flow and, 151
Systolic pressure, 101

T wave, 35
Tachycardia, cardioaccelerating area and, 120
  respiratory chemoreceptor stimulation and, 233
Temperature regulation, of cutaneous circulation, 157-158
Terminal bronchioles, 178
Terminal conducting fibers, 25

Terminology, 239
Tetanization, cardiac, 29
Thebesian veins, 150
Thoracic duct, 15
Thoroughfare channels, 11, *12*, 154
Threshold, of cell membrane, 23
Thromboplastin, 164
Tidal volume, 181, 199
    altering, 230-231
Tonic discharge, over vasoconstrictor fibers, 118
Total lung capacity, 181
Total peripheral resistance (TPR), 75
    arterial pressure and, 97
Trachea, 176, 177
Transmural pressure, 61-62
    of lungs, 188-189
    static, 65
Transpulmonary pressure, 188-189, *199*, 199-200
Transthoracic pressure, 194-195, *196*, 197
Transverse tubules, *41*, 43
Tricuspid valve, 5
Triple response of Lewis, 158-159
T-tubules, *41*, 43
Tube(s), collapsible, 69-73, *71*
    see also Starling resistor
    rigid, flow of fluid through, 68-69, *69*, 240-
        243, *241*
Tunica externa, 13
Tunica intima, 11, 13
Tunica media, 11

U wave, 35
Unipolar electrodes, 37
Unitary smooth muscle, 106
Unstressed volume, 63, 190
Urinary output, arterial pressure and, 166

V wave, of venous pulse, 57
Vagal receptors, 125-126
Vagotomy, coronary blood flow and, 152
Vagus nerve, 124
    coronary blood flow and, 152
    innervation of aortic bodies and, 232
    pulmonary vasculature innervation and, 148
    role in respiratory rhythm generation, 230
    stimulation of, 115, 117
    tidal volume and, 231
Valves, action of, *8*
    aortic, 5
    atrioventricular, 5, 53-54, 56
    heart sounds and, 54, 56-57
    mitral, 5
    pulmonic, 5
    semilunar, 5
    tricuspid, 5
    venous, 13, *15*
Vascular bed, 11, *12*
Vascular compliance, 64
    pulmonary, 66-68, 147
    systemic, 64-66
Vascular reservoir, 78
    venous return and, 81
Vascular resistance, 73, 75
    pulmonary, 75, *76*, 144, *144*, 145
        lung inflation and, 146

    systemic, 75, *76*
Vascular smooth muscle, distribution of, 106
    frequency of stimulation of, *111*, 111-112
    innervation of, 107
    structure and physiological characteristics of,
        105-108
    ultrastructure of, 105-106
    venous, 107
Vascular tone, defined, 105
    determinants of, 105-108
    local control of, 108-110
    neurogenic control of, 110-115
Vasoactive agents, vascular smooth muscle and,
        107
Vasoconstrictor innervation. *See also* Innervation
        of vascular smooth muscle, 110-112
Vasodilation, cold-induced, 158
    reflex, caused by lung inflation, 126
Vasodilator, universal, 110
Vasodilator innervation. *See also* Innervation
        of vascular smooth muscle, 112
Vasomotor tone. *See* Vascular tone
Vein(s), 11
    anatomy of, 13
    compliance of, 66
    coronary, 5, 150, 151
    elastance and resistance of, 78
    pulmonary, 5
    systemic, 5
    valves of, 13, *15*
Velocity of conduction, 28
Venae comitantes arteriae femoralis, 157
Venous admixture, 209
Venous pulse, 57
Venous resistance, for systemic and pulmonary
        venous systems compared, 147-148, 148t
Venous return, 81-84
    cardiac factors influencing, 89-90
    cardiac output and, 85
    pressure gradient for, 83-84
    pulmonary, 147-148
        lung inflation and, 146-147
    vascular reservoir and, 81
Venous return curves, 84
    right atrial pressure and, 87, *88*, 89
    varied systemic pressures and, *90*, 90-91
Venous-to-arterial anastomoses, cutaneous
        circulation and, 158
Ventilation. *See also* Ventilation-perfusion ratios;
        Ventilation-perfusion relationships
    alveolar, 218-219
    collateral, 179
    spontaneous, pressure-flow relationships and,
        197, 197-200, *199*
Ventilation-perfusion ratios, 208-209, *209*
    causes for, 220-221
    determining, 221, *221*, *222*, *223*, 224
    quantifying, 210-212
Ventilation-perfusion relationships, 247-255
    alveolar gas equation and, 249-251
    blood R lines and, 251, *252*
    distribution curve and, *253*, 254-255
    three-compartment model of pulmonary gas
        exchange and, 247-249, *248*
Ventral respiratory group, 229-230
Ventricles, 5, *7*
    ejection of blood from, 54, 56

pressure-volume curve of, 46, *46*, 47-48
Ventricular function curve, 46, 48-52, *49, 50, 51, 52, 53. See also* Cardiac function curve
Ventricular myocardium, fiber arrangement of, 5, 7
Ventricular performance, patterns of, 50-52
Ventricular pressure, cardiac cycle and, 53
Ventricular receptors, 126
Venules, 10-11, 78
  similarity to capillaries, 12-13
Vessels. *See also specific vessels*
  capacitance, 78
  lymph, 15
Vestibule, 177
Viscosity, coefficient of, 243-244
  hydraulics and, 243
Vital capacity, 181
Vocal folds, 177
Vocalization, anatomy and, 177
  as function of pulmonary system, 175
Volume. *See also* Lung volumes; Pressure-volume curve; Volume-pressure relationships
  of blood, 164-167
  of plasma, 166
  stroke, 47, 81, *82*
Volume-pressure hysteresis, 183-184, *184*
  alveolar surface forces and, 184-185
Volume-pressure relationships, 62, *63. See also* Pressure-volume curves
  basics of, 59-61

compliance and, 61-63
  of lung, 183-197, *187*, 187-190, *199*, 199-200
    chest wall compliance and, 190, *191*, 192-193, *196*
    compliance of lung plus chest wall and, 193-195, *195, 196*, 197
    functional residual capacity and, 193-194
    pulmonary compliance and, 185, 187-190
    static, *196*, 197
    volume-pressure hysteresis and, 183-184, *184*
  vascular, 64-68
    pulmonary compliance and, 66-68
    systemic compliance and, 64-66

Water, lung. *See* Lung water
Water reabsorption, plasma volume and, 166
Water-soluble molecules, diffusion of, 138-139
Weight, blood volume and, 164
Wheal, 159
White reaction, 158
Windkessel function of arterial system, 102, *102*
Windpipe, 176, 177
Work, of breathing, 205

Young's modulus, 60

Z lines, 40, *41, 42*
Zones, of lung, 142-144, *143*